A PLUME BOOK

EAT FAT, LOSE FAT

DR. MARY ENIG is a world-renowned biochemist and nutritionist, best known for her pioneering research on healthy fats and oils and her early protests against trans fats more than twenty-five years ago. A consultant and clinician, Dr. Enig is also the former contributing editor of the scientific journal *Clinical Nutrition* and a consulting editor of the *Journal of the American College of Nutrition.* Her work has been published in numerous journal publications, and she is a well-known lecturer at scientific conferences. Dr. Enig received her Ph.D. in Nutritional Sciences from the University of Maryland, College Park, and is a Fellow of the American College of Nutrition, a member of the American Society for Nutritional Sciences, and president of the Maryland Nutritionists Association. She is the author of the self-published "fats information bible," *Know Your Fats,* and coauthor with Sally Fallon of *Nourishing Traditions,* an expanded cookbook on traditional diets.

SALLY FALLON is the founder and president of the Weston A. Price Foundation, a nonprofit organization devoted to helping people put into practice the most health-promoting approaches to nutrition, based on the life-giving foods that have nourished humanity for centuries. The foundation has over two hundred chapters throughout the United States and abroad, and its website (www.westonaprice.org) is a popular Internet reference destination. Ms. Fallon is the editor of the foundation's quarterly journal, *Wise Traditions in Food, Farming, and the Healing Arts,* and she also directs the Weston A. Price Foundation's annual conference on nutrition and health. Ms. Fallon is a highly sought-after speaker, seminar, and workshop presenter, and she has been a guest of numerous radio talk-show hosts, including Dr. Robert Atkins, Robert Crayhon, Leyna Berman, Derek McGinty, and Terri and Joe Graedon of the People's Pharmacy. A gourmet cook, Ms. Fallon has recently applied her outstanding culinary skills to the discovery of many varied and wonderful ways to enjoy coconut.

Also by Sally Fallon and Dr. Mary Enig

Nourishing Traditions:
The Cookbook That Challenges Politically Correct Nutrition
and the Diet Dictocrats

Eat Fat, Lose Fat

The Healthy Alternative to Trans Fats

Dr. Mary Enig and Sally Fallon

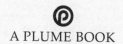

A PLUME BOOK

PLUME
Published by Penguin Group
Penguin Group (USA) Inc., 375 Hudson Street, New York, New York 10014, U.S.A.
Penguin Group (Canada), 90 Eglinton Avenue East, Suite 700, Toronto, Ontario,
Canada M4P 2Y3 (a division of Pearson Penguin Canada Inc.)
Penguin Books Ltd., 80 Strand, London WC2R 0RL, England
Penguin Ireland, 25 St Stephen's Green, Dublin 2, Ireland (a division of Penguin Books Ltd.)
Penguin Group (Australia), 250 Camberwell Road, Camberwell, Victoria 3124,
Australia (a division of Pearson Australia Group Pty. Ltd.)
Penguin Books India Pvt. Ltd., 11 Community Centre, Panchsheel Park, New Delhi – 110 017, India
Penguin Group (NZ), 67 Apollo Drive, Rosedale, North Shore 0632, New Zealand
(a division of Pearson New Zealand Ltd.)
Penguin Books (South Africa) (Pty.) Ltd., 24 Sturdee Avenue, Rosebank,
Johannesburg 2196, South Africa

Penguin Books Ltd., Registered Offices: 80 Strand, London WC2R 0RL, England

Published by Plume, a member of Penguin Group (USA) Inc. Previously published in a Hudson
Street Press edition.

First Plume Printing, April 2006
20 19 18 17 16 15 14

Copyright © Mary Enig and Sally Fallon, 2005
All rights reserved

℗ REGISTERED TRADEMARK—MARCA REGISTRADA

The Library of Congress has catalogued the Hudson Street Press edition as follows:
Enig, Mary G.
    Eat fat, lose fat : lose weight and feel great on the delicious, science-based coconut diet / Mary
Enig and Sally Fallon.
    p. cm.
    ISBN 1-59463-005-4 (hc.)
    ISBN 978-0-452-28566-8 (pbk.)
    1. Reducing diets.   2. Coconut oil.   3. Fatty acids in human nutrition.   I. Fallon, Sally.   II. Title.
RM222.2.E54 2005
641.5'635—dc22   2004016663

Printed in the United States of America
Original hardcover design by Eve L. Kirch

PUBLISHER'S NOTE
Neither the publisher nor the authors are engaged in rendering professional advice or services to
the individual reader. The dietary programs, recipes, resources, ideas, procedures, and suggestions
contained in this book are not intended as a substitute for consulting with your physician.
Consultation with your health practitioner is advised. The publisher and authors are not responsible
for your specific health or allergy needs that may require medical supervision, for any adverse
reactions to the dietary programs or recipes or products contained or referred to in this book, or
for any loss or damage arising or allegedly arising from any information or suggestions in this
book. While the authors have made every effort to provide accurate telephone numbers and
Internet addresses at the time of publication, neither the publisher nor the authors assume any
responsibility for errors, or for changes that occur after publication.

Acknowledgments

No one deserves more credit for making this book happen than Alison Rose Levy—it was her vision, her conviction, and her organizational and writing skills that set this project in motion and then wove our input together in a creative and timely fashion.

Stephanie Golden then worked ceaselessly to give us a structural and finished manuscript, always with an eye to clarity and consistency.

Janis Vallely of Janis Vallely Authors Group kept the project moving smoothly; her advice and suggestions have been invaluable.

And Laureen Rowland of Hudson Street Press created a remarkable alchemy—preserving our vision of what this book should be while molding it into a form that the public can embrace.

Many others contributed: Brian Shilhavy, with his coconut-info e-mail discussion board, provided important testimonials and feedback; members of the Weston A. Price Foundation, who were happy to provide their weight-loss and recovery stories; several creative cooks, who shared their recipes; and our own families, with their encouragement and support.

Finally, we must gratefully acknowledge Weston A. Price and many other scientists of integrity, willing to engage in the honest research that, although often unheralded, has provided guidelines to the use of coconut oil for weight loss, and whole foods for vibrant health.

Contents

Part One

The Truth About Fats

Chapter One

Facts Versus Fears About Fats

America's Anti-Fat Obsession

As the French maintain their trim physiques while consuming triple cream brie, steak au poivre, and béarnaise sauce, most American adults would barely dare to drink a glass of whole-fat milk. For the last 25 years, government recommendations, medical doctrine, food advertising, and so-called health experts have stressed low-fat and non-fat foods, cautioning people to avoid fats in general, particularly saturated fats from animal products and tropical fats, like coconut.

"Are you eating lots of foods high in fat (especially saturated fat)?" worries the American Heart Association website. "Choose a diet that is low in saturated fat and cholesterol," echo the current (2000) United States Department of Agriculture (USDA) food guidelines. A scant two to three daily servings of dairy or other animal foods—specified to be "low-fat or fat-free"—are recommended in the Food Pyramid (developed by the USDA and the U.S. Department of Health and Human Services). The National Heart, Lung and Blood Institute website offers "heart healthy recipes" with reduced fat content, such as Stuffed Potatoes made with soft margarine, low-fat cottage cheese, and low-fat milk.

Yet America, not France, is the nation with galloping rates of obesity, leading many people, and now many researchers, to wonder:

- Are the vegetable oils and trans fats contained in processed foods really healthier than the fats in natural foods, like butter and cream?
- Is coconut oil, a staple in countries with lower rates of chronic disease than ours, really so deadly?

How effective have the recommended low-fat diets and low- and non-fat foods really been, given that *97 million* Americans (that's 64 percent, an 8.6

percent jump from 1994 to 1999) are overweight, according to a study published in the October 2002 *Journal of the American Medical Association*.

And weight gain is not just a question of appearance. Obesity was number two on the Centers for Disease Control and Prevention list of preventable causes of death in 2004 (after smoking). According to government statistics, being overweight substantially increases the risk of hypertension, type II diabetes, coronary heart disease, stroke, gallbladder disease, osteoarthritis, and respiratory problems, as well as endometrial, breast, prostate, and colon cancers. Higher body weight increases mortality for all causes.

If you are among the overweight and want to avoid these diseases, you're caught in a vicious cycle. Once the pounds pack on, your energy plummets, making it harder to exercise. Even if you only need to lose a few pounds, or are not overweight at all, you may find that you suffer from low energy, chronic fatigue, food cravings, and depression. Why?

Based upon our collective experience—Dr. Mary Enig is a world-renowned biochemist and nutritionist, best known for her pioneering research on healthy fats and oils and her early protests against trans fats, and Sally Fallon is a food industry researcher, chef, and president and cofounder of the Weston A. Price Foundation—we believe that while you may be overweight, you are also likely to be *undernourished*, lacking vital nutrients that your body derives from fat. In this book, we offer you a dietary program that, depending on your needs, will help you lose weight (or gain weight if you need to), recover from debilitating health disorders, enhance your overall health and, last but not least, introduce you to a whole world of satisfying, delicious, wholesome foods that everyone in your family can enjoy.

Our three diet plans—Quick and Easy Weight Loss, Health Recovery, and Everyday Gourmet—are all based on eating adequate amounts of good, *healthy fat*, especially the valuable saturated fat of the coconut. Think "healthy fat" is a contradiction in terms? Read on.

Are You Fat Deficient?

Dutifully following the anti-fat recommendations, many people are mystified when they get results contrary to those they're led to expect. For example:

- Have you relied on fat-free foods and counted fat grams to lose weight, only to find that your weight has plateaued and you always feel hungry?
- Do you avoid red meats, butter, and eggs to lower your cholesterol, but lack sufficient energy to get through the day?
- Do you eat margarine because of a family history of heart disease, but feel listless and depressed?
- Do you eat so-called healthy meals (like a salad with no-fat dressing),

only to be overtaken by cravings that drive you to eat fatty foods, such as chips, french fries, doughnuts, or ice cream?

Or perhaps, like so many Americans, you suffer from one or more of these symptoms:

- Has your weight slowly been creeping up?
- Is it impossible to lose that last ten pounds no matter how hard you try?
- Have your energy and enthusiasm drooped?
- Do you still feel hungry after you've finished your meal?
- Do you crave fried foods, sweets, and sugary snacks?
- Do you experience a mid-afternoon "energy crash" and need caffeine or sweets to get through the rest of the day?
- Do sharp cravings for fattening foods overwhelm your best intentions to eat healthy, whole foods?
- Do you feel too fatigued to exercise, though you know you should?
- Do you blame yourself for your lack of "willpower"?
- Are you resigned to weight gain and fatigue?
- Do you suffer from a chronic illness like depression, chronic fatigue syndrome, hypothyroidism, digestive problems, or hormonal imbalances?

Every single one of these problems can signify a dietary fat deficiency. Instead of resulting in weight loss as promised, eating a low-fat diet can spark food cravings that lead to overeating. Instead of making you healthy, avoiding healthy fats can actually undermine your health because you *need* fats for countless bodily functions.

Creamy sauces, buttered vegetables, and ice cream taste good for a reason. It's not that your body is trying to torment you by making unhealthy foods seem delectable. Instead, your body is using your taste buds to signal what you need. That's why most of us enjoy rich foods, like succulent lamb chops, berries with heavy cream, and crispy turkey skin. But because we believe that fats are bad, *we are afraid to listen to our bodies.*

In fact, rich, delicious foods are nature's gift to us, in contrast to processed foods, the creations of the food industry. And helping people understand, prepare, and enjoy wholesome foods is the mission of the Weston A. Price Foundation. With 200 chapters around the world, the Foundation has helped thousands of people find their way to health and optimal weight while enjoying a wholesome, traditional foods diet.

Eat Fat to Lose Weight?

Our Eat Fat, Lose Fat program will put you back on the track that nature intended for efficient nourishment. Let go of the notion that you must suffer to lose weight. In fact, starving yourself is counterproductive, since it signals the body to *hold on* to fat. Instead, when you eat sufficient quantities of the right combinations of fats (as outlined in our recipes and menu plans), you'll notice that you can go for hours without eating and without experiencing cravings, because your body is satisfied and your blood sugar is stable. As a result, hunger pangs disappear and eating sensibly becomes easy!

Nutritional satisfaction signals your body that food is abundant, so it *releases* fat stores. This is the key to weight loss—but that's not all. On this diet, you'll be taking in good fats and over time releasing bad ones from your system. It's like upgrading to premium fuel. Efficient functioning and better health will result.

Through our work at the Weston A. Price Foundation, we've heard from hundreds of people who not only lost lots of weight but also healed a wide range of health problems precisely by following the eating programs that we're offering you in this book. Throughout the book, you'll find some of their stories in the sidebars. Though we've changed names and details to protect their privacy, the actual weight-loss and healing experiences described are all very real.

Along with other healthy fats, coconut oil is key to this diet. Saturated fats, such as those found in coconut oil, butter, cream, and red meat, can be good for you, as you'll learn throughout our book. And, among all the sources of saturated fat available, coconut is the most readily absorbed and utilized—not to mention the most likely to help you lose weight, which is why coconut is the cornerstone of the three dietary plans you will find in the following chapters.

Both of us bring many years of work in the field of nutrition to the eating

---

Janet's Story: Feeling Full

Our **Yogurt-Coconut Smoothie** (see page 205 for recipe) contains energy-boosting coconut oil and whole-milk yogurt, but when Janet went to prepare it she had neither on hand, so instead she used the low-fat yogurt she found in the fridge. An hour after eating the smoothie, Janet felt hungry and ate a "second breakfast" of French toast and syrup (loaded with high-fructose corn syrup). Good-bye, diet!

The next time Janet prepared the smoothie, she used whole-milk yogurt and added the 2 tablespoons of coconut oil that the recipe called for. Janet felt full after eating only half a serving. When lunchtime came, she didn't feel hungry. She finally ate the second half of the smoothie at 2 p.m. and experienced no desire for food until evening, when she ate a light but deliciously satisfying dinner of grilled chicken with skin, brown rice cooked in coconut milk, and vegetables with butter.

program offered here. Aside from being one of the world's most renowned nutritional scientists, Dr. Enig is the author of the highly regarded professional publication *Know Your Fats* (Bethesda Press, 2000), dubbed the "fat information bible" by Dr. Joseph Mercola, author of the bestseller *The No-Grain Diet* (Dutton, 2004). In the course of studying, lecturing, and teaching around the world for the last 20 years, Mary has both contributed to and kept abreast of all the scientific and medical literature on fats, and she became an early and articulate critic of the harmful type of fats we now know as trans fats. Against much opposition (as you'll see in Chapter 3), she began pushing for including the percentage of trans fats on nutrition labels decades ago. Mary is president of the Maryland Nutritionists Association and was recently honored by the American College of Nutrition for her pioneering work in calling attention to the dangers of trans fats.

As founding president of the Weston A. Price Foundation, Sally is a major spokesperson for wholesome nutrition. She travels the world, lecturing and teaching on healthy nutrition and traditional cuisine to thousands of people. We have also coauthored numerous articles on the complex subject of diet and health for various health publications.

Most recently, we have championed the use of coconut oil and other coconut foods. Mary has investigated the metabolism-enhancing properties of coconut

Satiation: The Key to Weight Loss

When you consistently use coconut oil (along with other healthy fats), you provide vital nourishment to every cell in your body, nourishment that supports optimal function of your nerves, brain, hormones, immune system, and metabolism. But beyond that, you trigger a powerful mechanism that is key to success in permanent weight loss: *satiation*.

How does your body register this? When you eat coconut (and other healthy fats like those found in butter, cream, nuts, meats, and eggs), your body actually produces a hormone in the stomach and small intestine that signals that you've eaten enough. When you feel satiated, cravings, and the persistent hunger you experience on most diets, are banished. An added bonus is that many health problems will resolve themselves and you will have more energy and a more optimistic attitude toward life.

Satiation is a truly revolutionary weight-loss concept. By feeding your body the healthy fats it needs, you won't feel hungry, you won't need to deny yourself, and you won't even *want* to overeat empty calories from foods like pizza, sodas, or commercially produced ice cream (which often contains gums, additives, and vegetable oils that negate the benefits of consuming cream).

oil, which contains special medium-chain fatty acids (MCFAs) shown to boost metabolism and stimulate weight loss, according to research carried out in France, Italy, Canada, Japan, and the United States over the past 14 years (Chapter 4 will go into this research in more depth). Meanwhile, Sally has applied her outstanding culinary skills to the discovery of many varied and wonderful ways to enjoy coconut, which you will experience yourself through the many traditional and coconut-based recipes from around the world featured in this book.

We know . . . you've heard that saturated fats are unhealthy. Who hasn't? Read on and you'll be surprised to learn about research published during the last 20 years in respected scientific and medical journals, like *The Journal of Lipid Research, Reviews in Pure and Applied Pharmacological Science,* and *The American Journal of Clinical Nutrition,* that shows that *just the opposite is true.* Your body needs not only fats, but *saturated fats,* to nourish your brain, heart, nerves, hormones and every single cell. Saturated fats form a key part of the cell membranes throughout your body. When you eat too many unsaturated fats, the kind found in polyunsaturated vegetable oils, these fats adversely affect the chemistry of those membranes.

How does this affect *you*? Overstocked with the *wrong* kinds of fats, and lacking sufficient quantities of the *right* kinds of fats to create healthy cells, your body becomes nutritionally deprived, and a host of health problems ensue. Your energy drops, your nerves don't fire efficiently, glands malfunction, your hormones and metabolism head south. With cells weakened from lack of necessary nutrition, weight loss is an uphill battle. Exactly what 95 percent of dieters have experienced up until now. You're tired, you're always hungry, *and* you gain weight!

Yet, for many people, the idea that your body *needs* fat seems hard to accept, when fat is what you're trying to lose. If you have flab under your arms, cellulite on your thighs, and a stomach that enters the room ahead of you, can you still be fat deprived? Yes! The fact is that your body's visible fat stores do not necessarily result from fat consumption. Nor do they indicate adequate levels of fat-derived nutrients. You could be 200 pounds overweight and still be undernourished and fat deprived.

Three Kinds of Fats

While most other diet plans tell you to leave certain foods *out* of your diet—such as fat, dairy, grains, meat, salt, or desserts—the Eat Fat, Lose Fat plan tells you how to *include* all these foods in your diet, exploring the science behind your need for them, how to choose healthy versions of them, and how to prepare them for maximum nutrient benefit and digestibility.

In order to understand how such a diet works, you need to know the differences among the three basic types of fats found in food. Then, you must be aware of the dangers of trans fat: an artificially produced fat found widely in processed and packaged foods.

Fats (also called lipids) are a class of organic substances that do not dissolve in water. They are composed of chains of carbon atoms with hydrogen atoms filling the available bonds and are called fatty *acids* because of their structure. Despite that terminology, they don't behave like acids in the way that water-soluble acids such as vinegar do.

Saturated Fats

Found predominantly in animal fats and tropical oils like coconut oil and in lesser amounts in all vegetable oils (and also made within your body, usually from excess carbohydrates), saturated fats are structured so that all available carbon bonds are occupied by a hydrogen atom, which makes them highly stable and also straight in shape, so that they are solid or semisolid fat at room temperature. As a result of their unique composition, they are less likely to go rancid when heated during cooking and form dangerous free radicals that can cause a litany of ills, including heart disease and cancer.

Monounsaturated Fats

The monounsaturated fatty acid most commonly found in our food is oleic acid, the main component of olive oil and sesame oil, as well as the oil in almonds, pecans, cashews, peanuts, and avocados. Your body can also make monounsaturated fatty acids from saturated fatty acids when it needs them for various bodily functions.

Chemically, monounsaturated fatty acids are structured with one double bond (composed of two carbon atoms double-bonded to each other). Because this bond causes the molecule to bend slightly, these fats do not pack together as easily as saturated fats, so they tend to be liquid at room temperature but become solid when refrigerated.

Like saturated fats, however, monounsaturated oils are relatively stable. They do not go rancid easily and hence can also be used in cooking.

Polyunsaturated Fats

Polyunsaturated fatty acids have two or more double bonds. The two polyunsaturated fatty acids found most frequently in our foods are linoleic acid with two double bonds (called omega-6) and linolenic acid, with three double bonds (called omega-3). (The omega number indicates the position of the first double bond.)

Because your body cannot make these fatty acids, they are called "essential" and must be obtained from foods. Polyunsaturated fatty acids have bends or turns at the position of the double bonds and hence do not pack together easily. They remain liquid, even when refrigerated.

Unpaired electrons located at the double bonds make these oils highly reactive. When they are subjected to heat or oxygen, as in extraction, processing, and cooking, free radicals are formed. It is these free radicals, not saturated fats, that can initiate cancer and heart disease. As such, industrially processed polyunsaturated oils, such as corn, safflower, soy, and sunflower oils, should be strictly avoided.

The Dangers of Trans Fats

Manufactured foods, such as baked goods, some frozen foods, margarine, chips, fast-food fries and countless other products, contain rearranged fatty acids called trans fats, which are produced artificially by bombarding poly-unsaturated oils with hydrogen, a process called partial hydrogenation. This process makes the normally twisty polyunsaturated fatty acids straighten out and behave like saturated fats in foods. As a result, trans fats have a longer shelf life. They pack together easily so they are unnaturally solid at room tem-perature and can be used as spreads and shortenings. Because they can be made so cheaply and because their inclusion helps packaged foods to last nearly for-ever, the food industry prefers to use trans fats made from cheap soy, canola, corn, or cottonseed oil rather than more expensive animal fats or tropical oils.

For years, as you will read in Chapter 2, medical experts, government agen-cies such as the Food and Drug Administration, and medical organizations such as the American Heart Association (AHA) urged Americans to abandon traditional saturated fats in favor of partially hydrogenated oils in order to re-duce the risk of heart disease. These organizations boosted margarine, for ex-ample, as healthier for the heart than butter.

Yet a large body of scientific research now demonstrates what Mary Enig's work showed long before the medical establishment was willing to acknowl-edge the facts: that these altered fats, which people are still told to eat to reduce their cholesterol levels, actually *increase* cholesterol and also the risk for heart disease. For example, the Nurses' Health Study, a long-term study of over 80,000 female nurses carried out by researchers at Harvard University, reported that substituting 30 calories of trans fats each day for 30 calories of carbohy-drates increased the risk of heart disease by a factor of nearly two. The direc-tor of the study, Dr. Walter Willett, professor of nutrition and epidemiology at the Harvard School of Public Health, claimed that saturated fats also increased the risk, although much less; but other commentators on the overall study, such as J. Salmeron in the *American Journal of Clinical Nutrition*, 2001, found no correlation between consumption of saturated fats and heart disease.

Trans fats also compromise many bodily functions, including hormone synthesis, immune function, insulin metabolism, and tissue repair. What's more, they promote weight gain. In fact, a person whose dietary fats are mostly trans fats is likely to weigh more than a person who does not consume trans fats, even if their caloric intake is the same. (One type of trans fat, called an isomer, occurs in small amounts in butter, beef, and lamb fat. But this isomer does not cause health problems. It is actually converted into a substance called CLA, which protects against weight gain.)

In 2002, the Institute of Medicine of the National Academy of Sciences concluded that there is *no* safe level of trans fat in the diet. In 2004, an FDA advisory panel concluded that trans fat is "even more harmful than saturated fat." (Actually, as we saw, saturated fats are not harmful.) Dr. Willett commented, "When partially hydrogenated vegetable oil was first used in foods many decades ago, it was considered safe. Now that studies have demonstrated that partially hydrogenated oil is a major cause of heart disease, it should be phased out of the food supply as rapidly as possible and replaced with more healthful oils."

In Chapter 3, we'll provide more details of how trans fats are detrimental to every system in your body.

Does This Product Contain Trans Fats?

You might assume that it's easy to avoid trans fats by reading nutritional labels on the food products you buy—but you'd be wrong. Until 2003, manufacturers were not required to list the trans fat content of foods on the label. That year, the FDA finalized a requirement that all food labels list trans fat content by January 1, 2006.

This regulation has led many food manufacturers to reduce or eliminate the amount of trans fats in their products. Frito-Lay, for example, no longer uses partially hydrogenated oils in most of its products. Kraft Foods has said it will reduce trans fat levels. Some smaller companies are moving in the same direction. Unfortunately, these manufacturers still are not using healthy, stable saturated fats, such as coconut oil, palm oil, lard, butterfat, or tallow (beef or sheep fat), and when they do use palm or coconut oil, it is usually also partially hydrogenated for a longer shelf life. Instead, they are primarily using liquid vegetable oils, which can also cause health problems, especially when consumed in large amounts or heated to high temperatures, as in frying.

The labeling requirement won't help you identify trans fats in restaurant meals, and most fast-food chains continue to use partially hydrogenated oils to fry foods. But not to worry: once you've begun eating wholesome, traditional foods, the idea of fast food won't tempt you in the slightest.

The Scientific Turnaround on Fat

Today, more physicians are beginning to admit that the anti-fat campaign hasn't won the health-and-weight-loss war. Dr. Frank Hu, also of the Harvard School of Public Health, cautioned that "the *exclusive focus on dietary fat has been a distraction* in efforts to control obesity . . ." (our italics). Speaking to the Dietary Guidelines Advisory Committee (DGAC), which is preparing the revised USDA Food Pyramid for 2005, Dr. Hu pointed out, "Conventional wisdom holds that the more fat you eat, the more likely you are to become obese. However, *the evidence does not support the conventional wisdom* . . ." He cited 16 long-term studies (6 to 18 months in duration) that showed "no evidence that a low-fat diet is more beneficial."

What's more, recent studies confirm that healthy fat consumption *promotes* sustainable weight loss (something we've been saying for years!). "Studies conducted in the past three years have found a moderately high-fat diet . . . to be more beneficial (than low-fat diets) in terms of adherence, weight loss, and weight maintenance, while also reducing cardiovascular risk factors," Dr. Hu affirmed.

With this new evidence, government and medical authorities will begin to readjust their dietary guidelines to include more fat. Yet they still subscribe to the false notion that saturated fats are bad, so the most prominent fats in the new food guidelines will be liquid vegetable oils, including soy, canola, and safflower, in spite of considerable evidence that a diet including only liquid fats can lead to serious health problems, including heart disease and cancer.

In *Eat Fat, Lose Fat*, we give you the straight story of what science says about the kinds of fats you should mostly be eating.

Healthy fats include omega-3 fatty acids (found in cod-liver oil, egg yolks, and flax oil), medium-chain fats (found in coconut oil, palm kernel oil, and butter), and long-chain saturated fats (found mostly in meat and dairy products). They'll help you lose weight, increase your energy, boost your immunity to illness, and optimize your digestion.

So the real, scientific way to lose fat is to eat fat—especially the fats you'll learn more about in this book.

Eat Fat, Lose Fat will take you beyond your fears about fat, to the facts about fat. The diet programs and menu plans in Chapters 6, 7, and 8 are based on Dr. Enig's pioneering work, in which she has courageously moved beyond prevailing assumptions and prejudices about fats to penetrate to the truth about how different fats affect us—a truth that the medical establishment is only beginning to understand. We'll lay out several strands of evidence to clear up prevailing misunderstandings about fats and their role in human health:

- **Historical:** World populations on four continents, subsisting on the coconut and other natural, wholesome foods (without heart disease, weight

A Closer Look at How Overweight Happens

Eating excess calories is only one reason for overweight. Listed below are the factors most commonly responsible for fat buildup, and how the Eat Fat, Lose Fat program addresses each one:

High-calorie, nutrient-empty foods: When you get all the healthy fats (and allied nutrients) that your body needs, you'll eliminate cravings that lead you to foods like soda, cookies, and breads.

Low thyroid function: When your thyroid is sluggish, you can't lose weight no matter how little you eat. On our program, you'll enhance thyroid function and upgrade your metabolism by consuming energy-boosting, thyroid-supporting coconut oil.

Excess sugar and carb consumption and insulin sensitivity (a condition in which your cells cannot process blood sugar properly): Emphasizing nutrient-rich protein, dairy, and vegetables, you'll bypass excess consumption of weight-inducing and insulin-activating sugars and grains.

Consumption of renegade fats such as trans fats: You'll cut out all trans fats, which interfere with numerous biochemical processes in the body and can contribute to weight gain.

gain, or other chronic illnesses), provide the world's longest epidemiological record of the safety of saturated fat.

• **Scientific:** Analysis of studies used to indict coconut oil and other saturated fats will reveal the faulty reasoning underlying the "lipid hypothesis," the theory that saturated fat and cholesterol cause heart disease. Other studies clearly demonstrate that saturated fats do not "cause" cardiovascular illness, and that coconut oil's medium-chain fatty acids actually make it an all-systems healer. (See Chapters 2 and 3.)

• **Anecdotal:** We'll provide case stories from a wide range of people who've used coconut oil and coconut products to lose weight and heal serious illnesses, including digestive disorders, diabetes, and hypothyroidism.

• **Nutritional:** We'll explain why the important nutrients contained in coconut and traditional fats like cod-liver oil and butter are vital to your health.

• **Culinary:** We'll show you how to use coconut in all its forms in recipes that satisfy your taste buds and put an end to food cravings and hunger. (See menu plans in Chapters 6, 7, and 8, and recipes in Chapters 9 and 10.)

Once and for all, *Eat Fat, Lose Fat* will clear away the misperception that fats are bad, and arm you with a concrete program and culinary tools that support this dietary change. Whether your goal is losing weight or gaining health, you'll get great results through eating coconut products and other sources of healthy dietary fats as part of an eating program based on wholesome, traditional foods.

Fats and Health Problems

Here is a brief overview of the ailments you can begin turning around by reintroducing healthy fats into your diet:

- **Chronic fatigue:** The medium-chain fatty acids in coconut oil provide energy and also fight pathogens in the digestive tract that contribute to fatigue.

- **Low energy:** The medium-chain fatty acids in coconut oil give quick energy, prevent low blood sugar, and support the thyroid gland; plus, cod-liver oil provides nutrients vital for vitamin and mineral absorption.

- **Anxiety:** The combination of fatty acids and nutrients in coconut oil and cod-liver oil helps prevent low blood sugar and helps the body make the adrenal hormones it needs to deal with stress. Trans fats (eliminated in our program) inhibit the production of these hormones, so removing these from the diet is another big step toward relieving anxiety.

- **Depression:** The nutrients in cod-liver oil have a proven record of helping relieve depression, and the saturated fats in coconut oil work synergistically with cod-liver oil.

- **Mood swings:** Plentiful fats in our diet help stabilize blood sugar swings that make your mood go up and down.

- **Thyroid imbalance:** Coconut oil alone improves thyroid function, but when used in conjunction with cod-liver oil, which supplies vitamin A (needed in high levels by the thyroid gland), the thyroid has the fats it needs to function properly.

- **Hypoglycemia:** Plenty of healthy fats at each meal help prevent drops in blood sugar.

- **Insulin resistance:** Trans fats interfere with insulin receptors in the cells. Replacing trans fats with coconut oil and other healthy fat is the number one step in preventing and reversing the insulin resistance so characteristic of type II diabetes.

• **Food cravings:** You experience cravings when your body isn't getting the nutrients it needs from food. Coconut oil is immensely satisfying, while cod-liver oil supplies vitamins A and D, needed to assimilate minerals and other vitamins.

• **Gallbladder ailments:** Coconut oil is the ideal fat for anyone suffering from gallbladder ailments because many of the fatty acids in coconut oil do not require bile for digestion.

• **Bacterial infections:** The antimicrobial medium-chain fatty acids in coconut oil, combined with vitamin A in cod-liver oil, provide the ideal combination for fighting bacterial infections.

• **Fungal issues, like candida:** Coconut oil has strong antifungal properties, both in the gut and when applied topically (on the skin). Eliminating refined carbohydrates while eating whole grains only when they are properly prepared can also help candida problems.

• **Viral infections:** The medium-chain fatty acids in coconut oil help kill the pathogenic lipid-coated viruses in the digestive tract.

• **Digestive problems, including irritable bowel syndrome and Crohn's disease:** The combination of medium-chain fatty acids in coconut oil and vitamin A in cod-liver oil enhances the immune system.

• **Gas and bloating:** The antimicrobial properties of coconut oil can help fight gas-producing bacteria.

• **Skin problems such as eczema, dry skin, scaly patches:** The synergistic combination of saturated fatty acids in coconut oil and very long-chain super unsaturated fatty acids in cod-liver oil helps maintain the right fatty acids in the cell membranes, thereby contributing to beautiful skin. Vitamins A and D in cod-liver oil are also very important factors in nourishing the skin.

• **Sagging, wrinkled skin:** Plentiful saturated fats in the diet are absolutely essential for avoiding wrinkles. Excess polyunsaturated oils make the cell walls "floppy," thereby contributing to wrinkles. Furthermore, these oils are invariably rancid and contain free radicals (reactive atoms or molecule fragments) that damage cells and contribute to aging.

• **Dandruff, lifeless hair:** The thyroid-supporting combination of coconut oil and cod-liver oil will result in shiny, healthy hair.

• **Liver support:** The combination of saturated fat in coconut oil, vitamin A in cod-liver oil, and bone broths (recipes provided in Chapter 10) that give you special amino acids the liver uses to detoxify provides excellent support for liver function.

See Chapter 7 for more about how and why our coconut and fat-enriched diet can help you address a wide range of health issues.

Our Three-Part Program

As you follow the Eat Fat, Lose Fat program, you'll reincorporate healthy fats (along with other wholesome foods) into your diet. Whether your goal is losing weight, or simply gaining energy, you'll find clear guidelines, complete menu plans, and delicious recipes, which hundreds of people have followed successfully.

You can select one of the following three diet plans:

• **Quick and Easy Weight Loss:** This streamlined program for weight loss, based upon weight-loss studies carried out during the last 15 years, features a moderate-calorie diet that contains about 50 percent or more of fats as medium-chain fatty acids (MCFAs) from coconut oil to jump-start your metabolism. Many people easily shed pounds with this satisfying diet plan, but for those wishing accelerated weight loss, we also provide a two-week calorie-restricted plan. Recipes and menu plans are designed to assure ease of preparation.

• **Health Recovery:** This program is for those with special health needs, such as chronic fatigue, allergies, and digestive disorders. It features high levels of all the healing fats to provide the optimal balance, along with vital nutrients from easy-to-digest foods that facilitate healing and assimilation. It's also ideal for those recovering from surgery or severe illnesses.

• **Everyday Gourmet:** A hearty maintenance program for life, one that the whole family can enjoy, featuring international cuisine. This plan provides a range of healing fats, as well as other traditionally prepared foods,

A Cautionary Note

There are no side effects from adding coconut products to your diet unless you are allergic to coconut. Even if you are, you can still probably take coconut oil, because the allergenic components of coconut are protein compounds found in the meat of the coconut, not in the oil. In that case, follow the Eat Fat, Lose Fat plans by using just the Traditional Recipes in Chapter 10 and taking coconut oil before meals in warm water or herb tea.

Did You Know ... ?

- The body can use coconut oil for energy more rapidly and efficiently than any other fat source. Special fats in coconut (called medium-chain fatty acids, MCFAs) are not normally stored in your body as fat. Instead, they're quickly converted to energy, making coconut ideal for weight loss.
- Small amounts of the MCFAs in coconut oil are used in the complex processes that enable cells to communicate with each other.
- Coconut improves thyroid function in people with hypothyroid disease.
- People in countries where coconut is an important part of the diet have lower rates of heart disease and cancer than Americans. For example, a 1996 report by the National Cancer Institute lists Thailand (with the highest coconut consumption of any country in the world) as having the lowest cancer rates for both men and women out of the 50 countries studied. (No other coconut-eating countries were included in the survey.) Inhabitants of the Philippines have some of the lowest rates of heart disease in the world, according to a study published in the *Philippine Journal of Internal Medicine,* 1992.
- Coconut oil is currently used in infant formulas and hospital invalid foods because it confers special health benefits. It's also used in sports drinks to help athletes produce lean body mass.
- The fats in coconut help fight infections of all kinds.
- Some dieters have even reported that coconut oil has helped them get rid of cellulite!

and introduces traditional culinary secrets to optimize the nutritional value of your food.

All three plans incorporate healthy fats into the diet in four ways:

- They increase beneficial coconut oil and coconut products.
- They use cod-liver oil (either in capsules or as recommended brands of oil that are processed to retain freshness) to obtain its vital fat-soluble vitamins and omega-3 fatty acids, and better absorb them as a result of synergy with saturated fats in coconut oil.
- They eliminate all harmful fats from your diet and from your body.
- They offer the benefits of wholesome foods, including other saturated fat sources such as butter, cream, whole milk, egg yolks, and meat fats.

This unique combination of diet components is designed to support thyroid function. Boosting your thyroid initiates a domino effect, revving up your

---

Margaret's Story: Cellulite Disappeared

Margaret is a thin, very active young mother who takes pride in her youthful figure. So she was upset when she developed cellulite on her thighs. Even regular swimming did not help, and she was too thin to lose weight. Then she started using coconut oil along with other traditional fats, while eliminating all commercial vegetable oils and trans fats from her diet. Within a year, her cellulite disappeared.

---

energy levels, speeding up your metabolic system, burning more calories per day, and sparking weight loss.

On all three food plans, you will use precise amounts of coconut and cod-liver oil (rich in thyroid-supportive vitamin A), along with other complementary foods to provide an optimal blend of fats and oils that boost metabolism and keep hunger at bay. Our calorie-restricted weight-loss plan shows you the exact number of calories per serving.

In Search of Nutritional Balance

How can we be ahead of the curve with this cutting-edge healthy fats program? Our work at the Weston A. Price Foundation is based on the pioneering research of Dr. Weston A. Price, a dentist who traveled the world as far back as the 1930s, studying and documenting the effects of both traditional and modern diets and identifying foods that produced enduring health, generation after generation (see sidebar). We've pored over the science and studied the foods eaten by healthy societies all over the world. Through our research and cross-cultural investigation, we've rediscovered the important role fats play in healthy nutrition. And through our website, westonaprice.org., our magazine, *Wise Traditions*, and over 200 local chapters, we have reached a wide network of people who have experienced the health benefits of traditional foods. Hundreds of people have followed the nutritional program you'll find in this book to achieve (and maintain) their optimal weight and to regain their energy, hormonal balance, and zest for life. Our program is effective in boosting energy and enhancing metabolism because we know the science!

In our bestselling cookbook, *Nourishing Traditions* (New Trends, 2000), we focused extensively on the foods and culinary techniques found by Dr. Price to support health. In *Eat Fat, Lose Fat*, we'll show you easy ways to use traditional natural ingredients and age-old culinary techniques. In his work, Price found that similar foods and preparation techniques evolved in many different cultures to provide the right kind of nutrients, prepared in a way that the human body could absorb. This is the foundation of the dietary program we'll offer in

Who Was Weston A. Price?

In 1932, Dr. Price, a Cleveland dentist, launched a unique investigation. He had grown increasingly concerned about the declining health of his patients. Observing rampant tooth decay and crowded and crooked teeth, he noted that people with these dental problems invariably suffered from other health problems as well. Price believed that these problems were not hereditary but nutritional. He was skeptical that the diets his patients were consuming, based on sugar, white flour, and vegetable oils, could support good health.

Having heard that isolated peoples consuming only local foods had excellent dental health, Price spent over ten years traveling to remote parts of the globe to study the health of populations untouched by Western civilization in order to discover whether nonindustrialized peoples indeed were healthy and, if so, what were they eating?

He visited sequestered villages in Switzerland, Gaelic communities in the Outer Hebrides, indigenous peoples of North and South America, Melanesian and Polynesian South Sea Islanders, African tribes, Australian Aborigines, and New Zealand Maori. In all, Price found 14 population groups that enjoyed beautiful, straight teeth free from decay, as well as fine physiques and resistance to disease, so long as they ate their traditional diets, which were rich in certain essential food factors.

On the other hand, whenever these traditional peoples began to eat devitalized Western foods, which Price called "the displacing foods of modern commerce," physical degeneration ensued. Health problems showed up immediately, and structural defects (namely, narrow jaws and crooked teeth) appeared in the next generation. Not surprisingly, widespread obesity often accompanied the transition to modern processed foods.

Eat Fat, Lose Fat, with a special emphasis on coconut oil and other healthy fats because of their unique ability to boost metabolism, build energy, and nurture health. The traditional foods our program uses are not unfamiliar: they're much like the scrumptious meals your grandmother used to make.

You'll find the whys, hows, and whats of healthy fat consumption in *Eat Fat, Lose Fat*'s three parts.

In Part 1, you'll learn why you should be eating traditional fats, why they are healthy, and why you've been told they aren't. Chapter 2 presents the history and science behind the anti-fat campaign, showing you how a different interpretation of the data leads to a totally different conclusion about fats. Chapter 3 explains in more depth why your body needs fats, and particularly why the kinds of fats you'll enjoy on our program are healthier than others. Chapter 4 provides the foundations of our nutritional philosophy and applies it to weight loss.

What Do We Mean by Traditional Foods?

We're talking about real foods: butter, cream, raw milk cheeses, steak, lamb chops, bacon and patés without additives, and hearty soups made with real stock. "Traditional" means the type of foods nonindustrialized peoples ate: foods in their natural, unprocessed form, from unconfined animals that feed on pasture. In our recipe section, you'll also learn traditional preparation methods, including fermentation, that make grains and vegetables healthier and easier to digest. You'll even learn how to make healthy soft drinks.

Hardship food? Hardly. These are all the basics you already know and love, plus new techniques that enhance digestion and absorption of nutrients.

In Part 2 you'll learn how to follow our program. Chapter 5 offers complete information about the traditional foods you'll learn to enjoy. Chapters 6, 7, and 8 present our three diet plans: Quick and Easy Weight Loss, Health Recovery, and Everyday Gourmet, each with a complete menu plan. In Part 3: Recipes and Resources, Chapter 9 presents those based on coconut, while the recipes in Chapter 10 show you how to prepare a variety of wholesome, traditional foods. Finally, our ample Resources section helps you locate sources of the products we recommend, explains the differences between brands, and offers a special treat: a list of coconut oil recipes for removing wrinkles, treating acne, and creating lustrous, smooth skin.

Right now, let's look further into one particular assertion about saturated fat: the charge that it's responsible for heart disease. Chapter 2 will show you otherwise—and also tell the story of the well-orchestrated campaign to hide the truth about saturated and trans fats from the American public.

Chapter Two

Fats, the Real Deal

We've seen thousands of Westerners dramatically upgrade their health by adopting a time-honored traditional diet while, on the other hand, traditional peoples who have abandoned that diet in favor of modern oils have experienced radical health *declines*, according to recent studies. For example, Indians experienced a dramatic increase in heart disease as they urbanized, according to an article in the *Journal of the Indian Medical Association*, 2000. The most likely reason? Their adoption of Western foods, especially switching to vegetable oils instead of using traditional ghee (clarified butter) for cooking.

If you're like most people we meet, when you hear about the benefits of coconut and other saturated fats, you may wonder, "If saturated fat is so great, why have I always been told it's bad?" The fact is that for the last four decades, saturated fats, including coconut oil, have been banned from general consumption, condemned and locked away for the *misdeeds of polyunsaturated fats, trans fats, and refined carbohydrates*, foods that are still at large wreaking havoc with American waistlines (not to mention our life expectancy).

If eating saturated fat caused heart disease and weight gain, then eliminating those fats should have resulted in a *decline* in heart disease and an *increase* in weight loss. But look around you. That's not what happened! While we Americans have been dutifully eliminating fat from our diet, eating low-fat foods, and avoiding saturated fats from tropical oils, butter, and red meats, obesity rates and the overall incidence of heart disease have *continued* to climb.

The truth is that the "diet police" condemned the wrong culprit. It wasn't saturated fat or coconut oil (a dietary staple in countries such as Thailand and the Philippines with consistently lower heart disease rates than our own) that caused our galloping heart disease rates. An entire body of research implicates refined grains and sugars (especially high-fructose corn syrup)—*not* saturated fats—as the cause of obesity, and vegetable oils and trans fats as key factors in heart disease. At long last, nutritional experts around the country agree and have called for a revision of the USDA Food Pyramid, which promotes excess consumption of the *real* culprits. (Although the new USDA guidelines do contain warnings about trans fats, they still condemn saturated fats.)

Let us repeat: *the very oils promoted as healthy* in place of saturated fats were, in fact, *accessories* (along with refined grains and sweets) to this nation's mounting weight gain and key contributors to heart disease. Recent research reveals that it is the polyunsaturated vegetable oils, *not* the saturated fats in coconut oil and animal foods, that *induce* changes leading to heart disease. For example, the work of Bernard Hennig, published in the *Journal of the American College of Nutrition*, 2001, indicates that an excess of omega-6 fatty acids (from commercial vegetable oils) contributes to pathological changes in the cells lining the arteries, and hence to heart disease. There is also much research demonstrating that the trans fats in many manufactured foods (the same foods people eat to avoid saturated fats) contribute to a wide range of illnesses, including cancer, heart disease, and obesity.

In particular, the entire ideology behind the indictment of saturated fats for increasing cholesterol, and cholesterol for causing arteriosclerosis, is faulty. But don't just take our word for it. To ensure that you feel comfortable following our healthy-fat, coconut-rich diet plans, this chapter will continue your "fats education" by laying out the history of the connection mistakenly made between saturated fats and heart disease, *and* explain why you never knew these facts until now.

We'll begin by examining the following core questions:

- Does saturated fat raise cholesterol?
- Does cholesterol cause atherosclerosis and heart disease?
- Does scientific evidence support or contradict the view that saturated fats raise cholesterol, thus causing heart disease?
- Are polyunsaturated oils "heart healthy," as we've been led to believe?

Next, we'll explain how we came to accept the theory that there's a link between saturated fats, cholesterol, and heart disease. This second part of the story is not scientific but historic, as we go back to the early 20th century to trace the evolution of the "lipid hypothesis," a theory that scientists held sacred for decades but are finally beginning to question as more and more contradictory evidence appears.

The Anti-Fat Campaign

The term "lipid hypothesis"—the theory that saturated fats and cholesterol in our food raise cholesterol levels in the blood, leading to heart disease—was coined in the 1950s by Ancel Keys, author of several epidemiological studies that, although in our opinion were severely flawed, are frequently quoted as supporting the theory that animal fats cause heart disease. (Another term, the "Diet-Heart Idea," was used by Dr. George Mann, who had participated in an important long-term study and became highly critical of the hypothesis.) This theory is so prevalent, so widely believed, and so fundamental to the modern treatment of cardiovascular illness, that up until now you've probably never heard that it is only *one* theory of heart disease, and that a different reading of the data, along with volumes of other research, supports a very different conclusion: that saturated fats do not contribute to heart disease and in fact actually protect us against this and many other diseases.

The lipid hypothesis grew out of scientists' attempts to grapple with a steep rise in heart disease, from less than 10 percent of all deaths at the turn of the 20th century to 30 percent of all deaths by 1950 (and almost 45 percent of all deaths today). Even more disturbing, most of the increase was due to a new phenomenon, myocardial infarction (MI) or heart attack, which did not exist before the 1920s. During the 1950s, Dr. Dudley White, the most famous cardiologist of his day (he was President Eisenhower's physician), noted that heart disease had increased as the consumption of liquid vegetable oils increased and the consumption of eggs and traditional fats like butter and lard declined. The use of margarine quadrupled, and that of vegetable oils more than tripled, between 1900 and 1950, while egg consumption declined by half.

What's more, after World War II, manufacturers began hydrogenating these liquid oils so that they could be used as a substitute for coconut oil and animal fats in baked goods. Thus more and more Americans were consuming products like Wesson Oil and Crisco, processed fats that had never been part of the human diet before. And these processed fats were being used in more and more processed products containing refined carbohydrates and many additives that gave them a long shelf life.

Dr. White and many others pointed out that these facts—heart disease increasing along with the use of polyunsaturated oils and partially hydrogenated oils in processed foods—suggested that Americans should eat traditional foods like meat, eggs, butter and cheese, and avoid the vegetable oil–based foods newly flooding the grocers' shelves. But other scientists suggested instead that *reducing* animal foods in the diet was the way to keep the heart healthy. They cited studies by a young researcher named David Kritchevsky, who discovered that feeding large amounts of purified cholesterol caused a type of atherosclerosis (a buildup of fatty plaques on the inner walls of arteries) in vegetarian rabbits.

By the early 1970s, the lipid hypothesis had become the ruling explanation for the rise in heart disease, accepted and promoted by leading medical experts such as Dr. Frederick Stare, head of Harvard University's Nutrition Department, respected organizations including the American Heart Association, government agencies such as the Food and Drug Administration (FDA), and of course the food manufacturers, especially the edible oil industry. (In fact, we have documented evidence that the edible oil industry worked behind the scenes to influence government policy to endorse the use of foods containing their products, and not traditional fats.)

What Is the Lipid Hypothesis, and How Has It Affected What You Eat?

In coronary heart disease (CHD), a buildup of fatty plaques in the artery walls causes a narrowing of the coronary arteries (which bring blood to the heart), leading to blockage of the blood flow to the heart. The result is angina (chest pain) and, often, heart attack. The lipid hypothesis describes coronary heart disease as a three-step disease process:

- **Step 1:** We eat a diet containing too much cholesterol and saturated fat, and as a result we develop a high level of cholesterol in our blood.

- **Step 2:** High blood cholesterol causes atherosclerosis.

- **Step 3:** Atherosclerosis obstructs the vessels that bring blood to the heart, resulting in coronary heart disease.

Each of these steps is like a link in a chain, connecting to form the lipid hypothesis. And yet extensive scientific evidence exists that contradicts each step in this "chain" of scientific theory, presented as fact for over five decades. This evidence has been around for years, but for various reasons—described by Dr. Mann as "reasons of pride, profit, and prejudice"—the media and the scientific community have not communicated this fact to the public.

Spokespersons from organizations promoting the lipid hypothesis don't understand the effects and benefits of dietary saturated fats (described in Chapter

What *Is* Cholesterol?

Cholesterol is often referred to as a fat, but it's actually a heavyweight alcohol with a hormonelike structure that behaves like a fat, being insoluble in water and in blood. Cholesterol, however, has a coating of a compound called a lipoprotein, which makes it water soluble so it can be carried in the blood.

Lipoproteins are described in terms of their density. Generally speaking, high-density lipoproteins (HDL) carry cholesterol away from the cells to the liver, and low-density lipoproteins (LDL) carry cholesterol to the cells. We speak of HDL as "good" cholesterol and LDL as "bad" cholesterol. However, both HDL and LDL play critical roles in body chemistry.

The Benefits of Cholesterol

- Your body uses cholesterol to make hormones that help you deal with stress and protect against heart disease and cancer.
- Your body needs cholesterol to make all the sex hormones, including androgen, testosterone, estrogen, progesterone, and DHEA.
- Your body uses cholesterol to make vitamin D, vital for the bones and nervous system, proper growth, mineral metabolism, muscle tone, insulin production, reproduction, and immune system function.
- The bile salts are made from cholesterol. Bile is vital for digestion and assimilation of dietary fats.
- Cholesterol acts as an antioxidant, protecting us against free radical damage that leads to heart disease and cancer.
- Cholesterol is needed for proper function of serotonin receptors in the brain. Since serotonin is the body's natural "feel-good" chemical, it's not surprising that low cholesterol levels have been linked to aggressive and violent behavior, depression, and suicidal tendencies.
- Mother's milk is especially rich in cholesterol and contains a special enzyme that helps the baby utilize this nutrient. Babies and children need cholesterol-rich foods throughout their growing years to ensure proper development of the brain and nervous system.
- Dietary cholesterol plays an important role in maintaining the health of the intestinal wall. This is why low-cholesterol vegetarian diets can lead to leaky gut syndrome and other intestinal disorders.
- Finally, the body uses cholesterol to repair damaged cells. This means that higher cholesterol levels are actually beneficial. Meyer Texon, M.D., a well-known pathologist at New York University Medical Center, points out that indicting fat and cholesterol for hardening the arteries is like accusing white blood cells of causing infection, rather than helping the immune system to address it.

1), nor do they comprehend the normal presence within the body of saturated fats—and their key role. Fundamentally, the war on saturated fats stems from a misperception about the effects of saturated fatty acids on cholesterol levels.

And, although there has been much alarm about cholesterol levels, in fact, the cholesterol found naturally in animal fats has many important functions (see sidebar).

We'll begin our critique of the lipid hypothesis by exploding four myths about the connection between saturated fat, cholesterol, and heart disease.*

*Much of the information disproving these myths comes from *The Cholesterol Myths: Exposing the Fallacy That Saturated Fat and Cholesterol Cause Heart Disease*, by Uffe Ravnskov, M.D., Ph.D., New Trends Publishing, 2000. Used with permission.

Myth #1: High-Fat Foods Cause Heart Disease

Since the 1950s, scientists, medical organizations such as the American Heart Association, and government agencies such as the FDA have issued dietary guidelines, which they claimed were based on scientific research, urging the public to consume fewer animal products and substitute vegetable oils for animal fats. The food industry followed suit with advertising campaigns touting the health benefits of products low in fat or made with vegetable oils.

Yet during the same time period, many studies were being carried out whose results directly contradicted the assumptions of the lipid hypothesis. Here is a selection of three such studies.

The Masai of Kenya

In the early 1960s, Dr. George Mann of Vanderbilt University studied the Masai people, cattle herders of Kenya whose diet consisted almost entirely of milk, meat, and blood. The Masai drank at least a gallon of milk per day, providing something like three-quarters of a pound of butterfat daily, and at festivals one person might eat four to ten pounds of meat!

Not only did Dr. Mann discover the Masai to be virtually free of heart disease; their blood cholesterol was extremely low, about 50 percent lower than that of most Americans. When Dr. Mann studied 50 hearts and arteries from Masai tribesmen of all ages, he found as much atherosclerosis as in those of Americans. However, the types of plaques that caused obstruction (by sticking out of the vessel walls) were rare. In fact, he found no evidence that any of the 50 hearts had experienced a heart attack.

Indian Railway Workers

In 1967, Dr. S. L. Malhotra published a study of Indian railway employees in the *British Heart Journal*. He found that heart disease was seven times more common among workers in Madras compared to those in Punjab. Yet the Punjabi workers ate ten to twenty times more fat (and smoked eight times as much) as those in Madras. And the Punjabi workers, eating their high-fat diet, also lived twelve years longer than the largely vegetarian workers in Madras.

The Framingham–Puerto Rico–Honolulu Study

In an even larger study conducted by the National Institutes of Health, 16,000 healthy middle-aged men in Framingham, Massachusetts; Puerto Rico; and Honolulu answered questions about their eating habits. Six years later, in 1981, the researchers compared the diets of those who had had heart attacks with those who had not.

The most significant finding was the fact that the heart attack victims had eaten *more polyunsaturated oils* than the other group. This result is clearly contrary to the assumptions of the lipid hypothesis.

Review of Many Studies

In 1998, the *Journal of Clinical Epidemiology* published a review of 27 studies, involving over 150,000 individuals, that looked at the relationship between diet and heart. In three groups, the patients had eaten more animal fat than the controls. In one group, they had eaten less. In all the other groups, researchers found *no difference* in animal fat consumption between people with heart disease and those without. What's more, in three groups the patients had eaten more vegetable oil than the controls. In only one group had patients eaten less vegetable oil than the control group.

Taken as a whole, then, this research did not—and does not—support the assumption that high-fat foods cause heart attacks. Nevertheless, in 1989 the American Heart Association and the National Heart, Lung, and Blood Institute

Should You Avoid Animal Fat If You've Had a Heart Attack?

The medical literature actually contains only two studies involving humans that compared the *outcome* (not just indicators like cholesterol) of a diet high in animal fat with that of a diet based on vegetable oils. Both studies showed that animal fats actually protect you from heart disease.

The Anti-Coronary Club project, launched in 1957 and published in 1966 in the *Journal of the American Medical Association*, compared two groups of New York businessmen, aged 40 to 59 years. One group followed a "Prudent Diet" consisting of corn oil and margarine instead of butter, cold breakfast cereals instead of eggs, and chicken and fish instead of beef. A control group ate eggs for breakfast and meat three times per day.

The final report noted that the average serum cholesterol of the Prudent Dieters was 220 mg/dl (milligrams per 1/10 liter), compared to 250 mg/dl in the eggs-and-meat group. But there were *eight* deaths from heart disease among the Prudent Dieters—and *none* among those who ate meat three times a day.

In a study published in the *British Medical Journal*, 1965, researchers divided patients who had already had a heart attack into three groups. One group received polyunsaturated corn oil, one got monounsaturated olive oil, and the third was given saturated animal fats.

After two years, the corn oil group had 30 percent lower cholesterol—but only 52 percent remained alive. The olive oil group fared little better: only 57 percent were alive. But among the group who ate mostly animal fat, *75 percent* were alive.

Unfortunately, the proponents of the lipid hypothesis have ensured that the many studies that refute the hypothesis do not get publicity, so that few doctors know about this research. As a result, heart attack patients in the U.S. are invariably told to avoid animal fats.

issued a joint statement that touted many of these same studies as "showing the link between diet and CHD." And, on that basis, they condemned saturated fats and promoted polyunsaturated oils.

Recent Studies Agree

One criticism of the studies cited focuses on the fact that they are old. But recent studies confirm the same. For example, the results of a study conducted by researchers in Denmark and published in the *European Journal of Clinical Nutrition*, 2002, indicated no association between dietary patterns and coronary heart disease. The study looked at the diets of patients admitted to the hospital for diagnosis of heart disease. Patients were divided into three groups: two groups ate diets that were "healthy" according to establishment standards—they avoided animal fats and frequently ate whole grains, fruit, and vegetables. The third group consumed a so-called Western diet with a lot of meat, butter, and white bread. Again, the study indicated no association between dietary patterns and coronary heart disease, *even though the otherwise healthy "Western" diet contained white bread.*

A Swedish study published in the *British Journal of Nutrition*, 2004, found that consumption of milk fat (that is, butterfat) was *negatively* associated with the risk factors for heart disease and also for actual heart attack. In other words, butterfat *protects* against heart disease.

Myth #2: High Cholesterol Causes Heart Disease

The idea that high levels of cholesterol in the blood cause heart disease is an axiom today. Yet if you look at the evidence—even evidence presented as proving the lipid hypothesis—you'll see that there is much data refuting it.

The Framingham Study

The first major government-sponsored study on heart disease was the 40-year Framingham Study, which began in 1948. Researchers looked at 500 residents of this Massachusetts town in an ongoing investigation of all the factors that might contribute to heart disease. An important early result of the study apparently indicated that high cholesterol was a risk factor for heart disease.

However, a follow-up study published 16 years later revealed that there was very little difference between the cholesterol levels of people who had heart attacks and those who did not. In fact, almost half of those who had a heart attack had *low* cholesterol.

Still another analysis, carried out 30 years after the original one, found that men older than 47 died just as often whether their cholesterol was high *or* low. Since most heart attacks occur in people over 47, this raises the question of whether cholesterol really makes any difference.

An even more startling result from this 30-year follow-up study was that people whose cholesterol had *decreased* over that period had a higher risk of dying than those whose cholesterol had *increased*. The researchers wrote that "For each 1 mg/dl drop in cholesterol, there was an 11 percent increase in coronary and total mortality." That is, deaths from heart disease and all other causes increased by *11 percent* for each 1 percent drop in cholesterol in the blood.

Yet a 1990 joint statement by the American Heart Association and National Heart, Lung and Blood Institute, published in the journal *Circulation*, claims that "The results of the Framingham study indicate that a 1 percent reduction . . . of cholesterol [corresponds to] a 2 percent reduction in CHD risk."

You may find this hard to believe, but it's true. And this is only one example of the way data that actually disprove the lipid hypothesis are frequently cited as supporting it.

The International Atherosclerosis Project

The lipid hypothesis could have been laid to rest as far back as 1968, with the publication of the results of the International Atherosclerosis Project in the journal *Laboratory Investigations*. Researchers performed detailed autopsies on 22,000 corpses in 14 nations. This study showed the same degree of atheroma (fatty plaques that block arteries) in all parts of the world—in populations that consumed large amounts of fatty animal products and those that were largely vegetarian; and in populations that suffered from a great deal of heart disease and in populations that had very little or none at all. Furthermore, the researchers found just as much artery blockage in people who had low levels of cholesterol compared to those whose cholesterol was high.

For Women: High Cholesterol Is Better

A truly surprising result of all studies involving women is the finding that in women, high cholesterol levels—even as high as 1,000 mg/dl—are *not* a risk factor for heart disease. In fact, for women low cholesterol is *more* dangerous than high cholesterol. This was the conclusion of a workshop that looked at every study involving cholesterol and women, held at the National Heart, Lung, and Blood Institute and published in the journal *Circulation* in 1992.

For example, a 1989 Parisian study published in *The Lancet* found that those who live the longest are old women with very high cholesterol levels. Women with very low levels had a death rate over five times higher!

And more recently, in the *British Medical Journal*, 2003, researchers at the University of British Columbia concluded that statin drugs, which lower cholesterol, offer no benefit to women for preventing heart disease.

Canada: No Link

Although there is a very slight association between high cholesterol and greater risk of heart disease among American men, this connection doesn't exist for Canadian men. This was the finding of the Quebec Cardiovacsular Study, published in the *Canadian Journal of Cardiology* in 1990. Researchers studied almost 5,000 healthy middle-aged men for 12 years. They explained away their results by claiming that more than 12 years were necessary to see the harmful effects of high cholesterol levels—even though the Framingham results showed clearly that this was not the case.

Russia: Low Cholesterol = Increased Risk

A study carried out by a research team from the Russian Academy of Medical Sciences in St. Petersburg and published in the journal *Circulation*, 1993, found that it was *low* levels of LDL (the "bad" cholesterol that we're always told to keep as low as possible) that were associated with *increased* risk of heart disease. Nor was this higher risk the result of lower levels of HDL (the "good" cholesterol), for the people with low LDL were the ones with the highest HDL levels.

The U.S. Government and LDL

We've described just a few of the medical studies reporting evidence that contradicts the lipid hypothesis. Yet *Diet and Health,* an official review of the research published by the National Research Council in 1990, asserts that LDL is the most important risk factor for heart disease, and in support of this statement, cites studies whose results do not, in fact, prove the relation between cholesterol and heart disease at all.

For example, *Diet and Health* cites a 1977 report from Framingham as evidence that high levels of LDL are dangerous. But one conclusion of this study is actually that "LDL-cholesterol . . . is a marginal risk factor" for people over 50. In fact, Framingham investigators found that women over 70 had a greater risk of heart disease if their LDL was *low.*

The Latest Research

The research cited in official government documents dates back to the early 1970s. What can more recent research tell us?

The Honolulu Heart Program A report published in *The Lancet*, 2001, as part of the Honolulu Heart Program, an ongoing study, looked at lowering cholesterol in the elderly. Researchers compared changes in cholesterol concentrations over 20 years with mortality from all causes. The results completely contradict the lipid hypothesis. Said the researchers, "Our data accords with previous findings of increased mortality in elderly people with low serum cholesterol, and show that . . . the earlier that patients start to have lower cholesterol concentrations, the greater the risk of death . . ." That is, when people maintain low levels of cholesterol in their blood over a long period of time—for example, by eating the kind of low-fat diet that government agencies recommend—their risk of death from all causes will *increase.*

No Benefit from Cholesterol-Lowering Drugs Studies carried out during the last 15 years have focused on the effects of cholesterol-lowering drugs. An analysis of 44 trials involving almost 10,000 patients was published in the *American Journal of Cardiology,* 2003. The investigators found that the death rate among three groups of patients—one taking Lipitor (a very strong cholesterol-lowering drug), one taking other cholesterol-lowering drugs, and one taking nothing—was identical.

Myth #3: High-Fat Foods Increase Blood Cholesterol

A key concept behind the lipid hypothesis is that cholesterol levels vary in different people because they eat different foods. This notion rests on the assumption that the levels of cholesterol in the blood are high in people who eat large amounts of food high in fats, especially animal fats.

Again, however, the results of a great deal of research completely oppose this idea.

Framingham: No Connection

During the early stages of the Framingham study, in the 1950s, researchers asked nearly 1,000 people about their eating habits. They found no connection at all between the food they ate and their cholesterol levels. The authors of the study noted that, although there was "a considerable range" of blood cholesterol levels among the participants, whatever might explain this variation, it was "not the diet."

We don't know why, but this part of the Framingham study was never published.

Tecumseh: No Connection

A study similar to the Framingham study was carried out in the small town of Tecumseh, Michigan, by researchers from the University of Michigan and published in the *American Journal of Clinical Nutrition,* 1976. They asked over 2,000 people about the food they ate during a 24-hour period, as well as about the ingredients in the food.

The study subjects were then divided into three cholesterol-level groups: high, middle, and low.

The results: there was no difference between the amounts that the three groups ate of any particular food item. What's more, the low-cholesterol group ate just as much saturated fat as did the high-cholesterol group.

British Bank Tellers: No Connection

In a report published in the *British Medical Journal,* 1963, researchers asked 99 middle-aged male bank employees in London to weigh and record everything they ate over a two-week period. Once more, the results showed no connection between what they ate and their cholesterol levels.

Just in case they had made an error, the researchers asked 76 of the tellers to do the whole procedure again for a week, at a different time of year: same results.

And finally, to be absolutely certain, the researchers reanalyzed the data from the men whose records were particularly detailed and accurate. Same result as before: no connection.

Israeli Civil Servants: No Connection

In a study published in the *Israel Journal of Medical Sciences*, 1969, researchers in Jerusalem studied the diets and blood cholesterol levels of 10,000 Israeli civil servants. These people came from many different backgrounds—Israel itself, Eastern, Southern, and Central Europe, Asia, and Africa—so their eating habits varied considerably. The amount of animal fat they ate ranged from 10 grams a day to 200, and their cholesterol levels ranged from high to low.

The researchers examined whether all the data from this extremely varied group of people indicated some kind of relationship between animal fat and blood cholesterol level, but they found nothing.

- They saw very low levels of cholesterol both in people who ate small amounts of animal fat and in those who ate the most animal fat.
- At the same time, they found high cholesterol in people who ate high, medium, and low amounts of animal fat.

Just to make sure, the researchers did a smaller study of 62 people using a method similar to that used in the British bank tellers study: they conducted a survey over several days and at different times of year, a method that gives the most accurate results. Nevertheless, they still found absolutely no correlation between the amount of animal fat consumed and blood cholesterol levels.

High-Fat Diet—Good Cholesterol

In a study published in the *Journal of the American College of Nutrition*, 2004, researchers at the State University of New York at Buffalo found that after 11 healthy adults ate a diet in which only 19 percent of calories came from fat for three weeks, their HDL or "good" cholesterol fell. Then they spent three weeks on a diet in which 50 percent of calories came from fat, and their HDL levels increased. Most important, the high-fat diet did not lead to an increase in LDL, the "bad" cholesterol.

Myth #4: Cholesterol Causes Plaque Buildup in Arteries

Another assertion generally taken as axiomatic is that high levels of cholesterol in the blood cause atherosclerosis, the buildup of the fatty plaques that obstruct arteries. Yet much research evidence indicates that high blood cholesterol has no relationship with degree of atherosclerosis.

Coconut and Cholesterol

Experts who promote the lipid hypothesis point to studies in which feeding coconut oil raised cholesterol levels in animals. However, the coconut oil used in these experiments was *fully hydrogenated,* that is, fully saturated with hydrogen, which turns all the fatty acids into saturated fats. (Partial hydrogenation creates mostly trans fatty acids, not all saturated fats.) The researchers were investigating the effects of essential fatty acid deficiency on the test animals, and full hydrogenation to eliminate all the essential fatty acids in the coconut oil. They used coconut oil because it is the only fat that can be fully hydrogenated and still be soft enough to eat.

As expected, the cholesterol levels in the animals went up, confirming other studies showing that essential fatty acid deficiency raises cholesterol levels. Yet, many commentators have pointed to this study as proof that coconut oil raises cholesterol levels, without mentioning that the researchers were not using natural coconut oil, but fully hydrogenated coconut oil that *created* the deficiency.

Other studies comparing various fats and oils found that natural coconut oil promoted the assimilation and storage of essential fatty acids, therefore *preventing* essential fatty acid deficiency. So it's the lack of essential fatty acids that created the health risk, not the coconut itself. And in these studies, an increase in cholesterol levels was simply a marker for another condition—not the *cause* of health problems.

Canadian Veterans

A team of researchers in London, Canada, conducted a long-term study of 800 war veterans confined to a hospital, published in *Circulation,* 1963. For years, the researchers analyzed the veterans' cholesterol levels and studied the arteries of those who died to determine the level of atherosclerosis for each veteran. They found that, although the levels of cholesterol varied considerably from one individual to another, each man's cholesterol remained more or less the same during the entire period of the study. That is, if a veteran had low cholesterol at the beginning of the study, it was still low when he died. Yet the men who had low cholesterol had just as much atherosclerosis as those with high cholesterol.

What About the Japanese?

The Japanese have low blood cholesterol, and their risk of heart attack is much lower than that of any other nation. According to the lipid hypothesis, atherosclerosis should be rare in Japan.

Two studies sought to confirm this. In the first, published in the *American*

Journal of Cardiology, 1985, researchers from Kyushu University looked at the aorta (the main artery of the body, which carries blood out of the heart) in 659 Americans and 260 Japanese, for signs of atherosclerosis. They found very little difference between the two groups, at all age levels.

The second study, carried out at the Geriatric Hospital in Tokyo and presented at the International Symposium of Atherosclerosis, 1977, examined the arteries of the brain in 1,408 Japanese and over 5,000 Americans. In every age group, the Japanese had *more* atherosclerosis in these arteries than the Americans did.

As for the coronary arteries—the ones involved in heart attacks—the Japanese have less atherosclerosis in these arteries than do Americans, which may be why they are less prone to heart attacks.

But if high cholesterol is what causes atherosclerosis, this should occur in all types of arteries, since the amount of cholesterol in the blood is the same in all parts of the body. It seems much more likely that something other than cholesterol causes atherosclerosis. Blood pressure, for example, does vary in different arteries and at different times, for example when you are under stress. But few scientists seem willing to look at these complicated details.

Cholesterol Lowering: No Effect on Plaque Buildup

A recent study, published in the *American Journal of Cardiology*, 2003, found that patients who successfully lowered their cholesterol levels did not reduce plaque buildup in their arteries. One group took a strong dose of a cholesterol-lowering drug while the other took a lower dose of the same drug. Researchers then measured the amount of blockage in their arteries. After more than one year, both groups showed a 9.2 percent *increase* in plaque buildup, suggesting that plaque buildup is not related to cholesterol level.

If This Is All True . . . Why Does the Lipid Hypothesis Still Rule?

In science, the burden of proof rests on the scientist. If even one study contradicts a hypothesis, then we must at the very least be open to reevaluating the hypothesis, even if many studies support it. We've just described *many* studies that contradict the lipid hypothesis, yet it remains the ruling theory of heart disease in modern medicine.

Why? Consider the fact that the widespread credence given to the lipid hypothesis certainly has helped a number of industries. For example, the hypothesis provides the pharmaceutical industry with a rationale for selling cholesterol-lowering drugs, which today is a multibillion-dollar business. The hypothesis has also been a boon for the food industry, since it justifies the use of inexpensive vegetable oils in processed food products, rather than more expensive coconut oil and animal fats.

The following pages tell the story of how, due in part to the exertions of these industries, the lipid hypothesis became the basis of government policy. Going back 60 years, we'll trace the evolution of this idea and the huge impact it has had on what Americans are eating today. And we'll tell the tale partly from a personal perspective, for an important participant in the struggle was Dr. Mary Enig.

The Lipid Hypothesis Gets Rolling

David Kritchevsky's 1954 studies, published in the *American Journal of Physiology*, July through September 1954, attracted the attention of scientists concerned about the emerging epidemic of heart disease because they appeared to support the lipid hypothesis. Kritchevsky's studies demonstrated that

- cholesterol caused atherosclerosis in vegetarian rabbits;
- polyunsaturated fatty acids could lower blood cholesterol levels in humans.

Kritchevsky's work *appeared* to show that by reducing the levels of animal products in their diet, Americans could avoid heart disease—as long as scientists ignored the many studies (including those we've described above) that contradicted Kritchevsky's findings. In fact, Kritchevsky's studies had no relevance to the lipid hypothesis for two reasons. First, the kind of plaque the rabbits developed was completely different from the kind of plaque humans develop. Second, the rabbits were fed purified cholesterol that was oxidized (damaged by processing), not the kind contained in ordinary food.

The lipid hypothesis was introduced to the American people in 1956, when the American Heart Association (AHA) aired a fund-raiser on all three major television networks. The panelists presented the hypothesis as the cause of heart disease and recommended the Prudent Diet, in which corn oil, margarine, chicken, and cold cereal replaced butter, lard, beef, and eggs. It was on this television show that cardiologist Dr. Dudley White, who served as one of the panelists, made his comments objecting to the lipid hypothesis and the Prudent Diet.

"See here," he remarked, "I began my practice as a cardiologist in 1921 and I never saw an MI patient until 1928. Back in the MI-free days before 1920, the fats were butter and lard and I think that we would all benefit from the kind of diet that we had at a time when no one had ever heard the words 'corn oil.'"

Despite these nationally televised comments, and in spite of the numerous contradictory studies already published in the scientific literature, the lipid hypothesis had already gained enough momentum to keep it rolling. (One such contradictory study was the Anti-Coronary Club project; see sidebar, page 27.) Both the food processing industry and the pharmaceutical industry could see the benefits of making patients out of healthy people, simply by making them afraid of cholesterol.

The following year, the food industry initiated advertising campaigns touting the health benefits of products low in fat or made with vegetable oils. A typical ad read: "Wheaties may help you live longer." Wesson recommended its cooking oil to consumers "for your heart's sake," while an ad in the *Journal of the American Medical Association* described Wesson Oil as a "cholesterol depressant." Mazola advertisements assured the public that "science finds corn oil important to your health." Medical journal ads recommended Fleishmann's unsalted margarine for patients with high blood pressure. Prominent physicians endorsed the use of vegetable oils as substitutes for saturated fat. Such claims continued well into the 1980s, after which they were quietly dropped when studies indicated that polyunsaturated oils contributed to cancer.

The American Medical Association at first opposed the commercialization of the lipid hypothesis, warning that "the anti-fat, anti-cholesterol fad is not just foolish and futile . . . it also carries some risk." The AHA, however, was committed to supporting the lipid hypothesis. In 1961, the AHA published its first dietary guidelines aimed at the public. The authors, Irving Page, Ancel Keys, Jeremiah Stamler, and Frederick Stare, called for the substitution of polyunsaturates for saturated fat, even though Keys, Stare, and Page had all previously noted in published papers that the increase in CHD was paralleled by increasing consumption of vegetable oils. In fact, in a 1956 paper, Keys had suggested that the increasing use of hydrogenated vegetable oils might be the underlying cause of the CHD epidemic.

These ongoing concerns about hydrogenated vegetable oils prompted the inclusion in a 1968 statement by the AHA on diet and heart disease of a carefully worded disavowal, making clear that the types of fats thought to lower cholesterol were not the same ones present in hydrogenated fats. The AHA statement implied that proponents of the lipid hypothesis could not claim that hydrogenated fats were heart healthy.

However, that disclaimer was never released. Among the likely reasons were the shortening industry's strong objections to the disclaimer and a letter from Fred Mattson, a researcher at Procter & Gamble, to Campbell Moses, medical director of the AHA, urging against its distribution, even though 150,000 copies had already been printed. The letter that Mattson wrote to Dr. Moses is part of the Congressional Record, for it was submitted as testimony during hearings held in 1977 by the McGovern Committee on Nutrition and Human Needs. The final recommendations to the public that the AHA did publish omitted the warning that partially hydrogenated (that is, trans) fats did not protect against heart disease.

Other organizations soon fell in behind the AHA in pushing vegetable oils instead of animal fats. By the early 1970s, the National Heart, Lung, and Blood Institute, the American Medical Association, the American Dietetic Association, and the National Academy of Sciences had all endorsed the lipid hypothesis and cautioned Americans to avoid animal fats.

Soon Congress jumped on the vegetable oil bandwagon. In 1977, George McGovern's Senate Select Committee on Nutrition and Human Needs published "Dietary Goals for the United States." Citing U.S. Department of Agriculture (USDA) data on fat consumption, the report stated categorically that "the overconsumption of fat, generally, and saturated fat in particular . . . have been related to six of the ten leading causes of death" in the United States. The report urged Americans to reduce overall fat intake and to substitute polyunsaturates for saturated fat from animal sources—margarine and corn oil for butter, lard, and tallow.

Opposing testimony included a moving letter—buried in the voluminous report—by Dr. Fred Kummerow of the University of Illinois, urging a return to traditional whole foods and warning against the use of soft drinks. In the early 1970s, Kummerow had shown that trans fatty acids caused increased rates of heart disease in pigs. A private endowment allowed him to continue his research, for government funding agencies such as the National Institutes of Health refused to give him further grants.

Enter Mary Enig

That same year, Mary Enig, a graduate student at the University of Maryland, began research on the levels of trans fatty acids in foods and the effects of dietary trans fatty acids on important enzyme systems in mice (mice react to drugs and other chemical carcinogens in a way similar to humans). When she read the McGovern Committee report, she was puzzled because she was familiar with Kummerow's research and knew that animal fat consumption was declining, not increasing. So how could the McGovern Committee find a connection between animal fat and heart disease?

Enig's own analysis of the same USDA data that the McGovern Committee cited pointed to very different conclusions: that people eating animal fat actually had *less* heart disease (as well as less cancer, another concern of the committee) than those who ate vegetable oil. She wrote a paper describing her findings, which was published in the Proceedings of the Federation of American Societies for Experimental Biology (FASEB) in July 1978. Her paper used the McGovern Committee's own data to refute its conclusions that animal fats cause heart disease and cancer. She noted further that the data pointed a finger at trans fatty acids as possible causes of these diseases. In conclusion, she called for further investigation.

Mary and the other University of Maryland researchers recognized the need for more research in two areas:

- The first question involved the effects of trans fats on cells once these fats became part of the cell membrane.

While some studies indicated that trans fatty acids posed no danger in a normal diet, Mary and her colleagues were not so sure. Some research indicated

Mary Enig Remembers

My paper rang alarm bells throughout the food industry. In early 1979, a representative from the National Association of Margarine Manufacturers came to see me. Visibly annoyed, he explained that both his association and the Institute for Shortening and Edible Oils (ISEO) kept careful watch to prevent articles like mine from appearing. My paper should never have been published, he said, since ISEO was supposed to be "watching out." As he put it, "We left the barn door open, and the horse got out."

He also challenged the data from the USDA that the committee and I had both used. He knew this data was incorrect, he told me, "because we give it to them." He didn't say the data was intentionally incorrect, but I had my suspicions.

A few weeks later, the same fellow met with me and the other members of the lipids group at the University of Maryland, this time accompanied by an ISEO adviser who also represented Kraft Foods, plus representatives from Central Soya and Lever Brothers (manufacturers of margarine and shortening). Clutching a two-inch stack of newspaper articles reporting on my article (including one in the *National Enquirer*), he shook them at me indignantly.

When I repeated this earlier admission that the margarine lobby had given the Department of Agriculture incorrect food data, his face flushed red with anger.

He also warned our lipids group that we would never get any more funding if we continued our current research: a survey of trans fats levels in supermarket foods. Incredibly, we were alone in attempting to gather this data since government databases at the time contained no reference to trans fats.

We continued nevertheless, and eventually published a paper on our findings, but the industry was true to its word. The lipids group at the University of Maryland never got another penny for trans fat research, and as the professors retired, the group's effort was gradually abandoned, except for some ongoing analysis for the USDA.

During his initial visit, the rather indiscreet National Association of Margarine Manufacturers representative also revealed that he had dropped in on the FASEB office in an attempt to pressure them to publish letters to refute my paper without giving me the chance to respond, as was customary. But the editors resisted the pressure and allowed me to reply to a series of letters criticizing my paper.

My reply stressed the correlation between vegetable fat consumption, especially trans fat consumption, and serious disease, including heart disease. I noted that the data warranted more thorough investigation, but no one was doing it.

that the trans fats contributed to heart disease. Mary's own research, published in her 1984 doctoral dissertation, indictated that trans fats interfered with enzyme systems in the body that made carcinogens harmless and increased enzymes that made carcinogens more toxic.

- The second question the researchers wanted to answer was: how much trans fat did the typical American consume?

At that time there was no data regarding the amount of trans fats in common foods. What's more, the data in U.S. government databases on any type of fat content in foods was often incorrect, Mary found.

To remedy this situation, Joseph Sampagna and Mark Keeney, lipid biochemists at the University of Maryland, applied to the National Science Foundation, the National Institutes of Health, the USDA, the National Dairy Council, and the National Livestock and Meat Board for funds to look into the trans fat content of common American foods. Only the National Livestock and Meat Board came through with a small grant for equipment; the others turned them down. One USDA official privately revealed that they would never get money as long as they pursued the trans fat work.

Nevertheless, they did pursue it. Sampagna, Keeney, and a few graduate students, including Mary, funded jointly by an existing USDA stipend for graduate students and by the university, spent thousands of hours in the laboratory analyzing the trans fat content of hundreds of commercially available foods. Mary herself, at times with a small stipend, at times without pay, helped direct the tedious process of analysis.

In December 1982, *Food Processing* carried a brief preview of the University of Maryland research. Five months later, the journal printed a blistering letter from Edward Hunter on behalf of the ISEO. Hunter was concerned that the Maryland group would exaggerate the amount of trans fat found in common foods. He cited ISEO data indicating that most margarines and shortenings contained no more than 35 percent and 25 percent trans, respectively, and usually considerably less.

Mary and her colleagues found that many margarines indeed contained about 31 percent trans fat (later surveys by others revealed that Parkay margarine contained up to 45 percent trans fat), but many shortenings found ubiquitously in cookies, chips, and baked goods contained more than 35 percent. She also discovered that many baked goods and processed foods contained considerably more fat from partially hydrogenated vegetables oils than was indicated on the label. This finding was confirmed by Canadian government researchers many years later, in 1993.

Mary's groundbreaking final results were published in 1983 in the *Journal of the American Oil Chemists Society*. Her analyses allowed University of Maryland researchers to confirm earlier estimates that the average American consumed at least 12 grams of trans fat per day—directly contradicting ISEO assertions that most Ameircans consumed no more than 6 to 8 grams per day. People who delibrately avoided animal fats typically consumed far more than 12 grams of trans fat per day, while vulnerable teenagers who ate a lot of processed snack foods typically took in 30 grams or more of trans fats a day.

Mary and her colleagues at the University of Maryland, opposed by the ISEO representatives, continued their debate in a form of cat-and-mouse game running through several scientific journals. The ISEO representatives peppered the literature with articles that downplayed the dangers of trans fats, used their influence to discourage opposing points of view from appearing in print, and responded to the few alarmist articles that did squeak through with "definitive rebuttals." For example, Hunter continued to object to assertions that average consumption of trans fat in partially hydrogenated margarines and shortenings could be more than 6 to 8 grams per day—a concern that puzzled Mary, since the ISEO also claimed that trans fatty acids posed no threat to public health.

As the debate continued through the 1980s, Mary testified before several expert panels. Early in 1985, for example, for the Federation of American Societies for Experimental Biology (FASEB), she reported on a series of University of Maryland studies indicating that trans fats might promote heart disease. Her testimony was omitted from the final report, although her work was listed in the bibliography, giving the impression that her research supported the assertions by other witnesses that trans fats were safe.

In other testimony, Mary pointed out that claims of trans fats' safety were based on flawed data. She argued that the percentages of trans fats should be included on food nutrition labels and cited the lack of information on trans fats in national food databases. Finally, she urged that Congress mandate correction of the databases and reevaluate dietary recommendations based on erroneous data.

Nevertheless, orthodox medical agencies remained united in promoting margarine and vegetable oils over animal foods containing cholesterol and animal fats. They maintained this position even though the official literature contained only a handful of experiments indicating that dietary cholesterol plays a major role in determining blood cholesterol levels. And many of these studies drew conclusions from flawed methodology that produced erroneous results.

In 1984, scientists who disputed the lipid hypothesis were invited to speak briefly at the NHLBI-sponsored National Cholesterol Consensus Conference, but their views were not included in the panel's report for the simple reason that NHLBI staff generated the report even before the conference convened. Dr. Beverly Teter of the University of Maryland's lipid group discovered this disquieting fact when she picked up someone else's papers by mistake just before the conference opened and found that they contained the report already written, with just a few numbers left blank.

In 1987, the National Academy of Sciences published a booklet containing a whitewash of the trans fat problem and a pejorative description of palm oil—

a natural fat high in beneficial saturates and monounsaturates that, like coconut oil and butter, has nourished healthy populations for thousands of years,
and, also like coconut oil and butter, competes with hydrogenated fats because
it can be used as a shortening.

The following year, the Surgeon General's Report on Nutrition and Health
urged that low-fat foods should be more widely available. Project LEAN
(Low-Fat Eating for America Now), sponsored by the J. Kaiser Family Foundation and a host of establishment groups such as the AHA, the American Dietetic Association, the American Medical Association, the USDA, the National
Cancer Institute, the Centers for Disease Control, and the NHLBI, announced
a publicity campaign to "aggressively promote foods low in saturated fat and
cholesterol in order to reduce the risk of heart disease and cancer."

Other scientists too were attempting to make the public aware of their concerns about partially hydrogenated fats. Fred Kummerow at the University of
Illinois, blessed with independent funding and an abundance of patience, carried out a number of studies published in scientific journals between the early
1970s and the present, indicating that trans fats increased risk factors associated with heart disease, and that fabricated foods such as Egg Beaters, which

Mary Enig Remembers

In 1989, I joined Frank McLaughlin, director of the Center for Business
and Public Policy at the University of Maryland, in testimony before the National Food Processors Association. It was a closed conference, for NFPA
members only. We had been invited to give "a view from academia." I presented a number of slides and warned against singling out classes of fats and
oils for special pejorative labeling. A representative from Frito-Lay took um-
brage at my slides, which listed amounts of trans fats in Frito-Lay products.
I offered to redo the analyses if Frito-Lay would fund the research. "If you'd
talk different, you'd get money" was the response. (Ironically, Frito-Lay now
claims that their products contain no trans fats.)

Next, I urged the association to endorse accurate labeling of trans fats in
all food items, but conference participants—including representatives from
most of the major food processing giants—preferred a policy of "voluntary
labeling" that was lax in alerting the public to the presence of trans fats in
their products. It has taken over 15 years for the FDA to mandate trans fats
labeling, and that was done only after a committee of scientists concluded
that processed trans fats are unsafe at any level. The new labeling is due on
January 1, 2006. It's good to have your research validated after all these
years—but we have a long way to go, because these agencies still condemn
saturated fats, saying they're "as bad as trans fatty acids."

are made with vegetable oils, cannot support life. George Mann, formerly with the Framingham project, possessed neither funding nor patience—he was, in fact, very angry with what he called the "diet/heart scam." His independent studies of the Masai in Africa, described earlier, had convinced him that the lipid hypothesis was "the public health diversion of this century . . . the greatest scam in the history of medicine." Mann resolved to bring the issue before the public by organizing a conference in Washington, D.C., in November of 1991.

"Hundreds of millions of tax dollars are wasted by the bureaucracy and the self-interested Heart Association," he wrote in his invitation to participants. "Segments of the food industry play the game for profits. Research on the true causes and prevention is stifled by denying funding to the 'unbelievers.' This meeting will review the data and expose the rascals."

The meeting did take place, but several speakers dropped out at the last minute, leading Mann to comment, "Scientists who must go before review panels for their research funding know well that to speak out, to disagree with this false dogma of Diet/Heart, is a fatal error. They must comply or go unfunded. I could show a list of scientists who said to me, in effect, when I invited them to participate, 'I believe you are right, that the Diet/Heart hypothesis is wrong, but I cannot join you because that would jeopardize my perks and funding.' For me, that kind of hypocritical response separates the scientists from the operators—the men from the boys."

By the 1990s, the United States had been transformed from a healthy nation consuming real foods, including traditional animal fats and tropical oils, into a decidedly unhealthy nation that ate mostly imitation foods based on vegetable oils. Consumption of butter was at an all-time low; use of lard and tallow was down by two-thirds. Prosperous Americans now consumed the same type of diet that Dr. Price observed in his Depression-era patients—and suffered from the same health problems he warned against.

Margarine consumption has changed little since 1960, perhaps because knowledge of margarine's dangers has been so slowly seeping into the public consciousness. However, most of the trans fats in the current American diet come not from margarine but from shortening used in fried and processed foods. And since the 1940s, the content of that shortening has gradually changed from mostly lard, tallow, and coconut oil to partially hydrogenated soybean oil. At the same time, shortening consumption shot up. By 1993, it had tripled to over 30 grams per person per day.

But the most dramatic overall change in the American diet was a 15-fold increase in the consumption of liquid vegetable oils, from slightly less than 2 grams per person per day in 1909 to over 30 in 1993.

In our view, the largely unrecognized power of the vegetable oil industry explains why myths about the "dangers" of saturated fat and cholesterol have dominated popular thinking about what constitutes a healthy diet. Fortunately, the wind of opinion has begun to shift. Even some old-line adherents of the lipid hypothesis may be tacking in a new direction.

The Evolution of Ideas

In 1998, a symposium titled "Evolution of Ideas About the Nutritional Value of Dietary Fat" reviewed the many flaws in the lipid hypothesis. One participant was David Kritchevsky, the same researcher whose early work helped launch the lipid hypothesis. He noted that the use of low-fat diets in a number of experiments "did not affect overall CHD mortality." And he concluded, "Research continues apace and, as new findings appear, it may be necessary to reevaluate our conclusions and preventive medicine policies."

Finally, it seems, scientists are waking up from their long infatuation with the lipid hypothesis. Eventually our government and medical experts will be forced to issue revised policies on saturated fat, just as they finally have had to admit that trans fats are dangerous. But there's no reason for you to wait for official government pronouncements to begin enjoying the health and weight-loss benefits of saturated fats. To learn more about why these fats are good for you, and more about the harmful effects of vegetable oils and trans fats, turn to Chapter 3.

Chapter Three

Know Your Fats—and Your Nutrients

In this chapter, you'll learn why you need the healthy fats you will consume on this diet. Second, we'll show you why eating unhealthy fats and low-fat products can sabotage your health and weight-loss goals. And finally, we'll explain the facts about your need for vital nutrients that you may not be getting if you're only consuming the USDA Recommended Daily Allowances (RDAs) of vitamins and minerals.

Why You Need the *Right* Kinds of Fat

In all three of the Eat Fat, Lose Fat programs, you will be consuming not only coconut oil, but also cod-liver oil supplements (which work in combination with coconut), as well as other healthy traditional fats such as butter, egg yolks, meat fats, and even lard. These fats provide key nutrients you need to maintain both optimal health and your desired weight.

Fats and Your Brain

Sixty percent of the brain is composed of fat. Phospholipids (which contain about *50 percent saturated fats*) help make up the brain cell membranes. They contain two fatty acids and one proteinlike component. Generally, the phospholipids in the cell membranes contain one saturated fatty acid and one unsaturated fatty acid. Thus you nourish your brain cells when you eat saturated fats, and when you don't eat enough saturated fats, the chemistry of your brain may be compromised. In a recent study, rats given vegetable oils low in saturated fats and omega-3 fatty acids had more strokes and shorter life spans.

Fats in the Cells

Saturated fats maintain cellular integrity everywhere in the body. Why? Because *every* cell membrane is ideally made up of about 50 percent saturated fat. When we eat too much polyunsaturated oil and not enough saturated fat (or carbohydrates that the body turns into saturated fat), our cells don't function correctly. Those cell membrane fatty acids need to be saturated for the cell to have the necessary "stiffness" or integrity and to work properly. When the cell walls do not contain enough saturated fat, they actually become "floppy" and cannot work properly.

Fats in Your Bones

A study published in the 1996 *American Oil Chemists Society Proceedings* found that for calcium to be effectively incorporated into the skeletal structure, at least 50 percent of dietary fats should be saturated. Why has osteoporosis become such a problem these days? One reason is the lack of fats like coconut oil and butter in our diets.

Fats and Your Liver

Open any biochemistry textbook and you will read that saturated fats protect the liver from toxins like alcohol and Tylenol. The tradition of eating butter or lard before a drinking bout is based on good science (although we do not recommend anything but very moderate alcohol consumption!). Today, as people shun saturated fats and eat more polyunsaturated oils, liver problems have become more common.

Fats and Your Heart

Saturated fats provide energy to the heart in times of stress. Studies have shown that saturated fats are the heart's preferred food, which is why there is a concentration of saturated fat in the tissues surrounding the heart. Moreover, two studies have shown that saturated fatty acids in the diet lower a substance in the blood called Lp(a), which (unlike cholesterol) is a good predictor of heart disease. Furthermore, saturated fats help reduce levels of a substance called C-Reactive Protein (CRP), an indicator of inflammation. Current theories hold inflammation responsible for many cases of heart disease.

Levels of total cholesterol, HDL (high-density lipoprotein, or "good" cholesterol) and LDL (low-density lipoprotein, or "bad cholesterol") are actually not good predictors of heart disease. And, as we saw in Chapter 2, heart disease is just as frequent in people with low cholesterol as in those with high cholesterol.

Fats and Your Lungs

The lungs cannot work without adequate saturated fats in the diet. This is because the fatty acids in the lung surfactant (a fluid that enables the lungs to work) are normally 100 percent saturated. When people consume a lot of partially hydrogenated fats and vegetable oils, trans fatty acids and polyunsaturated fatty acids are put into the phospholipids where the body normally needs saturated fatty acids. As a result, the lungs cannot work effectively.

Recent research suggests that consumption of trans fats and excess polyunsaturated oils contributes to the rising incidence of asthma in children, while children who consume ample amounts of butterfat have much lower rates of asthma. In fact, changes in fat consumption patterns over the past 30 years explain the rising incidence of all types of lung disease, including asthma and lung cancer.

Fats and Your Kidneys

Omega-3 fatty acids, saturated fats, and cholesterol all work together synergistically to maintain normal kidney function, which is critical for managing blood pressure and filtering toxins from the body. High consumption of polyunsaturated oils by the rats in the study mentioned on page 45 resulted in injury to the kidneys as well as the brain.

Coconut oil also enhances kidney function by providing a saturated fatty acid called myristic acid, which plays a vital role in the biochemistry of the kidneys. In a key reaction called myristolation, myristic acid is added to a protein. This process allows the cells of the kidney to communicate with each other.

Fats and Your Hormones

Hormones are the body's messengers, acting on the brain, nervous system, and glands and affecting thousands of bodily functions. Hormones require the right kinds of fats for proper functioning; your body cannot make stress and sex hormones without vitamin A, provided exclusively by fatty animal foods such as liver, shellfish, and cod-liver oil (taken as liquid or capsules). In contrast, the wrong kind of fats (the trans fatty acids) *inhibits* the production of stress and sex hormones, leading to problems with glucose balance, mineral metabolism, and reproduction.

Fats and Prostaglandins

Hormones that act locally, within the cells, are called prostaglandins. There are three major classes of prostaglandins, two of which are made from omega-6 fatty acids and one of which is made from omega-3 fatty acids. For the optimal production and balance of these prostaglandins, you need a good balance of omega-3 to omega-6 fatty acids, with no more than two or three times more omega-6 than omega-3. Unfortunately, in the modern diet, the ratio is more like 20 to 1, as a result of the high consumption of vegetable oils containing mostly omega-6 fatty acids.

While saturated fats play key roles in regulating the production of prostaglandins, trans fats interfere with this process, resulting in all sorts of imbalances that can lead to inflammation, weight gain, allergies, asthma, and even alcoholism and cancer.

Coconut oil in conjunction with other traditional fats supports the optimal production and balance of prostaglandins. So to redress this imbalance between omega-6 and omega-3, it is essential to avoid all commercial vegetable oils (which are composed largely of omega-6 fatty acids) and add coconut and traditional food sources of omega-3 fatty acids to the diet, such as wild salmon, egg yolks, from pastured chickens, and flax oil (added in small amounts to salad dressings).

Fats and Cell Communication

Both myristic acid from coconut and another saturated fatty acid called palmitic acid are involved in complex processes of cell communication. To adequately supply the body with the wide range of saturated fatty acids for these and the other functions we've described, it's important that the fats in our diet come from a variety of sources (including coconut oil).

All Fats Are Not Created Equal

We've already described the three basic types of fats and explained why saturated fats are *not* the culprits in the current epidemic of heart disease. Now let's explore in more depth the differences between saturated fats, especially coconut oil and polyunsaturated fats—particularly in relation to your health, weight loss, and well-being.

An oil's degree of saturation is determined by the climate in which it is grown. Vegetable oils from nuts and seeds that grow in northern climates contain mostly polyunsaturated oils. They are liquid at room temperature in a temperate zone. A temperate-climate plant like the olive tree produces a monosaturated oil that is liquid at warm temperatures but hardens when refrigerated. Vegetable oils from plants grown in tropical regions (like the coconut and palm) were designed by nature with increased saturation to help maintain their plant's leaf stiffness even in a hot climate where less firm oils would melt. That's why tropical oils are liquid in the tropics but hard as butter in northern climates.

Special Properties of the Coconut

Among saturated fats, coconut is queen because of its special properties.

Coconut Contains Abundant Medium-Chain Fatty Acids (MCFAs)

While longer-chain fatty acids, found in many foods, need to be digested by bile salts (secreted by the gallbladder), coconut's medium-chain fatty acids do not. That's why if you have trouble digesting fats, or are beginning to reintroduce fat to your diet, it's best to begin with coconut oil.

Coconut Contains High Amounts of Lauric Acid

The main MCFA in coconut oil is lauric acid, a proven antiviral, antibacterial, and antifungal agent that is also found in mother's milk. Converted in your body to a substance called monolaurin, it helps you defend against viruses, bacteria, and other pathogens and strengthens your immune system, protecting you from a wide range of diseases. Highly protective lauric acid should be called a "conditionally essential fatty acid," because it is made only by the mammary gland and not in the liver like other saturated fats. You can get it from just three dietary sources: in small amounts, butterfat, and in large amounts, coconut oil and palm kernel oil.

Coconut Is Synergistic with Essential Fatty Acids

Your body needs saturated fats to most effectively retain and use essential fatty acids (EFAs). When you consume lots of saturated fats, your body actually needs only a very small amount of essential fatty acids (both omega-3 and omega-6).

Coconut as Immune Booster

How do lauric acid and monolaurin boost your immunity? They have antimicrobial properties and will help your body fight disease organisms, including

- viruses, such as the herpes virus, measles virus, and HIV;
- bacteria, such as listeria (which causes food poisoning), staphylococcus, and streptococcus;
- protozoa (parasites), such as giardia lamblia (which causes gastroenteritis).

Did You Know . . . ?

Coconut is the most important nut crop in the world, grown on approximately 12 million hectares spread over at least 86 countries. The chief producers are in Asia: coconut is a key element in the economies of the Philippines, Indonesia, India, Sri Lanka, Malaysia, Thailand, and Vietnam. Coconut also grows throughout the Pacific Islands, in equatorial Africa, and in the Americas, especially Mexico, Brazil, Jamaica, the Caribbean islands, the Dominican Republic, and El Salvador.

Most of the world's coconut production comes from small farms. It is an ecologically sound crop, able to grow in difficult environments, such as atolls, or under conditions of high salinity, drought, or poor soil. It plays an important role in maintaining the fragile ecosystems of island and coastal communities.

Coconut trees produce between 50 and 100 nuts per year. Production begins when the palm is six years old, and the trees can live as long as 60 years.

About 70 percent of the coconut crop is consumed locally, as food, drink, and cooking oil. The fibers are used to make twine and rope. Western cultures have found other uses for the coconut, particularly in cleaning products and cosmetics. Any chemical compound containing "laureth" or "laurel" has been derived from the lauric acid in coconut oil.

Polyunsaturates: The Wrong Kinds of Fats

Remember all those television commercials singing the praises of polyunsaturated oils, like corn, safflower, soy, canola, and others? Well, they were just that: commercials.

Remember the warnings by leading doctors and medical authorities condemning saturated fats and encouraging polyunsaturates for heart health?

Perhaps not surprisingly, it turns out that many physicians were misled by the strategic influence campaign brought to you by industries that benefited financially from this (supposed) health message, as you've seen in Chapter 2.

Other Healthy Fat Sources

On our diet, in addition to coconut and cod-liver oil, you will be consuming other healthy fats from dairy, eggs, and meats. These are foods that, along with coconut, many doctors and government officials have told us not to eat. However, they contain many valuable nutrients and cofactors and should be part of your diet. The Eat Fat, Lose Fat programs include a number of healthy nutrients from milk products, eggs, and meats that you'll enjoy. Here's why you need them.

The Truth About Polyunsaturated Oils

The commercial oils that most Americans consume are extracted by toxic chemicals at high temperatures, a process that turns them rancid, destroys their nutrients, and produces free radicals (reactive molecule fragments that steal electrons from molecules in a process called oxidation, which damages cells). These free radicals can contribute to a host of diseases, including cancer, heart disease, premature aging, autoimmune disease, digestive disorders, and infertility.

Science has shown that even when cold pressed (as are many "natural health food" products), polyunsaturated oils consumed in anything but small amounts can contribute to many disease conditions, including increased risk of cancer and heart disease; immune system dysfunction; damage to the liver, reproductive organs, and lungs; digestive disorders; diminished learning ability; impaired growth; and weight gain.

Some experts tout these oils because they contain omega-6 essential fatty acids, but most Americans consume ample amounts of these fats from other foods (such as legumes, grains, nuts, green vegetables, olive oil, and animal fats), and excessive amounts can be harmful, resulting in an unhealthy ratio of omega-3 to omega-6 fatty acids.

Key Factors in Healthy Dairy, Eggs, and Meat

Let's face it, you can't live on coconuts alone. What you eat in addition to the coconut oil and other products on this diet is critically important. Coconut is a heavy lifter, but it can't do everything. That's why you'll be eating coconut as part of a nutrient-dense, satisfying traditional foods diet. The following foods contain key nutrients that support many essential functions in the body and are also found in other nutrient-dense foods that we recommend in Chapter 5. Together with coconut, they will provide all you need for vital metabolic functions.

Eggs and Liver These foods contain small but important amounts of arachidonic acid (AA), a very long-chain polyunsaturated fat that

- supports brain function;
- is used in your cell membranes;
- helps build one category of prostaglandins.

Some dietary gurus warn against eating foods rich in AA, claiming that it contributes to the production of "bad" prostaglandins that cause inflammation. But prostaglandins that counteract inflammation are also made from AA, so there is no problem including these foods in your diet.

Egg yolks also contain lecithin, which assists in the proper assimilation and

The Truth About Palm Oil and Palm Kernel Oils

Coconut oil comes from the nut of the coconut palm; palm oil and palm kernel oil come from the fruit of the oil palm. The coconut palm grows in coastal regions, while the oil palm grows in inland areas of tropical regions.

Palm oil is a healthy oil easily extracted from the oily palm fruit. It contains almost 50 percent saturated fat, mostly in the form of palmitic acid. It is widely consumed as a cooking oil in Africa and Asia, and European manufacturers are now using it in preference to trans fats in baked goods and snack foods.

Palm kernel comes from the seed of the palm fruit. It is a specialized oil, highly saturated, which is used mostly in candy making. Like coconut oil, palm kernel oil is rich in lauric acid, but it's more expensive.

metabolization of cholesterol and other fat constituents and trace minerals. Choline, another component of egg yolks, is critical to healthy nerve function.

Butter Butter contains lecithin, AA, omega-6 and omega-3 essential fatty acids, and short- and medium-chain fatty acids, which, like coconut oil, protect us against infection. Butter, as well as other animal fats, also provides palmitoleic acid, a monounsaturated fatty acid that has antimicrobial properties and is key for communication between cells. Butyric acid, a very short-chain saturated fatty acid, is practically unique to butter. It has antifungal properties as well as antitumor effects.

Butterfat (like the fats in meat and egg yolks) also contains many trace minerals, including manganese, zinc, chromium, copper, selenium, and iodine. In mountainous areas far from the sea, the iodine in butter protects against goiter. Butter is extremely rich in selenium, a trace mineral with antioxidant properties, containing more per gram than herring or wheat germ.

Beef and Lamb Omega-6 and omega-3 essential fatty acids occur in nearly equal amounts in the fat of beef and lamb. This excellent balance between linoleic and linolenic acid supports optimal prostaglandin production. The fat of pasture-fed beef and lamb, as well as butter made from pasture-fed cows, contains a form of rearranged omega-6 linoleic acid called conjugated linoleic acid (CLA), which has strong anticancer properties. It also encourages the buildup of muscle and prevents weight gain. CLA disappears when cows are fed even small amounts of grain or processed feed.

Whole Milk Glycosphingolipids, fats that protect against gastrointestinal infections, especially in the very young and the elderly, are found in whole milk.

Children who drink skim milk and thus don't get the benefits of glycosphingolipids have diarrhea at rates three to five times greater than children who drink whole milk.

The common denominator among all these foods is *cholesterol*, which the body needs to produce a variety of steroids that protect against cancer, heart disease, and mental illness. As we reported in Chapter 2, cholesterol is the precursor to the sex hormones, stress hormones, bile salts, and vitamin D. Mother's milk is high in cholesterol because it is essential for growth and the development of the brain and nervous system. No research has ever shown that cholesterol *in natural foods* causes heart disease.

Avoiding Toxins in Fats and Other Food

Despite their many healthy components, fats, like other foods, can accumulate environmental toxins. In particular, fats accumulate DDT and similar fat-soluble poisons. For this reason, some experts counsel avoiding fats. However, fats are not the only foods that can contain environmental hazards. Water-soluble poisons, such as antibiotics and growth hormones, accumulate in the water component of milk and meats, as well as in vegetables and grains.

The average plant crop receives ten applications of pesticides from seed to storage—while cows generally graze on pasture that is unsprayed. Aflatoxin, a fungus that grows on grain, is one of the most powerful carcinogens known. Unfortunately, all our foods, whether of vegetable or animal origin, may be contaminated.

Oxidized Cholesterol

Contrary to what you've heard, cholesterol is not the cause of heart disease, but rather a potent antioxidant weapon against free radicals in the blood. Naturally produced in the body and naturally present in the foods we eat, it's a repair substance that actually helps heal arterial damage.

However, heat and oxygen can damage cholesterol just as they do fats. Damaged, or "oxidized," cholesterol can injure arterial walls and lead to a pathological plaque buildup in the arteries. Both of these changes can result in heart disease.

That's why we recommend that you avoid foods that contain damaged cholesterol, such as powdered eggs and powdered milk (which manufacturers add to reduced-fat milk, yogurt, and other dairy products to give them body—without stating this fact on the label). Ironically, when you choose reduced-fat milks in order to avoid heart disease, you consume the very form of cholesterol that can *cause* heart disease.

The way to avoid environmental poisons is not to eliminate animal fats, which are essential to growth, reproduction, and overall health, but to seek out organic meats and butter from pasture-fed cows, as well as organic vegetables and grains. Organic produce and organic and grass-fed dairy and meat carry less risk of contamination from pesticides, hormones, and new strains of harmful disease than their conventionally produced counterparts. Organic products are becoming increasingly available in health food stores and supermarkets and through mail order and cooperatives (some listings are provided in our Resources section).

Your Need for Vital Nutrients

Did you know that the USRDAs for important nutrients are actually far *lower* than the amounts eaten daily by healthy primitive peoples? That's right, an Australian Aborigine or a South Sea Islander, eating a traditional diet, is much better nourished than the average American, who follows these misleading and market-driven guidelines.

On our meal plans, you'll receive ample amounts of all vital nutrients, with special emphasis on specific ones that jump-start weight loss. These include

- *calcium*, shown by studies to be a key factor in stimulating weight loss.

- *vitamin A*, which nourishes your thyroid gland and is vital for the production of adrenal hormones. It also guarantees calcium and mineral absorption, makes protein assimilation possible, and supports the endocrine system.

- *vitamin D*, which builds your bones, maintains proper calcium levels, helps your body deal with stress, and is needed to produce insulin and a variety of hormones.

Let's take a closer look at what each of these nutrients does for you on a weight-loss diet, and how much of them you *really* need:

Calcium

For an adult woman, the USRDA of calcium is currently set at 800 milligrams per day, even though respected scientists suggest at least 1200 milligrams per day. That's why, on this diet, you'll be eating lots of dairy (both raw cheese and raw whole milk), in addition to nutrient-rich bone broth, to boost your calcium levels into the necessary upper range. Our **Coconut Milk Tonic** (see page 220 for recipe) contains added calcium in the highly absorbable form of dolomite powder.

The January 2003 issue of the *Journal of Nutrition* devoted several articles to the importance of calcium for weight loss. Researchers have found that dietary

Myth: Plants Can Provide All the Vitamin A You Need

Truth: Many fruits and vegetables contain carotenes, substances that are the precursors to vitamin A, but not the true vitamin A. Although people can convert carotenes into true vitamin A through a complicated enzymatic process that occurs in the small intestine, it's actually quite difficult to obtain adequate amounts of true vitamin A in this manner. And some people are unable to make this conversion at all. Diabetics, people with thyroid problems, those suffering from various digestive disorders, and babies and children lack the enzymes needed to convert carotenes in plant foods into true vitamin A.

Yet another reason why cod-liver oil, so rich in vitamin A, is an essential component of the Eat Fat, Lose Fat food plans.

calcium plays a key role in reducing the number and size of fat cells, and dieters who included plenty of dairy foods were more successful at weight loss than those who did not. Interestingly, calcium from food—such as milk, cheese, and bone broth—worked better than most calcium supplements. Plentiful calcium also helps protect against bone loss, which is a real problem among dieters.

Vitamin A

This fat-soluble vitamin supports vision, bone growth, cell division and differentiation, and hormone production, as well as the integrity of the mucous membranes in the respiratory, urinary, and intestinal tracts. And that's not all: it's vital to the immune system's production of white blood cells. Make no mistake, it's a major player in bodily health.

Yet the National Institutes of Health assert that the USRDA for vitamin A for an adult woman is only 2330 IU. Is that amount really sufficient?

Weston Price found that primitive peoples eating much higher levels of this vitamin enjoyed optimal health and were free of the degenerative diseases that beset so many Americans. That's why, to bring you close to that optimal nutrition, in addition to vitamin A found in the other animal foods in our diet, you'll consume about 10,000 to 12,000 IU of vitamin A from cod-liver oil (which also provides 1000 to 1200 IU of vitamin D).

Vitamin D

Also found uniquely in animal fats, vitamin D is crucial to maintaining proper levels of calcium and phosphorous, and hence the health and strength of your bones. Although in this country the RDA of an adult woman under 50 is defined as 200 IU, your daily dose of cod-liver oil will give you 1000 IU, the

Vitamin D and Sunlight

We don't need to worry about getting vitamin D from food, because we get all we need from sunlight. That's been the mantra of orthodox nutritionists for the last two decades: just spend ten minutes in the sun every day, face and lower arms uncovered, and your body will make all the vitamin D it needs.

But recent research has demolished this unfortunate myth. Scientists have discovered that the body only makes vitamin D in the presence of UV-B light—and in temperate regions UV-B is only present when the sun is directly overhead, which occurs at midday during the summer months. If you sunbathe in bathing trunks or a bikini for half an hour every day when there is UV-B light, you will indeed make a lot of vitamin D—up to 10,000 IU, according to one estimate. But this is hardly practical for most of us, even during the summer, and of course impossible when the weather is cold. In fact, even in the tropics, where daily exposure to UV-B light is commonplace, people get lots of vitamin D from their food, including lard and other animal fats, organ meats, seafood, and even insects.

amount that current vitamin D researchers feel should be the RDA. If that sounds high to you, consider this: in a 1999 review of the data published in the *American Journal of Clinical Nutrition*, Canadian researchers concluded that the dose should actually be *4000 IU per day*. Even government researchers now recognize the fact that Americans suffer from widespread vitamin D defi-

Are You Nutrient Starved?

To find out whether you've been getting all the nutrients you need, ask yourself:

- Are you hungry between meals?
- Do you feel unsatisfied, even after eating?
- Do you crave sweets?
- Do you snack constantly?
- Is your skin dry, blemished, rough, or scaly?
- Are your hair and nails in poor condition?
- Is your energy low?
- Do you feel achiness or joint pain?

If the answer to any of these question is *yes*, incorporating the nutrient-dense "superfoods" that we'll describe in Chapter 5 into your diet is a safe and efficient way to redress these problems.

Douglas's Story: Good-bye to Junk Food

Douglas had been an active, athletic child, but in high school he began to eat a lot of junk food—pizza, commercial ice cream, french fries—and drink a lot of beer. He started to gain . . . and gain. Joining a fraternity in college didn't help. He ended up with 300 pounds on his six-foot-one-inch frame, and a huge beer belly. The extra weight made his feet hurt, so he stopped playing sports. He felt discouraged and depressed.

But Douglas reached a turning point when he moved out of his fraternity house and into an apartment. He embarked on a low-carb diet, eating only whole foods that he had prepared himself and avoiding all junk food, including beer, a distinctly high-carbohydrate food. He took coconut oil, which he learned about from a friend, before each meal, and added cod-liver oil to his regimen. Slowly but surely, the pounds came off, 50 in all, until his beer belly disappeared. Eventually, his muscles reappeared, and he could finally take pride in his strong physique.

Now Douglas could wear clothes many sizes smaller, and girls began to notice him. As an added bonus, his powers of concentration improved, and his grades went up. He began to enjoy life again—thanks to the healing powers of coconut oil and nutrient-dense foods.

---

ciency—without admitting the cause, namely, the low-fat diet that the USDA and FDA recommend.

Some diets offer only the USRDAs (or even lesser quantities) of vital nutrients. And often, on these plans, your nutrient sources are mainly synthetic vitamins. Such substances do not provide optimal nourishment since your body is less able to absorb them than the nutrients in *real* foods. As a result, you can only stay on those diets for a short while before your body's demands for nourishment overcome your willpower. But the nutrient-dense foods in our food plans will amp up your intake of real, readily absorbed nutrients, and help you break out of that vicious cycle.

As with Douglas, your cells may be starving for nutrients, and you may not know it!

Chapters 2 and 3 have shown you the truth about fats: why saturated fats actually are good for you, and why low-fat eating is not the great health benefit it's been cracked up to be. In the next chapter, we'll introduce you to our nutritional philosophy of consuming wholesome traditional foods for weight loss and explain exactly why a diet that includes *healthy* fats (especially coconut oil) will help you lose weight in a far more health-supportive and efffective way than today's popular low-fat diets. Then we'll compare the Eat Fat, Lose Fat program with other diets that are widely popular today.

Chapter Four

Our Nutritional Approach to Weight Loss

Science has progressed a great deal in the past century, but human beings remain basically the same. Your nutritional needs are really no different from those of the people Weston Price met in the Outer Hebrides, the Andes, Africa, Australia, or New Zealand in the 1930s and 1940s, and those people were eating the same way as did their ancestors over thousands of years.

The Eat Fat, Lose Fat diet takes into account the basic nutritional needs of the human organism, needs that modern food technologies usually fail to meet. These technologies produce foods that not only lack a full complement of nutrients but often contain harmful substances produced by industrial processing. On our diet, by contrast, you will be meeting your body's basic needs by consuming wholesome foods, prepared with methods that make all the nutrients more available.

There's another reason why Eat Fat, Lose Fat is better aligned with our natural life forces than many other diet plans. Because we emphasize organic fruits and vegetables and organic and grass-fed meat and dairy products, we are contributing to the health of the earth and the balance of our planet's resources. This method of agriculture honors and feeds the soil, the land and the earth itself, rather than despoiling the land with harsh chemicals and treating living animals without any care or respect. This form of agriculture and animal husbandry is called "sustainable," because it gives back to the land what is taken out and does not disrupt the environment.

Think about it! Although there are many causes of obesity, including genetics, a sedentary lifestyle, and overconsumption of processed foods, on the very simplest level the condition of overweight represents an imbalanced relationship between you and nature. Eating natural, sustainable foods, as you will learn to do on this diet, restores this native mutual interdependence, which is why this kind of diet, in and of itself, is healing—not only for overweight but for other health conditions as well.

Breaking the Boom-and-Bust Diet Cycle

The nutritional abundance we so fortunately enjoy today in the West, day in and day out, is an anomaly. In contrast to our plethora of food choices, most people who've lived on this earth (including the majority today) have gone through periods when food was scarce. In response, humans developed underlying patterns of energy use and fat storage. Even in this time of plenty, the body's tendency remains the same: to store fat for times of famine or want.

That's why going on any form of severely restrictive diet usually backfires: it triggers the body's biologically programmed tendency to store fat. Severe calorie restriction, fasting, or subsisting on juices gives your body the message that a food emergency lies ahead, creating a boomerang effect. When you return to normal eating, you find that your body stubbornly rebuilds its fat stores, ready for another crisis. This is the boom-and-bust cycle unwittingly engineered by other weight-loss programs. It's the reason why prolonged fasts and cleanses do not result in long-term weight loss or overall well-being. Instead, severe calorie restriction leads to *fat conservation, hunger, and bingeing*, as the body desperately seeks to obtain and retain needed nutrients.

When you nourish yourself well, impose a healthy (but not too harsh) discipline, and exercise, your body will start to feel confident that it can let go of that extra weight it's been carrying around for a rainy day. Follow our path, and you'll find successful weight loss ahead.

Our Three Diet Plans

All three Eat Fat, Lose Fat plans emphasize a balanced approach to eating, in order to provide your body with all the key nutrients it needs.

• **Quick and Easy Weight Loss** offers two phases, which provide health benefits along with weight loss in an easy-to-follow diet that minimizes time spent in food preparation for those on the go. Most people lose weight just by eating the recommended amount of coconut oil (along with other healthy fats) and cutting out unhealthy fats on Phase One, a moderate-calorie diet. If you still need to shed additional stubborn pounds, Phase Two is a more calorie-restricted (but still very satisfying) program.

• **Health Recovery** provides intensive health benefits, using greater quantities of coconut and other health-promoting foods in a highly nutritious diet that's more easily digestible for people with serious health problems such as hormonal imbalance, chronic fatigue, irritable bowel syndrome, and hypothyroidism.

- **Everyday Gourmet** is a complete ongoing maintenance diet that the whole family will love. It offers health benefits with a wider repertory of delicious traditional foods.

Quick and Easy Weight Loss in particular emphasizes four Core Principles that will help you attain health and release excess weight in a natural, nondisruptive way. They are as follows:

- Eat three meals per day, and always eat breakfast;
- Include traditional fats, especially coconut oil;
- Consume nutrient-dense foods, particularly those supplying calcium and vitamins A and D;
- Restrict calories moderately.

These Core Principles provide a synergistic environment that spurs weight loss, because this diet plan will communicate to your body

- that you have safely released it from the feast-or-famine cycle;
- that you will be providing it with what it needs, no more—but no less, either.

In response, your body will give you what *you* need—a slimmer, trimmer look, good health, and an abundance of energy. Imagine what it would be like to be in a stable, mutually satisfying, long-term relationship—with your very own body!

Why Diets with Healthy Fats Help You Lose Weight

The Zone and Atkins weight-loss diets have been popular because they provide adequate amounts of protein and, in the case of the original Atkins diet, plenty of saturated fats. However, on our weight-loss plan, you'll be eating a more balanced, well-rounded diet, consisting of a wider variety of higher-quality foods without the difficult restrictions on fat that characterize the Zone diet or the extreme limitation of carbohydrates of the Atkins diet. Our moderate-calorie diet adds the magic ingredient of coconut oil to kick-start your metabolism. We feature moderate protein (less than Atkins), lots of vegetables, small amounts of whole grains, and a wide variety of healthy fats, with coconut oil leading the pack.

Most people mistakenly believe that low-fat diets are the only way to lose weight. They do not realize that the right fats, such as coconut oil and other healthy oils in synergistic combination, not only encourage weight loss but also help you heal from a wide range of ailments. Built upon a variety of

James's Story: Returning to Simple Wisdom

James was a devotee of low-fat dieting. He had to be—he had so much weight to lose. And yes, he did lose a little weight, but nowhere near enough. Besides, he always felt hungry and weak. Frustrated, James decided to stop his low-fat regimen. He quickly regained the 50 pounds he had lost, and then some. In fact, he weighed over 400 pounds and was in terrible shape. Walking just a few feet was painful.

In desperation, James set forth to learn more about nutrition. He read books and learned medical and scientific jargon to uncover the real meaning behind published medical studies. What he discovered left him bewildered and angry, but also determined that he would no longer be a pawn of the food and pharmaceutical industries.

So James and his wife returned to the simple nutritional wisdom he had learned from his mother, an Alabama farm girl and avid gardener. They started their own garden to supplement the organic produce they bought. They ate organic meat as often as possible, and cut all prepared foods from their diet. They added healthy fats back into their diet, particularly coconut oil and lard (in order to avoid all additives and preservatives, they even rendered their own lard!).

The results were stunning. In less than a year, James lost 118 pounds, his wife lost 40 pounds, and they were healthier than they'd ever been. He walked and jogged eight miles a day three times a week and worked out in the gym three days a week. Their friends exclaimed, "We don't even recognize you anymore!" James himself was astonished that nothing more than eating wholesome foods, grown with care, and including healthy fats in his diet enabled him to lose weight and regain his health.

healthy traditional foods, our diet will provide the right combination of saturated and unsaturated fats to optimize health and weight loss.

Years of consuming trans fats, deep-fried foods, and other harmful fat sources can make it hard for some people to digest good fats, at first. But that's where coconut is key. Coconut oil is easy to digest because most of the fatty acids it contains don't require bile for digestion. What's more, the body turns these fatty acids directly into energy, making it terrific for losing weight. All this makes coconut oil the perfect oil for transitioning into healthy fats if you haven't been eating them up until now.

What the Research Shows

Our program rests on a large and growing body of research that demonstrates why coconut can help you lose weight and boost health. Recent studies show that eliminating fat is not an effective dietary strategy. The low-fat foods you eat instead are nearly always high-carb foods, which trigger the release of insulin, causing your body to *store* fat. What's more, carb consumption can cause blood sugar surges and drops. As a result, you lack sustained energy lev-

The Best of All Fats for Weight Loss

In 1998, researchers at the McGill University obesity research group discovered that, compared to other types of fatty acids, MCFAs (the type of fat found in coconut oil) actually use up energy when they are metabolized, and thus can act as weight-loss agents! That's right, eating these kinds of fatty acids can help you lose weight. This is because the amount of energy used by the body to oxidize them is greater than the amount of energy they provide. The most rapidly oxidized fatty acid, these scientists found, is the medium-chain fatty acid lauric acid. *Coconut oil contains almost 50 percent lauric acid.*

Coconut oil has a "thermogenic effect," which means that it raises your body temperature, thus boosting your energy and metabolic rate. A study in Japan, reported in *Journal of Nutritional Science Vitaminology*, 2002, found that consuming medium-chain fatty acids caused greater thermogenesis than did eating long-chain fatty acids, regardless of what kind of MCFA-containing food was eaten.

els and instead experience hunger. In contrast, the research confirms that eating the right fats at every meal keeps your blood sugar stable and maximizes your metabolism by providing a steady fuel supply throughout the day. You have more energy for work, exercise, and social activities, keystones of a healthy lifestyle.

A number of studies have found that obesity levels in animals decreased in

Genevieve's Story: High-Protein, Low-Carb Weren't Enough

Genevieve, a skilled jeweler, was co-owner of an Oregon jewelry store. Since her job was sedentary, weight gain crept up on her, until one day her business partner tactfully suggested she stick to designing and stay off the sales floor, because she presented a less than attractive appearance.

Resolved to lose the 40 pounds she'd gained, Genevieve decided to try a high-protein, low-carb diet. The weight started to come off slowly, until she read an article about coconut in a women's magazine. Inspired, she purchased coconut oil and added a couple of tablespoons of it to her morning smoothie.

Over the next three weeks, Genevieve was astonished to find that she lost 11 pounds without ever feeling deprived or hungry. She even started to power walk, something she never would have had the energy to attempt before. Now she walks effortlessly for 30 minutes after work. With renewed energy, she's been able to stick to her exercise and diet program, has lost all the weight she gained, and is back on the sales floor with customers.

direct proportion to the ratio of coconut oil in their diet. The more coconut they ate, the leaner they were. For example, in a study published in 1996 in the *Journal of Lipid Research,* animals fed a diet consisting of at least 50 percent MCFAs had significant weight loss—even though their diet was not otherwise designed to promote weight loss. In contrast, a control group fed the same diet with the same number of calories, but consisting of 50 percent long-chain fatty acids (LCFAs, found in other foods), lost no weight whatsoever.

Other studies confirm that MCFAs are oxidized (burned up and used for energy) instead of being stored in the fatty tissue of the body, as are the LCFAs. As a result, you generate more heat to burn calories, kick-starting the body into burning up existing fat stores.

Studies with humans confirm animal research:

- A report published in the *American Journal of Clinical Nutrition,* 2000, found that adult males oxidized 41 percent of lauric acid (the most common MCFA in coconut oil) but only 13 percent of stearic acid (a LCFA found in other fats). That means that you burn off coconut three times faster than other common fats.
- In a study published in *Life Sciences,* 1998, researchers at the McGill University obesity research group found that both animals and humans metabolize MCFAs and LCFAs differently. In humans, they found increases in post-meal energy expenditure after short-term feeding of MCFAs. They concluded that "MCFAs hold potential as weight-loss agents."
- Another study, published in the *American Journal of Clinical Nutrition,* 1991, found that humans consuming a meal containing 30 grams (2 tablespoons) MCFAs and 8 grams (about 1.5 teaspoons) LCFAs had a significant rise in temperature compared to those who ate the same meal containing 38 grams LCFAs. This rise in temperature indicates higher

---

Deborah's Story: Sluggish Metabolism

Deborah had been fighting hypothyroidism and a sluggish metabolism for ten years, gaining over 60 pounds. It seemed that her doctor increased her dose of thyroid medication with every visit, but to no avail. She continued to feel tired and to have trouble losing weight.

She decided to go on a low-carb diet and found that reducing her reliance on grains, sugars, and sweets produced weight loss. But she still was plagued by cravings and had trouble losing that last 15 pounds. Then Deborah learned about the benefits of coconut oil and tried adding two tablespoons, along with cod-liver oil and some whole foods, to her morning meal.

In three weeks, she lost 11 pounds. Two years later, she has retained her weight loss. She loved the fact that it was so easy to prepare wholesome foods that were delicious as well as satisfying, so she wasn't tempted to fall off the wagon.

Christine's Story: Thyroid Indicators Improved

Christine had suffered from symptoms of thryoid problems for years—she lacked energy and always felt cold. A lab test came back showing slightly abnormal thyroid function. She then added coconut oil to her diet. When she went back to repeat the test six months later, the results were within the normal range. Beyond that, Christine felt a lot warmer and had much more energy, especially when she woke up in the morning.

---

metabolic activity caused by better thyroid functioning, revealing how coconut oil helps your thyroid and boosts your metabolism.

Coconut and Your Metabolism

Hypothyroidism (thyroid deficiency, resulting in a low metabolic rate), which is characterized by weight gain, lethargy, dry skin, depression, and lack of mental clarity, is on the rise in America, affecting an estimated 12 million people. (Some endocrinologists suspect the condition affects many millions more.) Hypothyroidism is a serious condition in its own right, but also a precursor to other ailments, such as heart disease, breast cancer, and chronic fatigue. While no studies have investigated how coconut oil affects the thyroid gland specifically, the fact that it raises body temperature and causes weight loss indicate that it supports thyroid function. In fact, many dieters report that they are able to reduce or even eliminate their thyroid medications when they add coconut oil to their diet.

How Eating Coconut Makes Dieting Easy

In the coconut-based Eat Fat, Lose Fat weight-loss plan, we'll show you how to get your daily quota of coconut by using coconut oil, coconut milk, shredded coconut, and other products, in concert with other delicious whole foods. Sally, an acclaimed health-wise gourmet cook who developed all the recipes for our previous book, *Nourishing Traditions*, has created a rich cornucopia of easy-to-prepare international recipes, featuring Thai, Vietnamese, Indian, African, Indonesian, Brazilian, and South Seas cuisines, along with American standards, made the coconut way. Coconut's pleasing taste and aroma make it a natural ingredient in drinks, smoothies, breakfast foods, soups, sauces, curries, main dishes, desserts, and snacks.

Comparing Eat Fat, Lose Fat to Other Diets

To see why we—and countless people who have used it successfully— affirm that our coconut-rich diet is the best way to lose weight, let's consider

A Cornucopia of Coconut

The coconut provides a wealth of delicious foods, ranging in use from therapeutic to epicurean. Here's a list of coconut products available to Westerners. Please see our Resources section for more information on recommended brands and where to purchase them.

Coconut Oil: Used in the tropics for cooking and also topically (on the skin), coconut oil is white when solid, creamy colored when liquid. It melts at between 71°F and 76°F. High-quality coconut oil is now widely available in national supermarkets, such as Whole Foods, Trader Joe's, and Wild Oats, in health food stores, on the Internet, or by mail order. Look for virgin coconut oil, which means that it has been extracted by a careful method that does not involve high heat and harmful chemicals.

Coconut Milk: Coconut milk is a rich, creamy liquid that drips out of coconut meat when it has been pulverized in water and squeezed. Slightly thicker than cow's milk, it has a delicious, satisfying, slightly sweet taste. Use only whole coconut milk, which contains the oil, not "lite," in smoothies, cream sauces, curries, desserts, and soups. You can even use coconut milk to make our delicious **Coconut Milk Tonic** (see page 220 for recipe), formulated to have the same number of calories and the same amount of calcium as whole milk—a boon to those who are allergic to milk. Organic canned coconut milk is widely available in supermarkets and health food stores and on the Internet.

Unsweetened Desiccated Coconut: Tiny flakes of air-dried coconut can be used as a coating for sautéed shrimp or chicken, sprinkled on fruit, and added to macaroons and other desserts. Look for desiccated coconut in health food stores, but avoid the highly sweetened, additive-laden coconut flakes sold in commercial supermarkets.

Coconut Cream: When it contains no emulsifiers, coconut milk will separate into a cream (which rises to the top) and a more watery portion (often sold as "lite" coconut milk). The cream can be used in various desserts, even whipping up like cream. Coconut cream is not normally available in stores but can be purchased through the Internet or by mail order.

Creamed Coconut: Coconut meat that has been very finely ground and then pressed into blocks resembling very hard white butter is called creamed coconut. Sold in Asian markets in the refrigerated section, usually as 7-ounce rectangles, creamed coconut is a very useful, economical product. Add it to soups or curries, or mix it with water to make coconut milk. It has a stronger, more coconutty taste than canned coconut milk and a slightly gritty texture.

Coconut Water/Coconut Juice (Buko Juice): The water or juice from young coconuts is delicious and very rich in minerals, especially potassium, calcium, and magnesium, making it an excellent remedy for replacing electrolytes or rejuvenating the body on a hot day. Even better is cultured or fermented coconut juice, the ideal drink for athletes and convalescents. Coconut kefir—coconut juice cultured with a kefir culture—can be a very useful component of our Health Recovery diet. (Kefir is a fermented milk product, similar to yogurt but with more liquid.) During World War II, when IV solution was scarce, water from young coconuts was used as a substitute! In Asia, coconut juice is considered particularly beneficial for the kidneys.

Coconut juice is one of the best dietary sources of cytokinins, molecules that protect the cells as they undergo cell division. Cytokinins help cellular DNA replicate perfectly during cell division; without these molecules, mistakes occasionally occur. Thus cytokinins play a key role in fighting cancer and ensuring longevity.

Coconut juice can be obtained from young, live coconuts, frequently sold in Asian and Hispanic markets. You can also order packaged buko on the Internet.

Freeze-Dried Shredded Coconut: Delicious dried coconut flakes are made by quickly freezing deshelled coconuts and then evaporating the moisture with a vacuum. The product is much more flavorful and sweet than air-dried coconut—in fact, it's hard to believe it doesn't contain added sweeteners. Because of the low moisture content, freeze-dried shredded coconut does not require any preservatives. It's wonderful in desserts, puddings, and macaroons. You can buy it in specialty shops or by mail order.

Coconut Vinegar: Made from coconut juice, coconut vinegar has a delicious coconut flavor. It can be used for marinades, in salad dressings, and to make a great beverage called **Shrub** (page 222). It is available in Asian markets and through the Internet.

Coconut Rum: This is rum with coconut flavoring added—not exactly a traditional product but a terrific flavoring for ice cream and other desserts.

Coconut Sugar: Made by boiling the sweet water sap that drips from cut flower buds on the coconut palm, much as maple sugar is made by boiling and dehydrating the sap of maple trees, coconut sugar is a wonderful, nutrient-dense natural sweetener. It's pale in color and either soft or gooey, depending on how long the sap was reduced. The pale color makes it excellent for coconut desserts since it does not turn them brown.

some other popular diets you may have tried or heard about. We'll take a detailed look at how they work, what the science says about them, and where they fall short in delivering what you want: healthy, sustainable weight loss.

Atkins: Low-Carb, High-Protein, High-Fat

Many people have enjoyed real success with the Atkins diet because its high fat content calms hunger pangs, allowing dieters to go longer between meals and ultimately consume less food. The carbohydrate restriction on Atkins—as on Quick and Easy Weight Loss—is valuable because it ensures that you won't eat a lot of empty calories in the form of sugar and white flour.

However, some people find that when they restrict carbs too much, they develop cravings, indicating a possible B vitamin deficiency. This is why, on Quick and Easy Weight Loss, you will be eating small amounts of grains and carbs, carefully prepared to enhance digestibility and assimilation.

Another problem with the Atkins diet is that, as a shortcut, many people add additional protein in the form of soy-based protein powders and protein bars. Unfortunately, as we will see in Chapter 6, eating these foods can result in numerous deficiencies and create thyroid problems that lead to weight gain.

Some people have tried to "improve" on the Atkins diet by eating more protein and reducing the amount of fat it allows. High-protein, low-fat diets are especially dangerous because protein consumption rapidly depletes vitamin A stores. This is why we caution you against using protein powders or consuming a diet containing lean meat, egg whites, and skim milk. Children brought up on high-protein, low-fat diets often experience rapid growth. The results—tall, myopic, lanky individuals with crowded teeth and poor bone structure, a kind of Ichabod Crane syndrome—are a fixture in America. In adults, vitamin A de-

High-Carb Versus Low-Carb

In 1956, researchers at Middlesex Hospital, London, tested four different 1000-calorie diets: one consisted of 90 percent fat, one was 90 percent protein, a third was 90 percent carbohydrate, and the fourth was a normal mixed diet. Several subjects on the high-carb diet actually gained weight, even at only 1000 calories per day. Subjects on the very low-carb diet lost weight, even though they ate 2600 calories per day. But subjects on the high-fat diet lost much more weight than any of the others.

During the last 20 years, over a dozen studies have shown that low-carb diets result in more weight loss than high-carb diets. For example, in a ten-week study of obese women on 1700-calorie diets, the low-carb group lost more weight than the high-carb group, with significantly higher fat loss. The low-carb subjects also reported that they felt less hungry.

Stephen's Story: High-Protein—Low Vision

Stephen, a young electrician in Buffalo, New York, was a husky guy who struggled with weight gain all his life, until he married his childhood sweetheart and she turned him on to the Atkins diet. He lost 12 pounds in eight weeks and figured that at 230 pounds, and a height of 5 feet 10 inches, he had another 40 to go. Stephen was on a roll. He kept plenty of Atkins bars and drinks around, and munched on them in his truck.

After a while, though, he noticed sluggishness, along with a distinct decline in his night vision, making it hard to work past dusk. When he learned from the Weston A. Price website that night blindness can result from a vitamin A deficiency, Stephen wanted to consume more vitamin A. But why take a pill when you could eat real food? So he began taking liquid cod-liver oil, and decided to replace his habit of eating bars and meal replacements with two tablespoons of coconut oil before his Atkins meals. Soon the pounds came off a little faster.

Within three months, Stephen had lost 30 pounds. His night blindness also vanished, enabling him to take those income-building, night emergency calls again!

---

pletion can lead to autoimmune disease, immune system dysfunction, endocrine disruption, thyroid problems, and even cancer.

High-fat, high-protein, low-carb diets can also cause a condition called ketosis, in which the body burns fat instead of glucose as fuel, producing acidic substances called ketone bodies that can cause nausea, fatigue, and more serious problems, including dizziness and abnormal heart rhythms. The Eat Fat, Lose Fat plans, by contrast, provide enough carbohydrates to prevent ketosis from developing.

Another problem with the Atkins diet is its potential to cause calcium deficiencies. Atkins tells you not to drink milk since it's high in carbohydrates, so unless you make sure to eat cheese or use calcium-rich bone broths frequently, you won't be getting enough calcium on this diet.

If you're someone who loves the Atkins diet, not to worry. Our Eat Fat, Lose Fat diet is similar, but better. You'll lose weight just as well, you'll feel even more satisfied enjoying Sally's fabulous recipes—and you'll know that you're eating in the most health-supportive way possible.

Ornish: Low-Fat Vegetarian

Despite all you've heard, the very low-fat, low-cholesterol, vegetarian Ornish diet is actually nutrient *deficient, and* high in insulin-sparking carbohydrates. And because of its fat reduction, it produces no satiation. Instead, it prompts cravings and overeating. No wonder many people find this diet extremely difficult to stay on.

What's more, the steely-willed few who can remain on the Ornish diet long term are at risk for deficiencies of protein, vitamin A, vitamin D, vitamin B$_{12}$, zinc, and other key nutrients.

Nor, sadly, did Ornish find any real evidence that this diet lives up to its claim to protect you from heart disease. The study that launched the Ornish program, published in *The Lancet* in 1990, did not actually look at the long-term outcome of a severely fat-restricted diet. Instead, the researchers used a diagnostic technique called angiography to measure the diameter of the coronary arteries in a small group of patients (22 in the experimental group and 19 in the control group). They found that those on the low-fat diet had slightly more widening of the arteries. But no conclusions can be drawn from this finding because as arteries begin to get clogged, they actually widen a bit. It's only after the clogging becomes serious that the arteries narrow. Thus, the slight widening that the Ornish researchers measured could have resulted from the arteries becoming more clogged, not less!

Patients in the treatment group did at first report lessened angina (chest pain), but after five years there was no difference between the two groups in the frequency or amount of angina. Nor did the researchers follow up to see how the study group fared in the long term.

Another flaw of this study was that very few people could be persuaded to stay on the diet. Of the 53 initially selected for the experimental group, only 28 agreed to participate after the program was explained to them. Subsequently, a few more dropped out, and one died during heavy exercise. As a result, so few were left in the experimental group that the researchers could not draw any valid conclusions.

Ornish himself admits that his diet alone will not prevent heart disease. His program includes a number of strategies to reduce heart disease risk, including weight reduction, moderate exercise, smoking cessation, and stress relief. With all of these factors in place, it is difficult to determine whether the dietary component plays any significant role. In fact, from our point of view, Dr. Ornish's results might have been better if his patients were allowed to support their well-being and biology with more satisfying and nutritious food!

The Zone Diet: Moderate Carbs, High Protein, and Restricted Fat

Although this regimen is called a high-fat diet, in reality only 30 percent of its calories come from fat. According to its author, Barry Sears, if you maintain a strict ratio of 30 percent protein, 30 percent fat, and 40 percent carbs, you will enter the Zone, where "the mind is relaxed, yet alert and exquisitely focused . . . the body is fluid, strong, and apparently indefatigable." The Zone Diet is said to put one in "a metabolic state in which the body works at peak efficiency."

Unlike Ornish, who promises good health on low-fat meals, Sears agrees that the body needs fats, but only monounsaturated ones found in avocados, almonds, and olive oil. We should avoid saturated fats, he argues, and also too much of the long-chain fatty acid called arachidonic acid, found in foods like liver, eggs, and butter. Sears claims that his diet is satisfying, with lots of protein and "plenty of fat." But that's before you come up against the fuzzy math. Since fat contains 9 calories per gram, compared to 4 for proteins and carbohydrates, and since protein and carbohydrate foods contain a lot of water, whereas fats contain none, you can't add very much fat to meals before you surpass the 30 percent ratio.

In one Zone Diet meal, composed of 6 ounces of white fish for protein and 2 cups of steamed vegetables, plus 1 piece of fruit for the carbohydrates, the added fat amounts to 4 teaspoons of slivered almonds. Another Zone meal consists of 1 cup of low-fat cottage cheese and 1⅓ cups of cooked oatmeal, with fat supplied by 4 macadamia nuts. An omelet consisting of 6 egg whites and 1 ounce of non-fat cheese gets 1⅓ teaspoons of added olive oil.

If you have trouble keeping your ratios straight, or need a between-meal snack, you can eat a meal replacement bar that contains many processed products but has the correct ratio of 30/30/40. Ultimately, even with the synthetic vitamins in the bars, the Zone Diet is deficient in nutrients and carries the risks associated with diets in which high amounts of protein are not supported by adequate fats, as explained above in the discussion of the Atkins diet.

The Glycemic Index

Several popular diet plans advise people to limit their carbohydrate foods to those that have a low "glycemic index." The glycemic index indicates how quickly and how much a food raises the blood sugar. High-glycemic foods include grains (especially cold breakfast cereals), potatoes, corn, honey, and glucose (but not fructose, which has to be processed in the liver before it enters the bloodstream). Low-glycemic foods include legumes, non-starchy vegetables, and most fruits. The idea is that eating low-glycemic foods will help you last longer between meals by maintaining steady blood sugar levels.

Diets based on low-glycemic index foods usually overlook one important point: fats lower the glycemic index! Putting butter on a high-glycemic food like bread will lower its glycemic index, meaning that the food is absorbed more slowly into the bloodstream rather than in one quick burst. In fact, when testing foods for glycemic index, researchers found that a sugar-laden Mars bar had a lower glycemic index than cornflakes or potatoes . . . because the Mars bar contains lots of fat. That's why using butter as a spread, or including coconut oil in every meal, can further lower the glycemic effect of both high-glycemic foods, like potatoes, and low-glycemic foods, like vegetables.

The South Beach Diet: Low-Carb, High-Protein, Moderate Fat— but No Animal Fats

The South Beach Diet is a low-carb regimen that excludes, or keeps to a bare minimum, the usual carbs like bread (even whole-grain), sweets, fruit, fruit juices, rice, potatoes, and pasta. It emphasizes high-protein foods, non-starchy vegetables, and skim milk and other non-fat foods. White sugar is out, as well as the whole gamut of processed carbohydrate snack foods. While eliminating or greatly reducing your intake of carbohydrates and sugar is a great idea, this diet is full of shortcomings.

For one thing, low levels of dietary fat contributes to low blood sugar between meals, sparking a sudden need to eat. And that's not all. Despite its popularity, the South Beach diet may actually be one of the more dangerous diets out there. Because it's high in protein and excludes animal fats, it can rapidly deplete vitamin A stores, resulting in numerous health problems, as noted previously in the discussion of the Atkins diet.

Second, South Beach denies the dieter any source of vital saturated fats. As you now know, your body needs saturated fats to work properly—from the level of the organs right down to the cells. Our only good sources of saturated fat are coconut oil, palm and palm kernel oils, and animal fats; or high-carbohydrate foods like potatoes or grains that the body turns into saturated fat. The South Beach diet allows none of these, setting the hapless dieter up for numerous health problems—from lung disease to heart problems.

Lots of the South Beach recipes look inviting and tasty, but they're full of low- or non-fat ingredients. Non-fat sour cream and non-fat half-and-half are among the favorites, while the chicken is always skinless, to get rid of the sat-

Olive Oil Can Cause Weight Gain!

Several diet plans recommend monounsaturated oils such as olive and canola as the best oils for weight loss. Actually, these oils can contribute to weight gain! In a study published in *The Lancet*, 1994, researchers noted that the fatty acid they found most prominent in fat tissue was monounsaturated. That's probably why middle-age weight gain is so common in Mediterranean countries.

In the Eat Fat, Lose Fat plans, we reduce the amount of olive oil in salad dressings and mayonnaise by using Mary's Oil Blend, which is ⅓ olive oil, ⅓ sesame oil, and ⅓ coconut oil. We also do not recommend most nuts in the calorie-restricted phase of Quick and Easy Weight Loss. Nuts are a wonderful, nutritious food, but they tend to be high in monounsaturated fatty acids, the kind that your body accumulates when it gains weight.

urated fats that Arthur Agatston, the diet's creator, thinks are so lethal. (Actually, chicken skin contains mostly monounsaturated fatty acids.) Instead of butter, processed spreads, containing harmful trans fats, appear in many recipes and snack suggestions, as do margarine and egg substitutes.

Since Dr. Agatston is an orthodox cardiologist, he is firmly wedded to the lipid hypothesis and argues that saturated fats cause chemical changes in the bloodstream, raising so-called bad cholesterol, LDL, and leading to accelerated atherosclerosis and clogged arteries. In our opinion, however, his diet is a good example of how the lipid hypothesis leads to bad dietary advice.

Weight Watchers: Calorie Restriction

When you consider how many millions have tried this diet, it's certainly had very few successes. And when you take a closer look at how Weight Watchers really works, the reasons are pretty clear.

Weight Watchers relies entirely on calorie restriction, with no particular warnings against refined carbohydrates and no emphasis on healthy fats. Weight Watchers uses a point system, in which every food is given a value based on its calorie, fat, and fiber content—but not on its quality or nutrient content. Members choose their meals within a daily points range, depending on their current weight. Exercise also has a point value, which can be swapped for additional food points.

Because of the reduced calorie intake, Weight Watchers ends up being a low-fat diet, and most Weight Watchers wind up turning to unhealthy fats like margarine and vegetable oils. Plus, because it's low in fat, the diet leaves people unsatisfied, undernourished, and vulnerable to boomerang weight gain.

And that's not theoretical. A British therapist, Susie Orbach, the author of *Fat Is a Feminist Issue,* has accused Weight Watchers of false advertising, claiming that thousands of Brits have shelled out their money to the company, only to wind up fatter than they were before. Orbach further claims that the company's profits *depend* on the high failure rate. Watch out for Weight Watchers.

Sylvia's Story: The Perils of Low-Fat

Sylvia had struggled with her weight since her teenage years. She would go on low-fat diets that severely restricted calories. Several times she lost 20 pounds very quickly, but she invariably put them back on, plus extra, so she wound up heavier than when she started. While on these diets, she was prone to mood swings due to low blood sugar. The diets also depressed her metabolism, so that she always came to a point at which even the severest calorie restriction did not help her lose weight. Tired and discouraged, she would begin to eat again and quickly regained the pounds. Worse, over the years Sylvia developed hypothyroidism. She ended up 40 pounds overweight, sluggish, and constantly tired.

This diet rapidly leads to nutrient deficiencies and cravings, triggering binge-ing and splurging.

Juice Fasts

Numerous diet programs involve fasting on juices made from a variety of vegetables and fruits as a way to lose weight, provide enzymes, and "cleanse the colon, liver, and cells." Proponents claim that when we chew, we are turn-ing our food into juice, so juicing is therefore natural and healthy.

But the fact that foods made into juices are *not* chewed is actually one of the problems with juice fasts. Chewing actually begins the digestive process by mixing food (particularly carbohydrates) with saliva. The process of chewing and thoroughly tasting our food also sends signals to the digestive tract about what to expect in terms of nutrients and which enzymes will be needed to as-similate them. Juicing bypasses these mechanisms and can actually result in poor digestion!

Also, many foods that are juiced, such as green leafy vegetables and crucif-erous vegetables (members of the cabbage family), contain substances that block mineral absorption and depress thyroid function. When these vegetables are cooked, those substances are neutralized. In fact, cooking actually makes the minerals in vegetables much more available.

What's more, there are very few enzymes in most fruits and vegetables used in juicing recipes. Foods that contain a lot of enzymes are mostly foods that have been lacto-fermented, which we will describe in Chapter 5.

Traditional cultures did not have modern juicers, but they did crush certain foods to produce lacto-fermented beverages in a process akin to digestion that creates copious amounts of enzymes.

Those who claim that fasting on juices can cleanse the body lack a basic un-derstanding of biochemistry. The removal of toxins from the body is an ongo-ing process involving numerous enzyme systems that are supported mostly by nutrients from animal products. In fact, one of the best ways to help the body cleanse is to consume a lot of bone broth, which provides the liver with certain amino acids involved in the process of clearing the residues of metabolism.

Finally, juice fasts can create the same problems as low-fat diets—they lead to low blood sugar and serious deficiencies in nutrients normally provided by animal protein and fat. Even with added coconut oil, the body is likely to in-terpret a juice fast as starvation, slow down the metabolism, and put the pounds back on very quickly as soon as the fast is over.

The Right Nutritional Strategy

To summarize, all these modern diets depend on some degree of calorie re-striction, with different proportions of macronutrients. The original Atkins diet is the best, both for achieving weight loss and for satisfying your body's

What's in Your Mayonnaise?

If you reach for the Miracle Whip as you're preparing tuna salad, you'll be eating soybean oil, modified food starch, artificial color, and sodium caseinate (a synthetic ingredient made from milk protein). Contrast this with our easy-to-make **Mayonnaise** (see page 238 for recipe), which keeps well in the fridge and provides many key nutrients from real foods, including MCFAs from coconut oil.

nutritional requirements. But like the others, the Atkins diet can lead to cravings, vitamin A depletion, and calcium deficiency (if you don't eat cheese).

None of these programs take advantage of the metabolism-boosting powers of coconut oil along with the thyroid-supporting powers of cod-liver oil (whose many virtues we'll explain fully in Chapter 5). As a result, all of them can lead to lowered metabolism, either through the body's feast-or-famine reaction, or through vitamin A depletion that undermines your thyroid function, or both. And once you head in that direction, no matter how severe your calorie restriction, *you won't lose weight.*

That's why our diet emphasizes a well-rounded array of healthful foods with all the right nutrients to support your health, improve thyroid function, and permit safe, sustainable weight loss.

Our approach, based on the way healthy people eat in countless traditional societies, is above all balanced. However, your ability to eat in a natural, wholesome, balanced way has been undermined by decades of constantly changing advice from so-called experts. Nor can you regain a sense of balanced eating from following carefully calibrated numerical prescriptions, like those of the Zone Diet, or the larger quantities of protein in the newer version of the Atkins diet. But you can regain it by eating moderate amounts of traditional food combinations, many of which you already know and love (and some of which will be new), since they all inherently have this balance.

So accustomed are we Americans to the convenience of fast-food restaurants and manufactured foods that many of us have forgotten how real food tastes. Is it any surprise that meals made of lab ingredients (like the trans fats in nearly all packaged and baked goods) fail to nourish or satisfy you, leading to overeating, bingeing, and splurging, and ultimately to disease?

In Part 2 of *Eat Fat, Lose Fat,* we'll reintroduce you to creative yet simple steps to restore some of the traditional foods your body longs for (specific menu plans and recipes are in Part 3). In the next chapter you'll learn about the wholesome, traditional foods, including healthy fats, that you can begin adding to your diet right now. Be prepared for a nutritional plan you'll love!

Getting Used to Coconut Oil and a Traditional Diet

If you have been on a low-fat diet for many years, you may need to transition slowly into a higher-fat traditional diet. Occasionally, someone reports a feeling of nausea, especially after taking the one to two tablespoons of coconut oil that we recommend before meals. This is probably due to the body's inability to produce enough fat-digesting bile after so many years of not needing it. (The short- and medium-chain fatty acids in coconut oil don't require bile for breakdown; but coconut oil contains smaller amounts of longer-chain fatty acids that do require bile for digestion, and butter and other animal fats require even larger amounts.)

If this is the case, simply cut back on the amount of coconut oil you are taking. Start with one teaspoon and build slowly from there to the suggested one to two tablespoons. You can also take the coconut oil with your meal instead of twenty minutes before. And, be sure to eat three meals a day at regular intervals so that the body learns to produce bile on a predictable schedule. Some dieters have actually reported that they want a very slight feeling of nausea because it suppresses their appetite.

In a similar vein, several individuals have reported that they gained weight at first when they started taking coconut oil. They persevered because they liked the increased sense of energy they experienced. Then after a few weeks, they found that they had started losing weight. Of course, moderate restriction of calories and carbohydrates is also important for successful weight loss.

Part Two

Real Foods—
for Healing and Health

Chapter Five

Real Food, the World Over

While coconut oil and other healthy fats are significant additions to your diet, you'll gain the most benefit from this program if you also incorporate traditional foods and methods of food preparation, which you'll learn more about in this chapter. While some of these foods may be new to you, many will already be familiar and will remind you of foods your grandmother might have made. Although modern dietary myths may have scared you away from eating them, this chapter will explain the scientific evidence that supports the consumption of nutrient-dense traditional foods, and encourage you to enjoy them. Consumption of traditional foods, prepared according to traditional methods and including plenty of healthy fats, has been the basis of our nutritional philosophy in all our writings, as well as of Dr. Enig's nutritional practice.

We owe tremendous gratitude to Dr. Weston A. Price, the dentist who studied the diets of healthy nonindustrialized peoples and reported his findings in his classic work, *Nutrition and Physical Degeneration*. He was ahead of his time in identifying health problems—including tooth decay, crowded and crooked teeth, tuberculosis, arthritis, growth problems, and fatigue—arising from the modern diet based on sugar, white flour, and vegetable oils, and for discovering and articulating basic dietary principles for building strong, healthy bodies. At the Weston A. Price Foundation, which we founded in 1999, we use Dr. Price's guidelines to sort through the many conflicting nutritional claims to foundational foods that build health. The Foundation is dedicated to publicizing the scientific validation for the health benefits of traditional diets, which Price was the first to describe.

Dr. Price explained that vitamins A and D are catalysts to mineral absorption and protein utilization. Without them, you cannot absorb minerals, no matter how abundant they may be in your food. In addition, Price discovered another fat-soluble nutrient, a potent catalyst for mineral absorption that he

Weston Price's Nutritional Discoveries

In analyzing the key factors in the foods traditional, nonindustrialized peoples ate, Dr. Price was surprised to learn that, in comparison to the American diet of the 1940s, these traditional diets provided at least *four times* the water-soluble vitamins, calcium, and other minerals, and at least *ten times* the fat-soluble vitamins. The fat-soluble vitamins Price found to be so important—A and D—are uniquely provided by certain animal foods: shellfish, fish eggs, oily fish, fish liver oils; butter, egg yolks, and organ meats of ruminant animals raised outdoors and on pasture; and the fat of birds and pigs raised outside and on pasture. Yes, the very cholesterol-rich foods now shunned by the American public as unhealthful were a critical source of health for diverse populations around the world.

labeled Activator X. It was present in all the diets he studied. Dr. Price identified Activator X in fish liver oils, fish eggs, organ meats, blubber of sea animals, and butterfat from cows eating rapidly growing green grass in the spring and fall. Unfortunately, there has been no research on this nutrient since his death in 1948.

In describing the essential factors of nutrition, Dr. Price provided an overarching nutritional perspective that is proving timeless and far more universal than passing food theories and fads.

As we saw in Chapter 2, the USRDAs for important nutrients are lower than the amounts of these nutrients your body actually needs. What's more, modern food fads and theories (along with modern agricultural practices) have substantially reduced the nutrient value of most foods. While traditional diets in his time provided about ten times more fat-soluble vitamins than the American diet of the 1940s, today this ratio is probably higher (we don't know for certain, since this research is not being done), since Americans have deliberately reduced animal-fat consumption. What's more, fats from animals raised in confinement (as they are nowadays) are not as nutritious. The average American child eats vitamin-rich foods like shellfish and organ meats rarely, if at all, while sources prized by other societies, like blubber and insects, are obviously not part of our Western diet. Unfortunately, we have also demonized butter, eggs, and cream, which *are* traditional Western sources of these healthy nutrients. When we do eat these foods, they usually come from animals raised in confinement, so their nutritional value is compromised.

Comparison of Traditional and Modern Diets

Traditional diets *maximized* nutrients, while modern diets *minimize* nutrients.

TRADITIONAL DIETS	MODERN DIETS
Foods grown on fertile soil	Foods grown on depleted soil
Organ meats (liver, marrow, heart, tongue, brain) preferred to muscle meats	Muscle meats (steaks, chops, roasts), few organ meats
Animal fats	Vegetable oils
Animals on pasture	Animals in confinement
Dairy products, raw and/or fermented	Dairy products, pasteurized
Grains and legumes, soaked/fermented	Grains, refined and/or extruded
Bone broths	MSG, artificial flavorings
Unrefined sweeteners (honey, maple syrup)	Refined sweeteners
Lacto-fermented vegetables	Canned vegetables
Lacto-fermented beverages	Modern soft drinks
Unrefined salt	Refined salt
Natural vitamins in foods	Synthetic vitamins added to foods
Traditional cooking methods	Microwave, irradiation
Traditional seeds/open pollination	Hybrid seeds, GMO seeds

If any two words can sum up the characteristics of healthy traditional diets, they are *nutrient dense*. In this chapter, we'll survey some of the common nutrient-dense foods that Dr. Price discovered formed the basis of the health and well-being of people in traditional cultures.

Rediscovering Nutrient-Dense Foods

Below you will find descriptions of the traditional foods that, together with coconut, make up the basis of our diet plans. Some, such as butter, eggs, and milk, will already be familiar to you, although you may never have tasted them in the traditional, far healthier—and tastier—forms we recommend. These foods will provide the vitamins, beneficial fatty acids, and other nutrients in the right combinations for both weight loss and enhanced health.

Principles of Healthy Traditional Diets

- Eat whole, unprocessed foods.
- Eat beef, lamb, game, organ meats, poultry, and eggs from pasture-fed animals.
- Eat wild (not farm-raised) fish, shellfish, and fish roe from unpolluted waters.
- Eat full-fat milk products from pasture-fed cows, preferably raw and/or fermented, such as raw milk, whole yogurt, kefir, cultured butter, whole raw cheeses, and fresh and sour cream.
- Use animal fats, especially butter, liberally.
- Use traditional vegetable oils only—extra-virgin olive oil, expeller-expressed sesame oil, small amounts of expeller-expressed flax oil, and the tropical oils—coconut oil and palm oil.
- Eat fresh fruits and vegetables—preferably organic—in salads and soups, or lightly steamed with butter.
- Use whole grains, legumes, and nuts that have been prepared by soaking, sprouting, or sour leavening.
- Include enzyme-enhanced lacto-fermented vegetables, fruits, beverages, and condiments in your diet on a regular basis.
- Prepare homemade meat stocks from the bones of chicken, beef, lamb, and fish and use liberally in soups, stews, and sauces.
- Use filtered water for cooking and drinking.
- Use unrefined salt and a variety of herbs and spices for food interest and appetite stimulation.
- Make your own salad dressing using raw vinegar and natural, traditional oils.
- Use natural sweeteners in moderation, such as raw honey, maple syrup, date sugar, coconut sugar, dehydrated cane sugar juice (sold as Rapadura or sucanat), and stevia powder.
- If you drink alcohol, use only unpasteurized wine or beer very moderately with meals.
- Cook only in stainless-steel, cast-iron, glass, or good-quality enamel—don't use aluminum cookware.
- Do not use a microwave oven.
- Use only natural, food-based supplements.
- Get plenty of sleep, exercise, and natural light.
- Think positive thoughts and practice forgiveness.

Eggs

Eggs contain every nutrient the body needs except vitamin C. Egg whites provide the highest-quality protein of any food, and the yolks provide special fatty acids necessary for nerve function. If the chickens are raised on pasture, their yolks will provide generous amounts of vitamin D and also vitamin A (although not as much as liver or cod-liver oil).

In a study carried out in 1929—almost 70 years ago yet extremely relevant to the modern era of confinement agriculture—researchers in Kansas found that the second most potent source of vitamin D was egg yolk (number one was cod-liver oil) and that the amount of the vitamin varied depending on how the chickens were raised. Only those exposed to bright sunlight (containing UV-B light) or to a UV-B lamp produced eggs with sufficient levels of vitamin D. Egg yolks from chickens kept under glass or in cages were so low in vitamin D that rats fed on them developed rickets.

Egg yolks also supply choline and the long-chain fatty acid DHA, both important for nerve function. Perhaps that's why eggs are considered a brain food in China, where a pregnant or nursing woman will eat up to ten eggs per day if she can afford them, to ensure that her child is intelligent.

Organic Versus Pasture-Fed Many people have heard about the horrors of confinement egg production and are buying organic eggs instead. However, you may not be aware that chickens producing organic eggs are also raised in confinement. It's true that conditions are vastly better for organic chickens than those producing regular commercial eggs; the chickens are not confined to cages, which is why their product can be labeled "free-range." However, organic chickens rarely have access to bright sunlight, and their diet is highly artificial, lacking the green plants and insects that chickens are designed to eat. In fact, the USDA organic standards *forbid* feeding animal foods to chickens— yet the chicken is an omnivore, not a vegetarian!

Many far-thinking farmers are now raising chickens on pasture by using moveable hen houses. The chickens get fresh green pasture and plenty of bugs every day. This is the only method that ensures that the egg yolks will contain vitamins A and D as well as DHA. That's why we encourage you to find pasture-raised (as opposed to free-range) eggs. Many health-conscious consumers make a big effort to purchase eggs directly from farmers, or at stores that obtain their eggs directly from farmers. (See Resources for sources.)

In our recipes and menu plans, you will find many ways to consume eggs. Raw egg yolks from pastured hens are mixed into smoothies, mayonnaise, and other foods. (There is no danger of salmonella from the egg yolks of hens raised out of doors, without antibiotics. Egg yolks from organic eggs are also safe to eat raw. However, we do not recommend eating the yolks of supermarket eggs raw.) The whites should mostly be eaten cooked, as they contain enzyme inhibitors that can interfere with protein digestion. Although many diet books advise you to eat "egg white omelets," we don't recommend this, because you need the vitamin A in the yolks to assimilate the protein in the whites. In fact, it's better to eat the yolks without the whites than vice versa.

The Anti-Egg Scare Once called nature's most perfect food by nutritionists, eggs fell into disfavor and their consumption began to plummet after 1950. The average number of eggs consumed in the United States per person per year has dropped from a high of 389 in 1950 to only about 185 today. Tragically, many people, including many children, never eat eggs.

Why this turnaround? Since eggs contain high levels of cholesterol, various authorities promulgated the hypothesis that eating eggs raises cholesterol levels and thus contributes to heart disease.

Surprisingly, there are very few published papers on the relationship between egg consumption and heart disease, but the little research that has been done indicates that egg consumption creates no risk. One study, published in the *Journal of the American Medical Association*, 1999, found that consumption of one egg per day carried no risk of increased heart disease or stroke among healthy men and women.

During the period when egg consumption in the United States went into decline, rates of heart disease and other chronic diseases soared. Yet negative publicity creating fears of egg consumption has drowned out all the evidence that eggs are good for you. In fact, the food industry has created imitation egg products like Egg Beaters, promoted as a healthy alternative. But a University of Illinois study published in the journal *Pediatrics*, 1974, refutes this claim. One group of lactating rats was fed exclusively on fresh eggs, while another group ate Egg Beaters. The rats who ate eggs thrived, grew normally, and enjoyed perfect health, while those on Egg Beaters were stunted, had a variety of physical abnormalities, and all died long before reaching maturity. In this case, as in countless others, efforts to improve on Mother Nature are not real improvements.

Proving the folk wisdom of the Orient, unpublished research carried out during the 1990s at the University of California at Berkeley divided 80-year-old men into two groups: those who were senile and required constant care, and those with their faculties intact who were able to care for themselves. All filled out dietary surveys. Researchers found only one difference between the dietary habits of the two groups: the group that was mentally alert ate at least one egg per day.

Butter

In his study of traditional diets, Dr. Price found that butter was a staple among groups that kept herds, and no native peoples at that time consumed polyunsaturated oils. Most highly valued (and especially beneficial for children and expectant mothers) was the deep yellow butter produced by cows feeding on rapidly growing green grass. When Dr. Price analyzed this deep yellow butter, he found that it was exceptionally high in all fat-soluble vitamins, particularly vitamin A. He called these vitamins "catalysts" or "activators" because they are needed for mineral metabolism and for the absorption of water-soluble vitamins. When cows are kept in barns and fed dry feed, the amount of vital fat-soluble vitamins is greatly diminished.

Most of us don't keep herds these days, but the value of vitamins A and D is indisputable with respect to growth, healthy bones, proper development of the brain and nervous systems, and normal sexual development. Many studies have shown the importance of butterfat for reproduction; substitutes based on vegetable oils have led to infertility. As butter consumption in America has declined, sterility rates have increased. In calves, butter substitutes are unable to promote growth or sustain reproduction, according to an unpublished study submitted to the McGovern Committee on Dietary Goals in the early 1970s.

Although long demonized by the vegetable oil industry and the industry's spokespeople in the universities, government agencies, and the medical establishment, butter is actually one of the healthiest fats on the planet, and certainly the most important fat in traditional Western diets.

Looking more closely at butter, we see that it has a perfect fatty acid profile. Most of the fats in butter are saturated or monounsaturated, making it very stable. You can sauté foods in butter, even at relatively high temperatures, and it will not break down. Like coconut oil, butter contains medium-chain fatty acids, although in lower amounts. Uniquely, butter contains short-chain fatty acids with immune-stimulating and antimicrobial properties. Butter also contains the right amount and the perfect balance of omega-3 and omega-6 fatty acids.

Despite butter's many health benefits, Americans have been taught to avoid it because it supposedly raises cholesterol. Instead, people have been told to consume margarine. Is that a healthy change? Margarine actually provokes chronic high levels of cholesterol and has been linked to both heart disease and cancer, studies show. *And do not be fooled by the new soft margarines or tub spreads.* Although they are lower in partially hydrogenated fats than their predecessors, they are still produced from rancid vegetable oils and contain many additives.

On the Eat Fat, Lose Fat program, you can feel free to add butter (ideally an organic, grass-fed variety) to vegetables. Spread it on sprouted whole-grain bread or crackers. Add it to meat dishes and sauces. This will help ensure proper assimilation of the minerals and water-soluble vitamins in the vegetables, grains, and meat you eat—and also make your food satisfying and great-tasting!

Cream

Cream should be avoided at all costs, according to so-called food experts; instead, they tell us to use "non-dairy creamers," imitation foods based on vegetable oils. The anti-cream campaign has been so successful that it's actually

Traditional Forms of Butter

"In the high mountain and plateau district in northern India, and in Tibet, the inhabitants depend largely upon butter made from the milk of the yak and the sheep. . . . The butter is eaten mixed with roasted cereals, is used in tea and in a porridge made of tea, butter, and roasted grains. In Sudan, Egypt, I found considerable traffic in high-vitamin butter which . . . was being exchanged for and used with varieties of millet grown in other districts. . . . Its brilliant orange color testified to the splendid pasture for the dairy animals. The people in Sudan had exceptionally fine teeth with exceedingly little decay." (Weston A. Price, D.D.S., *Nutrition and Physical Degeneration*)

difficult to find good thick cream these days. Supermarkets often sell only thin, ultrapasteurized stuff, or cream with artificial thickeners added. (Fortunately, there are still a few brands of good cream available—see Resources for brand names.)

Like butter, cream is a supremely healthy food, containing all the vitamins and minerals of butter plus smaller amounts of nutrients found in the whey (water fraction) and milk solids. Price describes Swiss athletes drinking "bowls of pure cream" to fortify them during athletic contests. Cream is infinitely versatile in the kitchen—the perfect addition to soups, sauces, and gravies, a wonderful base for salad dressings and casseroles, and the essential ingredient for puddings, icings, and cakes. And what would fruit be without whipped cream? Finally, cream is the base for the planet's most delicious dessert—ice cream.

Dishes made with cream are uniquely rich and satisfying. When you use cream in your cooking, you feel satisfied, even with small amounts, and do not overeat—the food "sticks to your ribs" and you don't need to raid the fridge between meals.

Liver

Liver is a sacred food in many cultures. In China, it is served at weddings. Dr. Price noted that among African tribes, "The liver is so sacred that it may not be touched by human hands." The inhabitants of the South Seas prized the livers of various sea animals, including the shark. The inhabitants of the Isle of Lewis in the Outer Hebrides valued cod's liver. Cod's head stuffed with oats and chopped cod's liver was an important dish for growing children.

Europeans and Americans traditionally ate calf's liver once a week. They also consumed liver and other organ meats in various sausages and patés. Until recently, pregnant women were advised to eat liver several times a week—now pregnant women are told not to eat liver, due to misplaced concerns about vitamin A overdose (see below).

Today, unfortunately, this nutrient-dense food is shunned, with doctors claiming that it contains toxins. In fact, toxins such as heavy metals and pesticides are generally stored in the fatty tissue, not the liver itself. The livers of animals raised in clean conditions, out of doors and eating green grass, are both safe and healthy to eat.

Another needless warning is that liver contains dangerously high amounts of vitamin A. Studies showing that synthetic vitamin A in large amounts can cause health problems such as bone loss and birth defects have led authorities to mistakenly condemn healthy foods containing natural vitamin A. In fact, natural vitamin A protects against bone loss and birth defects. For example, a 1999 study carried out in Rome found no congenital malformations among 120 infants exposed to more than 50,000 IU of vitamin A per day, while a 2002 study at the University of Wisconsin found that men taking 25,000 IU of vitamin A from cod-liver oil for six weeks had no alteration of bone-loss indicators. According to the authoritative *Merck Manual*, natural vitamin A from healthy animal sources is not toxic except in very large amounts (100,000 IU per day).

Vitamin A is essential for optimal health, and liver is a premier source of this vital nutrient, supplying between 16,000 (for chicken liver) and 36,000 IU (for beef liver) of vitamin A per 100-gram serving. Liver also supplies minerals and B vitamins in abundance. It's our best source of vitamin B_{12}, along with special long-chain fatty acids.

That's why liver is the *number one traditional nutrient-dense food*. While it's essential for athletes and those suffering from chronic fatigue, it should also be included in everyone's diet at least once a week. And there are many ways of enjoying liver, ranging from sautéed calf's liver, to patés, liverwurst, and spreads. (Chapter 10 provides recipes, if you are unaccustomed to preparing it.)

And don't worry—if you just cannot stomach liver (even as a delicious paté), you can take desiccated liver tablets (see Resources).

Whole Raw Milk

Designed to nourish the young, real milk—full-fat, unprocessed, and from pastured cows—is a fully "self-sufficient" food, containing numerous enzymes that, when exposed to the specific pH of the intestinal tract, become active and assimilate the milk's various components, making it easy for you to digest. But when pasteurization destroys these enzymes, your body must work hard to supply its own to break down the milk protein, sugars, and fat.

During the 1920s and 1930s, as health officials encouraged universal pasteurization of milk, scientists researched the effects of this new process.

- In one study, pasteurized milk resulted in anemia, while raw milk did not.
- Due to raw milk's antibacterial effects, children fed raw milk became more resistant to tuberculosis, while those given pasteurized milk were more likely to develop it.

- A study from 1937 found that children drinking raw milk were less likely to have tooth decay than those drinking pasteurized milk.
- Scientists found that pasteurization decreases the factors in raw milk that promote healthy bone growth. In one study, pasteurized milk was much less effective than raw milk in inducing height increases in children.
- A study from 1933 showed that adults who drank raw milk absorbed more calcium from the milk than did those drinking pasteurized milk. This study also stated that milk from barn-raised cows contained less available calcium than milk from pasture-raised cows.
- Pasteurization destroys or reduces many nutrients in milk, including vitamins A and C and the B complex vitamins. Rats fed pasteurized milk developed nerve disorders, while those on raw milk did not, one study showed. In another study, the offspring of rats fed pasteurized milk died young or failed to thrive.

Sadly, no published research comparing the nutritive value of raw versus pasteurized milk has appeared since these studies from the 1930s and 1940s, but the laws of biochemistry haven't changed, so these findings are still valid.

Many people don't realize that pasteurization was originally proposed as a temporary solution to the problem of dairies that existed side by side with breweries in the inner cities during most of the 1800s.* In these "swill dairies," cows lived in confinement in incredible filth and were fed nothing but the swill (refuse) from the breweries. There were no standards of hygiene for milking, storing, or transportation. The milk was not only extremely dirty but thin and watery, lacking the nutrients that normally occur in milk. Some dairies even added chalk to the milk to make it whiter! Not surprisingly, the death rate among inner-city children dependent on this milk was as high as 50 percent.

Pasteurization was implemented around the same time that the swill dairies were outlawed and the invention of refrigeration made it possible to bring milk from the country safely into the city. When the children's death rate dropped, pasteurization took the credit, but it's more likely that the removal of cows to pasture and the introduction of more sanitary dairying methods were responsible.

By the late 1940s, increased knowledge about how to produce healthy milk and advances in technology made pasteurization completely unnecessary, but it was just then that lobbying for mandatory pasteurization began in earnest. Why? Because investors and businessmen realized that mandatory pasteurization was the easiest way to consolidate the industry. Tens of thousands of small, pasture-based dairy farms are still being put out of business as the dairy

---

*This information comes from Ron Schmid, N.D., *The Untold Story of Milk*, New Trends Publishing, 2003.

industry has become more centralized and monopolistic, with milk production increasingly transferred to huge confinement operations where cows are fed soy feed, bakery waste, citrus peel cake, and even the swill from ethanol manufacture—anything but the green grass they need to make healthy milk.

Where to Find Raw Milk Although raw milk has been difficult to find for the last 20 years, it is now becoming increasingly available. In California, Connecticut, New Mexico, and some parts of Pennsylvania, you can buy it in stores. In many other states you can purchase raw milk directly from farmers, or through a "cow share" program (see Resources).

If you are obtaining raw milk from a farmer, be sure that the milk comes from healthy cows that have tested as disease-free. The cows should graze on unsprayed pasture for most of the year and be fed unsprayed hay or silage during the winter months when they must be in the barn. The milk should be extracted by a milking machine and stored in chilled stainless-steel tanks. To find out whether such milk is available in your area, visit realmilk.org or contact a local chapter of the Weston A. Price Foundation (you can find them listed at the "Local Chapters" link on our website, westonaprice.org). These local chapters have played a key role in finding conscientious grass-based dairy farmers and setting up cow-share programs.

Coconut and Kosher Kitchens

Coconut oil is ideal for those who keep a kosher kitchen. You can use coconut oil as a substitute for butter in baked goods and **Mary's Oil Blend** (see page 188 for recipe) as a substitute for animal fat in frying. You can also use coconut milk in place of cow's milk and coconut cream in place of dairy cream. In our shrimp and pork recipes, substitue fish and kosher meats, respectively.

Jewish cookbooks dating back 150 years recognized the nutritional value of traditional fats, including butter, tallow, goose fat, and egg yolks, and called for coconut oil as an ingredient in many baked goods, especially those that were to be served with meat.

Jewish housewives were an early target of the vegetable oil industry. A 1913 recipe book published by Procter & Gamble specifically recommended Crisco vegetable shortening to Jewish housewives as a substitute for butter in kosher cooking.

With the advent of margarines and shortenings, and the demonization of coconut oil, healthy and delicious coconut alternatives to dairy fats disappeared from Jewish kitchens.

What About Organic Milk? Several brands of organic milk are now available in health food stores. Yet this milk is always processed. In fact, most of it is ultrapasteurized, a process that gives milk a very long shelf life but completely deadens it. You can't make yogurt with ultrapasteurized milk, for it will not support microbial life—and it's unlikely to support human life, either.

Raw milk sold in stores is almost always organic, but farmers selling raw milk directly usually don't bother to get organic certification. More important than the organic label is how the farmer feeds his cows, as described earlier.

If you can't find raw milk, we recommend not using milk at all. But don't worry—milk is not critical to any of our diet plans. Instead, eat raw cheeses (available in many stores and on the Internet) and good-quality yogurt (which is cultured to put at least some of the enzymes back into the product). A good substitute for raw milk is our **Coconut Milk Tonic** (see page 220 for recipe), which is formulated to contain approximately the same amount of fat, calories, and calcium as whole milk.

Raw Cheese

Today, many people rely on "energy bars" and "meal replacements" for their convenience; they don't spoil easily, require no preparation, and can be taken on outings and trips. Unfortunately, though touted as "complete," these bars are made with chemicals and many processed ingredients, such as high-fructose corn syrup, soy protein isolate, and refined and hydrogenated oils. Anything but complete, they lack many nutrients, especially calcium and fat-soluble vitamins.

From our perspective, the ideal convenience food is cheese, a delicious, concentrated food that travels easily and provides all necessary nutrients, including adequate calcium, along with the whole gamut of vitamins and minerals, including vitamin C if the cheese is made from unheated milk.

Unlike raw milk, raw cheese is available in most towns and also on the Internet (see Resources). Remember: we're not talking about processed products like Velveeta, nor even the type of cheese sold in supermarkets. Look for raw cheese from cows raised naturally, such as cheddar, feta, and blue cheese, which has been processed on or near the farm—the label will tell you that it is made from "raw" or "unpasteurized" milk. The range of taste and textures of such cheese is extraordinary. (See Resources for sources and brand names.)

Fish Eggs

Fish eggs were a sacred food in widely diverse cultures, Dr. Price found. The Eskimos in Alaska dried salmon roe "so they could have healthy babies." South American Indians living high in the Andes Mountains, the people of the South Sea Islands and the islands north of Australia, the Gaelics in the Outer Hebrides, and the coastal Peruvian Indians all used fish eggs during pregnancy. Roe was prized in the Orkney Islands and among all peoples who consumed seafood. Even today, caviar is considered an aphrodisiac.

Roe is truly a nutrient-dense food, containing components key to healthy reproduction, including vitamins A and D, vitamin E, zinc, iodine, and the special long-chain fatty acids DHA and EPA. In our menu plans, we recommend salted cured roe spread on buttered whole-grain bread or crackers and a delicious fish roe spread made with **Mary's Oil Blend**, which contains coconut oil (see page 188 for recipe).

Shellfish

Populations eating seafoods had the best bone structure—the widest palates and thickest skulls, Dr. Price noted. And chief among sea foods were shellfish, easy to gather and often eaten raw. Oysters, clams, conch, abalone, shrimp, crab, lobster, crayfish—all were considered sacred foods, rich in vital factors needed for good health and successful reproduction. Shellfish are particularly rich in vitamin D, but they also provide vitamin A, the gamut of minerals and fatty acids.

Shrimp and oysters are particularly important. Shrimp is very rich in vitamin D, and throughout Africa and Asia little dried shrimp form the basis of condiments and sauces. And oysters are our best source of zinc (essential for male reproductive health), which is probably why they're considered an aphrodisiac.

Nuts

Nuts are an extremely nutrient-dense food, supplying high levels of minerals, as well as B vitamins, some protein, and lots of fat. The fat content of nuts ranges from 40 to 70 percent, most of it monounsaturated. A few varieties of nuts, particularly walnuts, are a good source of omega-3 fatty acids. Nuts are very satisfying and make a great snack food. But be warned: they are calorie-dense, and their monounsaturated fats can contribute to weight gain. So nuts are great if you lead an active life or don't need to lose weight (or even need to gain weight). But they're not for you if you need to take pounds off.

Many traditional cultures used nuts, from the acorns eaten by the California natives to the Queensland nuts (macadamias) used by the Australian Aborigines. But these groups instinctively realized that nuts contain many irritants and toxins, such as enzyme inhibitors and tannins. That is why they prepared nuts very carefully, usually by soaking, then sun-drying. Roasting also eliminates some of the anti-nutrients.

The best preparation method is to soak raw nuts in salt water for 6 to 8 hours, then drain and dehydrate in a warm oven or dehydrator until completely dry and crisp. We call these **Crispy Nuts** (see page 259 for recipe.)

A word of caution: Do not buy nuts from open bins—they are often rancid. Purchase nuts in airtight packages.

Whole Grains/Tubers/Legumes

Proponents of traditional foods, including Loren Cordain, author of *The Paleo Diet*, theorize that ancestral diets did not include high-carbohydrate foods. However, an in-depth look at traditional diets refutes this notion. Even Paleolithic peoples had access to carbohydrate foods. Native Americans consumed tubers called *wapatos* that thrived in swampy areas. Tubers such as the taro root were a staple in South Sea diets. South Americans ate various types of potato. Grains and legumes were consumed in Australia, Africa, and both North and South America.

However, traditional peoples did not eat these foods hastily prepared, as we do. They usually prepared starchy foods by long soaking or fermentation, which greatly increased their nutrient values and minimized their anti-nutrient content, as well as making them much more digestible.

In Chapter 10, you'll find many recipes using these ancient methods, which give whole-grain foods a light taste and make them easy to digest. Genuine sourdough breads, fermented to neutralize the phytic acid and enzyme inhibitors, are also available for purchase. (See the Resources section for sources.)

Lacto-Fermented Foods

To recover from digestive disorders, many people today take probiotics, supplements containing healthy bacteria for the digestive tract. Traditional people did not take probiotics. They got beneficial bacteria from lacto-fermented foods such as sauerkraut and other pickled vegetables and fruits.

Toxic Breakfast Cereals?

All but a few brands of cold breakfast cereals—even so-called organic health food cereals—are produced by a process called extrusion that subjects the grains to very high pressure at high temperatures (Grape Nuts is one exception—it is not extruded but baked). Analysis of the grains after extrusion indicates that this industrial process breaks up the carefully organized proteins they contain, creating neurotoxic (damaging to nerves) protein fragments.

Unpublished animal studies described by Paul Stitt in his book *Fighting the Food Giants* indicate that animals fed extruded grains rapidly develop serious anomalies of the digestive and nervous systems and die before animals given nothing but water. And, since organic whole grains are high in protein, extruded health food cereals are likely to contain higher levels of these toxic protein fragments than the cereals sold in supermarkets.

That's why it's so much healthier to prepare your own grain dishes, making sure to soak and ferment the grains. So we've provided two delicious recipes for soaked, then baked, cold breakfast cereals (see page 209 and 258).

All traditional cultures consumed fermented food, from fermented fish in Arctic regions to fermented tubers, such as poi (fermented cassava), in the tropics. Coconut meat and coconut juice can also be fermented.

Sauerkraut, cabbage that has been preserved by lacto-fermentation, is familiar to most Westerners. Traditionally, it's never made with sugar or vinegar, nor is it canned or pasteurized. Instead, the cabbage is pounded and mixed with salt, to encourage the growth of lactobacilli, bacteria that produce lactic acid, which acts as a preservative. Fermented dairy products, such as yogurt and kefir (a sour, fermented milk beverage), also act as probiotics.

Another big topic today among health-conscious people, one that encourages sales of a lot of supplements, is enzymes. Enzymes in our food aid digestion, saving the body a lot of work. Some people assert that all our food should

Raw Versus Cooked

How much of your food should be cooked? Proponents of the newly popular raw food diets claim that cooking ruins vitamins and enzymes, making food difficult to digest and therefore contributing to disease.

But all traditional peoples cooked some or most of their food. Even in the tropics, where people did not have to build fires to keep warm, they built fires every day to cook. In addition to cooking grains and legumes, they usually cooked their vegetables, the very foods some recommend that people eat raw.

Why cook? Cooking helps neutralize many naturally occurring anti-nutrients and irritants in food, also breaking down indigestible fiber. Many foods, such as beans and potatoes, are indigestible until cooked.

While cooking—especially at very high temperatures—does destroy some nutrients, it makes minerals more available; and a surprising benefit of cooking is the fact that it makes proteins more digestible by gently unfolding these large molecules so that the digestive enzymes can latch on and do their work.

Though cooking does destroy enzymes, many foods we cook do not have many enzymes to start with. Consuming lacto-fermented condiments and beverages will more than compensate for enzymes lost in cooking.

Raw Foods You Should Eat

Interestingly, all traditional cultures consumed at least some of their animal foods raw. Cooking destroys vitamin B_6, derived from animal foods, and greatly reduces milk's nutrients. That is why we've included several raw meat and fish dishes in this book. *Note:* It's important to freeze meat that will be eaten raw for 14 days before using, to ensure that parasites are destroyed. Fish to be eaten raw is marinated in an acidic medium, equally effective for getting rid of parasites.

be raw, because enzymes are destroyed in cooking (see sidebar). But all traditional cultures cooked some or even most of their food; they got their enzymes from moderate amounts of fermented foods. We like to think of fermented foods as "super-raw," because they contain very high levels of enzymes (formed during the lacto-fermentation process) that more than compensate for the enzymes destroyed by cooking. Consumed as condiments, these fermented foods help digest cooked foods.

Fermented foods also contain high nutrient levels. For example, the vitamin C content of cabbage increases up to tenfold in the process of making sauerkraut. B vitamin content also greatly increases, and the minerals in the foods become more bio-available.

Lacto-Fermented Beverages

Traditional cultures made healthy lacto-fermented beverages (either non-alcoholic or slightly alcoholic) out of palm sap, coconut juice, herbs, roots, tubers, and fruit. They drank these beverages to provide quick energy and aid digestion.

Soaking grains is one form of lacto-fermentation, while making lacto-fermented beverages from grains increases their nutritive value even further. North Americans made a sour corn beverage, while Africans made beer from sorghum, a type of cereal grass. These beverages supplied abundant vitamins, enzymes, beneficial bacteria, and lactic acid, all of which contribute to intestinal health.

Lacto-fermented beverages are an important feature in Health Recovery and optional (although strongly suggested) in Quick and Easy Weight Loss and Everyday Gourmet. They are delicious and actually more nutritious than the raw vegetable juices recommended in some diets. Think of lacto-fermented beverages as soft drinks that are good for you! There's a tremendous need for beverages that provide a healthy alternative to commercial sodas, and these traditional sparkling beverages—especially our **Kefir Sodas** (see page 262 for recipes) flavored with fruit and ginger—can really help people kick the soft drink habit.

We've included several recipes for easy-to-make lacto-fermented beverages. But if you don't have time even for that, you can buy them ready-made (see Resources)—or just add a pinch of sea salt and a squeeze of fresh lemon, lime, or grapefruit to sparkling water to provide important trace minerals and aid digestion.

Broth

Traditional diets contain only two good sources of calcium—dairy products and bones. In very primitive cultures, the bones of small animals are ground with water to make a paste. In more advanced cultures, the bones are cooked in water to make broth or stock. In cultures that do not consume milk

A Glossary of Lacto-Fermented Beverages

Here are descriptions of less familiar lacto-fermented beverages that are especially healthful and useful for the Eat Fat, Lose Fat program.

Beet kvass: A fermented Russian beverage made out of beets (see page 263 for recipe). It requires **Homemade Whey** (made from yogurt, see page 227 for recipe), but once you have the whey, beet kvass is actually very easy to make. The taste is somewhat medicinal but not unpleasant.

Coconut kefir: Many people report complete recovery from digestive problems using coconut kefir. You make it by adding a culture to fresh coconut water, the liquid from inside the immature coconut. Many markets now carry immature (white) coconuts. It's easy to make a hole in these relatively soft coconuts to extract the juice, or you can buy packaged coconut water by mail order. To make coconut kefir, simply add the culture (which comes in powdered and grain form) to the fresh coconut juice and leave at room temperature for about two days, then transfer to bottles and refrigerate. The taste of coconut juice and coconut kefir is somewhat medicinal. Some people can't stand it, but others love it. Many swear by it as a key factor in recovering health.

Ginger ale: We provide a recipe for fermented ginger ale that uses a kefir culture (see page 262 for recipe). This is a really delightful way to take your lacto-fermented beverage—ginger tastes great and also is good for the digestion.

Kombucha: This extremely healthy fermented drink, made by adding a culture from the kombucha mushroom to sweetened tea, is from Russia. The culture transforms the sugar into many beneficial acids that aid digestion and actually help the liver detoxify. You can either make your own (see page 264 for recipe) or purchase ready-made kombucha (see Resources).

and cheese, bone broths play a key role in supplying calcium, as in the Asian diet, where a bone broth is consumed with every meal, even at breakfast. Miso soup, so popular in Japan, is actually a fish broth to which miso has been added (see page 233 for recipe).

In the "good old days," your grandmother purchased meat differently than you do today. The neighborhood butcher sold her meat on the bone rather than as individual fillets. She bought whole chickens rather than boneless breasts. Our thrifty ancestors made use of every part of the animal by preparing stock, broth, or bouillon from the bony portions. Almost all traditional cuisines—French, Italian, Chinese, Japanese, African, South American, Middle

Eastern, and Russian—use meat and fish stocks to produce nourishing and flavorful soups and sauces, but this practice has almost completely disappeared from American cooking.

Bone Broth or Stock Properly prepared, meat stocks are extremely nutritious, containing the minerals of bone, cartilage, marrow, and vegetables in a form that is easy to assimilate. Acidic wine or vinegar added during cooking helps to draw minerals, particularly calcium, magnesium, and potassium, out of the bone and into the broth. Dr. Francis Pottenger, a doctor and researcher and author of *Pottenger's Cats*, wrote extensively on the benefits of gelatin; he once stated that the stockpot was the most important piece of kitchen equipment anyone could own.

Gelatin in meat broths can help treat many intestinal disorders, including hyperacidity, colitis, and Crohn's disease. Although gelatin is not a complete protein, it allows the body to more fully utilize proteins from other foods.

Many people today fear that bones—or even gelatin, for that matter—might be a source of mad cow disease. We have reviewed the evidence, and we do not believe that mad cow disease can be transmitted to humans by using or consuming either meat or bones. Mark Purdey, a British farmer and researcher, published studies in *Medical Hypotheses* in 1996 and 1998 indicating that the

---

MSG: A Surprising Cause of Weight Gain (and Worse)

Since making broth is a time-consuming process, the food industry instead uses MSG (monosodium glutamate), along with synthetic flavorings, to give a meatlike taste to soups, sauces, and gravies.

You probably know that MSG can cause all sorts of neurological problems, from headaches to seizures, the so-called Chinese restaurant syndrome. But you may not realize that MSG can also cause weight gain! In animal studies, rats fed MSG became obese (and also blind). In fact, the way scientists induce obesity in laboratory animals is by feeding them MSG! It appears that MSG causes injury to the hypothalamus, an area of the brain that controls appetite, thyroid function, and the endocrine system.

This is yet another reason why it's crucial to avoid processed food: nearly all of it contains MSG, even though the label may not say so. In fact, if the label lists "spices," "flavorings," "natural flavorings," citric acid, or anything "hydrolyzed" or "autolyzed," the food probably contains MSG. Canned and dehydrated soups, frozen dinners, bottled sauces and sauce mixes, soy foods, commercial salad dressings, and even many spice mixes are loaded with MSG.

The Magic of Broths

The wonderful thing about fish and meat stocks is that, along with conferring many health benefits, they also add immeasurably to the food's flavor. In European cuisines, rich stocks are the base of delicious sauces that add flavor to so many dishes. This flavor comes from the stock, made with as much care as the final dish.

Visiting the kitchens of fine restaurants in France, you will always find pots of pale broth simmering on huge cookstoves. When this liquid is reduced by boiling down, the flavors are concentrated, resulting in a sauce that is both nutritious and delicious. Making meat stocks on a regular basis will confer innumerable health benefits (and earn you a reputation as an excellent cook). You'll find complete recipes for stocks in Chapter 10.

most likely cause of mad cow disease is the use of neurotoxic pesticides and overload of certain neurotoxic minerals such as manganese, both of which occur in today's confinement animal facilities. Avoidance of these unhealthy procedures is one of the reasons we recommend pasture-fed or at least organic meat. But while there are many problems with today's industrial animal foods, we believe that they pose no risk of causing mad cow disease in humans. Purdey notes that there have been no cases of the human variant (Creutzfeld-Jakob disease) in the Shetland Islands, where the volcanic soil frequently causes scrapie in sheep (scrapie is similar to mad cow disease) and where the national dish is raw sheep brains!

Chicken Broth In folk wisdom, rich chicken broth—the famous "Jewish penicillin"—is a valued remedy for the flu. The 12th-century physician Moses Maimonides prescribed chicken broth as a treatment for colds and asthma. Modern research has confirmed that broth helps prevent and moderate infectious diseases. Using gelatin-rich broth often, or even every day, can protect you against many health problems.

Fish Broth Stock made from the carcasses and heads of fish is especially rich in minerals, including all-important iodine. Even more important, stock made from the heads, and therefore the thyroid glands, of fish supplies substances that nourish your thyroid gland. Four thousand years ago, Chinese doctors rejuvenated aging patients with a soup made from the thyroid glands of animals. According to ancient texts, this treatment helped patients feel younger, gave them more energy, and often restored mental abilities. Another traditional belief is that fish-head broth contributes to virility.

In the Victorian age, prominent London physicians prescribed special raw thyroid sandwiches to failing patients. Very few of us could eat such fare with relish, but soups and sauces made from fish broth are absolutely delicious.

According to some researchers, it's possible that up to 40 percent of Americans suffer from (often undiagnosed) thyroid deficiency, with its accompanying symptoms of fatigue, weight gain, frequent colds and flu, inability to concentrate, depression, and a host of more serious complications like heart disease and cancer. We would do well to imitate peoples from the Mediterranean and Asian regions by consuming fish broth as often as possible. We've provided a recipe for **Quick Fish Stock** (see page 226 for recipe) so you can make fish soups and sauces with little effort. If you don't have time to make your own stock, some excellent brands of traditionally made stock are now available (see Resources).

Salt

With few exceptions, all traditional cultures use some salt. Isolated peoples living far from the sea burned sodium-rich marsh grasses and added the ash to their food.

Today, however, medical orthodoxy advises restricting salt intake, claiming that salt raises blood pressure. Some early research did correlate salt intake with high blood pressure, but a large 1983 study conducted in Japan found that dietary salt did not significantly affect blood pressure in most people. In some cases, salt restriction actually raised blood pressure. A similar study in Connecticut, published in the *Journal of the American Medical Association* that

Refined or Unrefined? How Salt Is Processed

Most salt is highly refined through an industrial process that uses chemicals and high temperatures to remove valuable magnesium salts and natural trace minerals, while putting in several harmful additives, like aluminum compounds and potassium iodide in amounts that can be toxic to some people. Processors also add dextrose, which turns the salt a purplish color, and then must add a bleaching agent to make it white again.

Although sun-dried sea salt is best, some brands labeled "sea salt" are produced by industrial methods. The most health-promoting salt is extracted by the action of the sun on seawater in clay-lined vats. Its light gray color indicates a high moisture and trace mineral content. This natural salt contains only about 82 percent sodium chloride; it also contains about 14 percent magnesium and nearly 80 trace minerals.

The best and purest commercially available source of unrefined sea salt is the natural salt marshes of Brittany, where the salt is "farmed" according to ancient methods (see Resources). Unrefined salt mined from ancient sea beds is also acceptable. You can find it in many health food stores.

same year, concluded that "dietary salt intake has a clinically insignificant effect on blood pressure in the majority of individuals. . . ."

Salt is essential to health, activating enzymes needed for brain development and enzymes needed to digest carbohydrate foods, as well as helping your body produce hydrochloric acid for the digestion of meat. Salt also supports adrenal function.

Different people do need different amounts of salt. Those with weak adrenal glands lose salt in their urine and must replace it, but for others, excessive salt causes the excretion of calcium, contributing to osteoporosis. Excessive dietary salt also depletes potassium.

Let your taste buds be your guide as to how much salt you need, but it's also important to pay attention to the kind of salt you use. Though we're advised to consume iodized salt to prevent thyroid problems, Americans are plagued with thyroid problems despite its universal availability. That's because the iodine added to refined salt is harder to absorb than natural iodine in unrefined salt. A further danger of iodized salt is iodine overdose, since too much can be as harmful as too little.

Natural Vitamins

Vitamins found naturally in foods differ from vitamins in pill form. When vitamins occur naturally in whole foods, food concentrates, and superfoods like nutritional yeast, desiccated liver, bee pollen, and cod-liver oil, they come with many cofactors—such as related vitamins, enzymes, and minerals—which ensure that the vitamins are absorbed and properly used.

By contrast, most commercially produced supplements contain vitamins that are either crystalline or synthetic.

- Crystalline vitamins have been separated from natural sources by chemical means.
- Synthetic vitamins are produced "from scratch" in the laboratory.

Both types are fractionated concentrates that act more like drugs than nutrients, disrupting body chemistry and causing many imbalances. An additional danger is that synthetic vitamins often occur as the mirror image of the natural vitamin, thereby causing the opposite effect. Synthetic forms of fat-soluble vitamins can be especially dangerous.

For example, synthetic vitamin B_1 derived from coal tar did not cure beriberi in Korean prisoners-of-war, but rice polishings containing natural vitamin B complex did. In scientific studies, synthetic vitamin C is not as effective in curing scurvy as fresh citrus juice, and synthetic beta carotene given to smokers actually increased their risk of cancer. And finally, research indicates that synthetic vitamin D_2 has the opposite effect of natural vitamin D, causing softening of the bones and hardening of soft tissues such as the arteries. The dairy

Why Eat Sweets?

Surprisingly, most traditional diets included some sweet foods. Many traditional people ate honey. Native Americans ate maple syrup and maple sugar. Residents of the tropics dehydrated cane sugar juice in the sun to make a mineral-rich sweetener. Naturally sweet sap from coconut flower buds can also be turned into a sugar.

These sweet foods were quite different from the refined sugars we eat today, for two reasons:

- They were unrefined and concentrated, hence loaded with nutrients, especially minerals, while white sugar, fructose, and other refined sweeteners are completely devoid of nutrients.
- They were expensive or rare, so people did not consume them in large amounts as we do today.

Our natural taste for sweets can be satisfied with sweet foods that also provide nutrients. If we restrict sweets entirely, cravings develop.

So although we urge caution, we don't forbid sweeteners in our food plans, unless you're trying to lose weight. But on Everyday Gourmet, you can enjoy small amounts of natural sweeteners such as Rapadura or Sucanat (dehydrated cane sugar juice), raw honey, maple sugar, or maple syrup, coconut sugar, and molasses (the mineral-rich residue of white sugar manufacture). And one of the wonderful things about coconut is that it can be made into such delicious desserts! The naturally sweet dessert recipes we provide are great for children—they won't feel deprived of sweet things on this diet.

Several recipes in Quick and Easy Weight Loss contain stevia powder, made from the leaves of a naturally sweet South American herb. This non-caloric sweetener is perfectly safe in small amounts.

Important note: Even worse than refined sweeteners (which actually use up the nutrients we take in from other foods) are the artificial sweeteners, such as aspartame (sold as Equal or Nutrasweet), used in so many "diet" foods. Like MSG, aspartame is toxic to the nervous system and can cause weight gain. Sucralose (Splenda), xylitol, and other newfangled sweeteners have caused digestive problems and immune system dysfunction in laboratory animals. Avoid them all by preparing your own desserts as occasional treats.

industry used to add D_2 to milk but quietly dropped it in favor of the less toxic (but not completely natural) D_3 when they realized how dangerous it was. Yet D_2 is still added to many products, including soymilk and rice milk.

We believe that synthetic vitamins are not necessary. If you follow our diet plans and also use the superfoods described below, you will be getting all the nutrients you need.

Superfoods—Better Than Vitamins

Superfoods—as opposed to vitamins or supplements—are whole foods that naturally concentrate important nutrients. Unlike dietary supplements or vitamins taken in isolation, superfoods provide many nutrients that support each other and work synergistically, preventing the imbalances that often occur when vitamins are taken singly. Superfoods are real foods. The body recognizes them and more readily incorporates their important nutrients.

Do you need superfoods? In theory, if your diet is good, you should need nothing more; but in actuality no one has a perfect diet. First of all, most foods today are grown in soil depleted of minerals and other vital nutrients. Furthermore, at one time or another, you, like most other Americans, have consumed harmful ingredients like artificial additives, sugar, refined carbohydrates, and rancid vegetable oils. Superfoods can help redress whatever deficiencies these unhealthy foods may have created. And for those unwilling or unable to give up bad habits like caffeine, alcohol, or smoking, a daily supply of superfoods is essential.

The following list is not exhaustive; it provides just a few examples of superfoods that can, in general, be taken by everyone. To purchase hard-to-find superfoods, see Resources.

The most important superfood is cod-liver oil, which we recommend for all three diet plans. The others may be incorporated on an individual basis, as needed, especially if you are following Health Recovery (see page 159 for our Health Recovery supplement plan).

Cod-Liver Oil

Cod-liver oil supplements are critical for redressing the widespread deficiencies in vitamins A and D in the modern diet. Unless you have access to whole dairy products from pastured cows and also eat liver several times per week, you will not be getting the levels of fat-soluble vitamins that Price found in the diets of healthy traditional peoples.

Traditional peoples made a practice of consuming special nutrient-dense foods before conception and during pregnancy and lactation and of giving them to growing children, to ensure the health of everyone in the village or tribe, generation after generation. For modern Westerners, then, taking cod-liver oil for several months *before* conception is particularly important for

How Much Cod-Liver Oil Do I Need?

An optimal maintenance dose of cod-liver oil provides 10,000 IU of vitamin A per day for adults and 5000 IU of vitamin A per day for infants and children. Those recovering from illness, accidents, or surgery should take 20,000 IU a day. Miraculous cures from various conditions, especially cancer and hormonal imbalances leading to menstrual and fertility problems, have been reported by people taking even larger doses for several weeks or months. High-vitamin cod-liver oil is perfect for weight loss, since it provides the maximum amount of A and D for the minimum number of calories.

How to Buy It

Cod-liver oil comes in several potencies, both as capsules and in liquid form. You can get 10,000 IU from about 1 teaspoon high-vitamin cod-liver oil or 2 teaspoons regular cod-liver oil. For capsules, look at the label to see how many capsules equal 10,000. (Note: The high-dose capsules are quite large.) Many people find the capsules easier to take, but they are more expensive, and some report difficulty in digesting them or even have allergic reactions to the capsule material itself.

There are also some very low-potency brands from which vitamins A and D have been largely removed due to misplaced concerns that these vitamins are toxic. For recommended brands, see the Resources section.

Note: Fish oil contains very little vitamin A or D. You should take fish *liver* oil (oil from the liver of cod or of other fish such as haddock, shark, or burdot, a type of freshwater cod), because only oil from the liver supplies generous quantities of these vitamins. Buy cod-liver oil in dark bottles and store in a cool, dark, dry place. If your kitchen is very warm, keep it in the refrigerator.

women *and* their male partners, as well as for women during pregnancy and lactation, to ensure the optimal development of the child and prevent birth defects. Growing children will also benefit from a small daily dose.

Cod-liver oil is also rich in DHA and EPA, the long-chain fatty acids critical to neurological health and many other processes in the body. Cod-liver oil should be part of a diet that contains ample saturated fats from butter, coconut oil, and other sources because the very unsaturated fatty acids in cod-liver oil work synergistically with saturated fats. To increase its effectiveness in treating serious medical conditions, Dr. Price always gave cod-liver oil along with high-vitamin butter oil (see the section on butter oil below).

How to Take It

Many people have very unpleasant memories of taking cod-liver oil—a smelly, oily dose of medicine on a spoon. And indeed, that's a very off-putting way of taking it. Instead, try mixing it with a small amount of water or fresh juice. Just stir and take it in one gulp, bypassing the taste buds and avoiding the oily sensation. Even most children have no difficulty taking cod-liver oil this way.

Modern processing methods now give us a very fresh product, which means the fishy smell is greatly reduced. However, if the smell bothers you, try adding a few drops of lemon oil or purchasing flavored cod-liver oil (see Resources).

If you still find taking liquid cod-liver oil too unpleasant, you can always take the capsules.

Is It Safe?

Many people are concerned about pesticides and mercury concentration in fish products. However, cod-liver oil sold in this country (all of which is imported, mostly from Norway) is highly tested; it contains undetectable levels of pesticides and no mercury (mercury is water soluble and resides in the protein part of fish).

Acerola Powder or Amla Tablets

Acerola and amla are fruits rich in vitamin C and numerous cofactors, including bioflavonoids and rutin, that optimize the body's uptake and use of ascorbic acid. The fruits themselves are very tart but make an excellent source of vitamin C in the form of powder and tablets.

Vitamin C, the most important dietary antioxidant, was popularized during the 1970s and 1980s by Linus Pauling, who recommended taking pure ascorbic acid in amounts up to 15 grams a day for a variety of ailments, including allergies, cancer, and heart disease. But large quantities of vitamin C may be harmful to the kidneys and can lead to deficiencies in bioflavonoids. Small quantities of natural vitamin C can provide the same protection as large amounts of pure ascorbic acid, without the side effects.

A maintenance dose of acerola powder or amla tablets should provide about 50 milligrams of vitamin C per day. Take more—up to 250 milligrams per day—divided up throughout the day, if you suffer from allergies, hay fever, or asthma or are under a lot of stress.

Desiccated Liver

If you don't like the taste of fresh liver, consider taking dried liver capsules on a daily basis, particularly if you're an athlete or you have chronic fatigue. Look for products that have been freeze dried rather than processed at high temperatures. A good maintenance dose is four capsules per day.

Bitters

Herbal extracts of bitter, mineral-rich herbs are a traditional tonic for stimulating the bile and increasing digestion and assimilation of fats. Bitters often are the best remedy for calming a queasy stomach and are good for curing constipation. They supply nutrients from bitter leaves that are often lacking in the Western diet. Many cultures, including the Chinese and Hindu, value bitter herbs for their cleansing, strengthening, and healing properties.

If you have difficulty digesting fats, take ½ teaspoon bitters mixed with a little warm water morning and evening.

High-Vitamin Butter Oil

Deep yellow butter oil from cows feeding on rapidly growing green grass in the spring and fall, produced by a low-temperature centrifuge process that concentrates the vitamins in the oil, supplies not only vitamins A and D but also Activator X. Dr. Price made butter oil and prescribed it to his patients, reporting the miraculous results in many journal articles and in his book *Nutrition and Physical Degeneration*. He used it with cod-liver oil to treat diseases such as bone loss, arthritis, tooth decay, and fatigue.

High-vitamin butter oil is part of the Health Recovery plan since it has proven very beneficial for digestive problems and convalescence. Even if you don't suffer from serious health problems, you may want to include this remarkable superfood in your diet. The recommended dose is ½ teaspoon per day. The best way to take it is with your cod-liver oil.

Note: High-vitamin butter oil is not the same as ghee. Ghee, or clarified butter, is butter from which the milk solids have been removed. It is a wonderful fat for cooking because it does not burn as easily as regular butter and also has a delightful flavor and color. However, it's not a superfood since its nutrients are much less concentrated than those of high-vitamin butter oil.

Since Dr. Price's retirement in the mid-1940s, butter oil has not been available until recently. Several years ago an enterprising farmer named David Wetzel developed a method to grow new green grass year-round, plus a way to centrifuge the butter at low temperature. Now that high-vitamin butter oil is again available (see Resources), many holistic doctors are recommending it to their patients and reporting the same results Dr. Price described.

Wheat Germ Oil

Expeller-expressed wheat germ oil is an excellent source of natural vitamin E, which provides our best antioxidant protection for the cell membrane. The Shute brothers, Canadian doctors known for their research on heart disease during the 1950s, demonstrated that vitamin E supplements are an effective protection against cardiovascular problems. In their studies they used wheat germ oil, not synthetic vitamin E preparations. Wheat germ oil is recommended for people who are predisposed to heart disease and those who have consumed a great deal of polyunsaturated oils, which deplete vitamin E. A suggested maintenance dose for both groups is two capsules per day.

Nutritional Yeast

Dried nutritional yeast is an excellent natural source of B complex vitamins (except for B_{12}) plus a variety of minerals, particularly chromium, so important for the diabetic. Nutritional yeast does not contribute to candida, as has been claimed. Candida feeds on refined carbohydrates, not yeast.

During the 1950s and 1960s, many holistic doctors treated cases of chronic fatigue with nutritional yeast supplements. (Nutritional yeast is different from brewer's yeast since it is usually grown on molasses or the residue of sugar beets, both of which are rich in minerals and vitamins.) Unfortunately, most commercial brands of nutritional yeast contain MSG, which is formed from the glutamic acid naturally present in the yeast when it is subjected to high temperature and chemicals during processing. (Actually, high levels of natural glutamic acid in yeast make it an excellent superfood for alcoholism and sugar cravings.) Look for yeast that has been processed at low temperatures. It should be a light yellow color and dissolve easily. A recommended dose is one heaping tablespoon mixed with water, taken every morning.

Even though your diet may not contain all the foods that traditional peoples prized, by adding superfoods to it, you can be sure that you're obtaining all the nutrients you need for optimal health. And if you're struggling with overweight, the combination of superfoods plus ample amounts of the traditional foods described in this chapter will satisfy your body and successfully banish the cravings, bingeing, and splurging that are the downfall of so many dieters. Turn to the next chapter to get started on the last weight-loss program you'll ever need!

Chapter Six

Quick and Easy Weight Loss

Now that you understand how healthy fats, particularly coconut oil, can help you lose weight, and how a diet of nutrient-dense whole foods is absolutely critical for maintaining good health and optimal weight, you're ready to put all this knowledge into practice!

This chapter presents our two-phase Quick and Easy Weight Loss plan. It begins with a Start-Up Week schedule that leads you through preparations for launching the diet—clearing out your kitchen cupboards, buying ingredients, and preparing a few key recipes. A two-week menu plan then follows for each phase.

Phase One

This initial two-week menu plan is composed of delicious, slightly calorie-restricted meals, along with additional coconut oil and cod-liver oil. Although refined carbohydrates (such as sugar, white flour, and white rice) and potatoes are limited, there is plenty of variety, from hearty breakfasts to satisfying lunches to delicious two-course dinners. As you move through Phase One, you may be among the many people who discover that they lose weight while eating approximately 2500 calories per day, without any additional calorie restriction.

Some people are delighted to find that they lose a pound or two per week, even though the diet provides plenty of calories. Others may notice that their clothes are looser, even though the scales do not change. If you're satisfied with your weight loss on Phase One, you don't need to move on to Phase Two.

Phase Two

If you don't lose weight after two weeks on Phase One, or you find that Phase One doesn't help you get rid of those last pesky pounds, you can move to Phase Two, which restricts you to about 2000 calories per day.

Note: Even if you're sure you'll need Phase Two, we encourage you to begin with Phase One so that you can become familiar with traditional foods and the three-meal-a-day schedule. You will find that you can more readily adapt to Phase Two's extra level of calorie restriction after having incorporated coconut and other healthy fats into your diet in Phase One. Because of these fats, you are not at risk for triggering the feast-or-famine cycle.

Phase Two features what we consider the optimal macronutrient ratio for efficient but healthy long-term weight loss: about 10 percent protein, 60 percent fat, and 30 percent carbohydrate. About half the fat calories are provided by medium-chain triglycerides, mainly from coconut oil, since studies indicate that this is the ideal ratio for weight loss. As part of this diet, therefore, you'll consume three to six tablespoons of coconut oil daily, depending

High-Fat, Low-Carb Really Works

Although the medical establishment is generally skeptical about high-fat diets for weight loss, a study conducted in 2003 (not published, but presented at a conference of the Association for the Study of Obesity) provides persuasive evidence in favor of our plan.

Researchers at the Harvard School of Public Health divided 21 overweight volunteers into three groups. The first group consumed a low-fat, high-carb diet; the second, a high-fat, low-carb diet. Both diets provided 1500 calories for women and 1800 calories for men. A third group also ate a high-fat, low-carb diet but got an extra 300 calories per day. Both high-fat diets consisted of 5 percent carbohydrate, 15 percent protein, and 65 percent fat, proportions very similar to our Quick and Easy Weight Loss plan. All the food was prepared for the volunteers, so the researchers knew exactly what they were eating.

By the end of the study, everyone had lost weight. The people on the lower-calorie, high-fat, low-carb diet lost 23 pounds, while those on the low-fat, high-carb diet, eating the same number of calories, lost only 17 pounds. But the volunteers getting the extra 300 calories per day and eating high-fat, low-carb foods lost 20 pounds—more than the low-fat group.

Here's scientific evidence that the type of diet we're offering you—high-fat, low-carb, and relatively generous with calories—really works. The difference is that we've added coconut oil—which will make your weight loss even easier.

on your size. (Three tablespoons of coconut oil are counted as part of the 2000 daily calories.)

Once you've reached your desired weight, you can move on to our Every-day Gourmet plan, detailed in Chapter 8, then continue that plan to maintain your weight loss (although you should eat desserts only on special occasions).

How Much Weight Do I Need to Lose?

No one wants to be overweight, but punishing your body to live up to un-reasonable standards of thinness will only undermine your metabolism and hurt you in the long term. That's why it's important to establish a realistic weight-loss goal before beginning your weight-loss program.

In a 1990 bulletin, the USDA and the U.S. Department of Health and Human Services provided a very sensible range of appropriate weights for adults ages 19 and over (see sidebar).

In recent years, unfortunately, "ideal" weight guidelines have become more stringent. Those based on the concept of body mass index (BMI), for example, define a maximum healthy weight at about 20 pounds less than the guidelines in the sidebar. Such guidelines do not take into account differences in bone density, body shape, and age, and generally are unrealistic for most people. Some people who wear a size 14 (the average size in the United States) but have heavy bones have found themselves categorized as "obese"!

Please go by the 1990 guidelines in the sidebar to determine your ideal weight. The wide range of acceptable weights shown in this chart takes into

Appropriate Weights for Adults 19 and Older	
Height	**Total Range**
5'3"	107–152
5'4"	111–157
5'5"	114–162
5'6"	118–167
5'7"	121–172
5'8"	125–178
5'9"	129–183
5'10"	132–188
5'11"	136–194
6'0"	140–199

account the natural variations in people's body type and metabolic rate. Generally, the lower weights in the chart are applicable to women and the higher weights to men, but there is a large overlap. Some women have heavy bones, heavy muscles, and no fat; for them a healthy weight is in the upper range. Some men have never fully developed their muscles and have light bones, so their healthy weight would be at the lower end of the range for their height.

Remember, too, that it's normal for women to gain some weight at menopause. This extra weight means more muscle, stronger bones, and increased estrogen-producing fat around the midriff. If you are 50 and wear the same size as you did in high school, you are probably too thin for your age. Thinness at a later age also translates into thinner bones and more wrinkles. Women who let themselves gain a little weight at menopause usually have smoother skin. Many of us (like Katherine, in the sidebar) do not actually need to lose weight, but rather to tone our bodies, gain energy, and improve immune function.

So, consult the chart to see the range of healthy weights for someone of your height. Then use that range to figure out your approximate ideal weight, based on your body structure and age.

The important thing to remember is: *Don't assume that you're overweight just because your weight is at the top end of the range for your height!*

Core Principles of Quick and Easy Weight Loss

Our weight-loss program is based on four Core Principles:

1. Eat three meals per day, and always eat breakfast.
2. Eat traditional fats, including coconut oil.
3. Eat nutrient-dense foods, particularly those supplying calcium and vitamins A and D.
4. Restrict calories moderately.

Principle One: Eat Three Meals a Day

On this diet, you will eat regular meals three times a day, with no in-between snacks. This schedule puts the body on a rhythm of satiety and hunger. Overeaters Anonymous has found that this is the surest way to achieve weight loss and to stick to your diet long term.

One reason you may be continually tempted to overeat now is that you never really allow yourself to sense the difference between the feeling of hunger and the feeling of satiation. Instead, you become more psychologically attuned to when you *want* to eat, not when you *need* to. As a result, you eat at odd times . . . or snack constantly. This undermines both your health and your attempts to lose weight:

- First, you never give your body a needed rest from digestion, freeing your energy for other life tasks.
- Second, your body loses touch with key signals that help you know when you've had enough.
- Third, you begin to eat according to psychological or emotional responses, rather than physiological ones.

Our diet's high-fat content will help balance your blood sugar, preventing cravings, energy dips, and mood swings. If you happen to be hypoglycemic, suffering from bouts of low blood sugar, you need higher levels of fat and lower levels of carbs at each meal in order to avoid drops in blood sugar. Extra fats will slow down digestion time, allowing you to go longer between meals.

Why you must always eat breakfast: Breakfast is the most important meal and must not be skipped in general, but certainly not on this plan. In a study published in *Obesity Research* in 2002, researchers found that eating breakfast was a key factor in maintaining successful weight loss. Another study, in the *Journal of Pediatric Psychology,* 2002, found that overweight adolescents were less likely to eat breakfast than those whose weight was normal. And a 1992 article in the *American Journal of Clinical Nutrition* reported that dieters who eat breakfast lose more weight and are less likely to engage in impulsive snacking.

On this diet, we make sure that you're satiated in the morning, eating a nourishing and satisfying breakfast, such as:

Katherine's Story: Do I Really Need to Lose Weight?

Katherine was a petite, stylish woman in her 50s who prided herself on her trim figure. At five foot one, she weighed 100 pounds and wore a size 4. Yet she had a slightly protruding belly (which is completely natural at her age) and wanted to get rid of it. She embarked on the Quick and Easy Weight Loss plan and immediately noticed she had more energy. But when she weighed herself a week later, she found she had actually gained weight! Why? Because Katherine was too thin to begin with. Her weight gain actually showed up as better muscle tone—Katherine's measurements did not increase, nor did her clothes become tight.

Katherine had heard that being too thin is associated with osteoporosis and fatigue, and she had experienced low energy for many years, so she put her fears aside and continued on the diet. She gained several more pounds before stabilizing at 110 pounds, feeling much better. An added bonus: her skin did not look so dry and wrinkled.

Katherine's problem was not overweight, but a mistaken *body image.* Fortunately, the benefits of Eat Fat, Lose Fat helped her overcome her fears of gaining a small amount of weight. She ended up with better muscle tone, so that the extra bit of fat around her midriff became less noticeable.

- Scrambled eggs with buttered toast or bacon
- A smoothie containing coconut oil and whole-milk yogurt
- Nourishing oatmeal with butter or cream
- A cheese omelet
- Smoked wild salmon with toast and butter or coconut oil

Principle Two: Eat Traditional Fats

After years of hearing about the low-fat credo, it may at first feel strange to incorporate healthy fats into your diet. Yet increasing your fat intake in order to lose weight is the second Core Principle of this diet. Healthful fats, like coconut oil, butter, and cod-liver oil, deliver major benefits: as we explained in Chapter 3, they actually boost your metabolism and encourage weight loss.

Studies have shown that the body does not easily store the medium-chain fatty acids (MCFAs) from coconut oil, but mostly uses them for energy shortly after they are consumed. And as we've explained, in addition to upping the rate at which you burn your food, the fats in Quick and Easy Weight Loss create a feeling of satiation. It's easy to stay on the plan, even though the portions are small, because you come away from your meals feeling full. These healthful, essential fats will help you go the distance toward weight loss.

Your brain, nerves, hormones, and all your body's intracellular communication systems require the right kind of fats to function. In addition, fats act as carriers of the key fat-soluble vitamins D, E, K, and especially A, which boosts thyroid function and helps maintain a healthy metabolism. Thousands of years of evolution have trained your body to seek and absorb these nutrients from food, not vitamin pills. These vitamins are found mostly in animal fats; in fact, as we explained earlier, the only source of true vitamin A is animal fat.

Polyunsaturated vegetable oils are usually rancid (even if they taste fine), do not contain these vitamins, and have other harmful side effects as well. But if you've ever wondered why you crave fried foods, doughnuts, ice cream,

---

Judy's Story: Skipping Breakfast

Judy always began her day with the best of intentions. She never ate breakfast, assuming that breakfast calories would make her gain weight. For lunch she would have a salad and a diet drink at her desk at work. But by midafternoon, desperately hungry and tired, she'd run off to the vending machine for potato chips or a candy bar. When she returned home, she was often so tired that she just warmed up a frozen dinner.

It was after dinner, when her body's nutritional needs were still not met, that the bingeing and splurging occurred—ice cream, chips, cakes, and pastries, anything to take away the gnawing hunger and symptoms of low blood sugar. Then to bed, waking up with the best of intentions (but not hungry enough for breakfast after an evening of bingeing)—and so the cycle continued.

Special Weight-Loss Tip: Drink Your Oil

Want a surefire way to escalate weight loss? Twenty minutes before each meal, take some coconut oil!

By mealtime, coconut's satiation effect will be in full force, so that you won't feel hungry. You may even feel full before finishing your meal, so that you eat less and lose weight.

The easiest way to take your coconut oil is to make a Coconut Infusion: place 1 to 2 tablespoons of softened coconut oil into a mug and add hot water (or hot herbal tea), allowing the oil to melt before drinking. Use the following formula to determine the amount:

- If you weigh 90–130 pounds, take 1 tablespoon coconut oil before each meal, for a total of 3 tablespoons per day.
- If you weigh 131–180 pounds, take 1½ tablespoons coconut oil before each meal, for a total of 4½ tablespoons per day.
- If you weigh over 180 pounds, take 2 tablespoons coconut oil before each meal, for a total of 6 tablespoons per day.

To keep coconut oil soft during the winter months, put it on top of your refrigerator, above your stove, or in a warm cupboard.

chips, and a host of other greasy foods, the reason is simple. These cravings are your body's desperate attempt to get the fats and fat-soluble vitamins it needs to function smoothly. If you were eating good-quality fats containing these nutrients, you would not crave unhealthy foods containing the wrong kinds of fats.

Principle Three: Eat Nutrient-Dense Foods

Although most people don't realize it, obesity is actually a symptom of nutritional *deficiencies*. That's why food *quality*—not just quantity—is key to successful weight loss—and why eating nutrient-dense foods is the third Core Principle of Quick and Easy Weight Loss. As you know from the previous chapter, these foods provide complete protein, healthy fats, and unrefined carbohydrates, plus the vitamins and minerals your body needs to build, maintain, nourish, and heal all the cells in all your systems.

We recommend that you always consume real foods, as opposed to isolated vitamins or even multivitamins. Instead of synthetic vitamins, we recommend the superfoods described in Chapter 5—including cod-liver oil, acerola or amla tablets, bitters, high-vitamin butter oil, desiccated liver tablets, wheat germ oil, and nutritional yeast—which naturally concentrate many important nutrients

25 Ways to Enjoy the Benefits of Coconut

1. Coconut oil melted in warm water
2. Coconut oil melted in hot tea
3. Morning eggs cooked in coconut oil
4. Coconut oil plus Coconut Sprinkles on hot oatmeal
5. Coconut oil in your morning smoothie
6. Coconut Milk Tonic
7. Chicken stock with coconut milk
8. Coconut milk added to any type of creamy soup
9. Coconut oil spread on sourdough toast
10. Coconutty Butter spread on toast
11. Vegetables sautéed in coconut oil
12. Coconut milk added to gravy
13. Curry made with coconut milk
14. Coconut-crusted chicken or fish
15. Coconut kefir
16. Coconut Orange Julius
17. Coconut milk added to sautéed vegetables
18. Mayonnaise made with coconut oil mix
19. Salad dressing made with coconut oil mix
20. Whipped Coconut Cream on fruit
21. Coconut Sprinkles on fruit
22. Coconut oil in mashed potatoes
23. Fish or shrimp sautéed in coconut oil
24. Peanut Coconut Sauce on chicken or beef
25. Coconut Rice

You'll find recipes for many of these coconut delights in Chapter 9.

that support each other, preventing the imbalances that often occur when vitamins are taken singly. These foods will give your body plentiful amounts of the nutrients it needs to run at maximum efficiency and health.

Although you can derive great benefit from Quick and Easy Weight Loss with or without superfoods, when you make the additional effort to incorporate them, you'll be surprised to see your energy soar *and* those pounds melt away. To understand why, just remember our simple axiom:

The higher the nutrient content of your food, the less you need to eat to satisfy your basic nutritional needs.

The Burden of Nutrient-Poor Food

- Running on low-octane foods starves your cells.
- Your body must work harder to digest food that gives little back.
- Nutrient-poor foods may contain toxic substances (like trans fats or MSG and other additives) that block life energy.
- Your body stores nutrient-poor foods as fat—and your energy declines.

Like Julia, you probably associate diets with deprivation. Unless you're suffering, you couldn't be eating healthy, right? Wrong! For many years, as the consumption of trans fats, empty carbs, and fast and processed foods has expanded American waistlines, many people have incorrectly assumed that the antidote is some form of fasting diet. But the solution to a nutrient-poor diet is to restore nutrients, not take even more of them away. As Julia discovered, when your body has ample amounts of needed nutrients, it *releases* fat.

Julia: Cleansing and Fasting Didn't Work

As the receptionist in the executive suite of a Fortune 500 corporation, Julia had a sedentary but hectic job. Hoping to deal with creeping weight gain and shake off her lethargy, she decided to try a cleansing diet of fruits and vegetables, foods she loved. Although she felt really good for a few days, she lost no weight.

Then she decided to fast. She did the first ten days of a Master Cleanse fast, drinking nothing but water with lemon juice, maple syrup, and cayenne pepper. Her body felt cleansed, but she felt hungry, a little tired, and out of focus. Nevertheless, she persisted and after completing the cleanse was delighted to see that she had lost six pounds.

Unfortunately, neither her delight nor her weight loss lasted very long. Julia went off the cleanse and returned to regular meals, emphasizing salads, tofu, and a little brown rice. To her horror, after two weeks of this boring diet, she had not only regained all the weight she'd lost, but had put on an additional three pounds.

Then Julia learned about the dietary benefits of coconut and began taking a tablespoon of coconut oil before each meal.

During her first days on the coconut oil, she maintained her meager diet, but soon began to enjoy modest portions of richer foods, such as omelets, beef, and full-fat cheeses, and she was amazed to discover that by taking the coconut oil, she could eat only small portions. After a week of taking coconut oil with a diet she considered "bad," Julia weighed herself and was amazed to discover that she had lost four pounds. A week later, she dropped another two, and her pants felt loose.

Five weeks later, Julia had maintained her new way of eating, as well as her weight loss.

Principle Four: Restrict Calories Moderately: A Little but Not Too Much

Why do we recommend modest calorie restriction? Research consistently shows that lowering your caloric intake (and/or increasing exercise) is the most direct route to weight loss. Calorie restriction ensures that you don't take in more energy than you expend, but instead begin to use up your body's stores of fat. On the other hand, to restrict the amount of calories even more than the amount we specify is to deny your body what it needs to breathe, beat the heart, and perform other vital functions. Extreme calorie restriction is tantamount to starvation. The body responds with cravings and, as a result, you may wind up bingeing or eating undesirable foods. Even if you have the willpower to maintain the calorie restriction, your body may react to this perceived emergency by storing fat and altering your metabolism for the worse.

That's why, on our diet, you'll offset calorie restrictions by eating a moderate amount of protein and, compared with other diets, a relatively high amount of fat to induce satiation.

You'll also cut back on carbohydrates from sweets and refined grains. As shown in the groundbreaking book *The No-Grain Diet* by Joseph Mercola with Alison Rose Levy, refined grains convert to sugars in your body and set off the same insulin reaction as sweets. You feel energized for a while, but then you sag—and reach for another snack to make up for it. On Quick and Easy Weight Loss, you'll be eating *healthy* carbs, prepared in a way that makes them tasty, digestible, and very satisfying.

What's the Right Level of Calorie Restriction? The degree to which you can safely and effectively restrict calories to lose weight depends on two factors:

- About two-thirds of the energy produced in the body by the food we consume is needed to support basic body functions: of the lungs, heart, liver, and kidneys.

This basic requirement ranges between 1100 and 1800 calories, depending on your size, build, and sex. A woman who weighs 132 pounds, for example, needs about 1300 calories just to support basic body functions; one who weighs 154 pounds requires 1500 calories. She'll need about 500 to 700 additional calories for normal light activities, and much more if she is very active.

If you eat so little that the number of calories in your food drops below the amount required for these basic functions, your body starts to think it is starving, and its alarm bells go off.

- The exact point at which you start to lose weight also depends on your metabolism.

What's Wrong with Soy?

Today, many dieters try to meet their health requirements by eating foods based on soy, promoted as beneficial in many popular books and weight-loss plans. However, soybeans contain several natural toxins, and high-temperature chemical processing adds many more. As early as 1972, a soy-industry textbook (*Soy Beans: Chemistry and Technology*) listed a number of well-documented toxic effects from soybeans—everything from endocrine disruption to undesirable changes in many organs.

The most serious problem with eating soy while you're trying to lose weight is that soy is a *goitrogen*, that is, it depresses thyroid function. When your thyroid gland malfunctions, you tend to gain weight even when you eat very little. Dr. Dan Sheehan and Dr. Daniel Doerge, government researchers at the National Center for Toxicological Research, discovered that the antithyroid component of soy is the isoflavones or phytoestrogens, which inhibit the synthesis of thyroid hormone. All soy foods, including tofu, soymilk, protein bars, and meal replacements, contain these thyroid-inhibiting isoflavones. In 1999, these researchers actually wrote a letter urging the FDA to require a health warning on soy foods, rather than the health claim that the agency eventually approved.

What's more, the effects of soy foods can be deceptive. Dieters who rely heavily on soy often report initial weight loss and energy increase, since at first the thyroid gland works harder to counteract the effects of soy isoflavones. But after a time, the thyroid gives out, with hypothyroidism the result. The dieter rapidly regains the lost weight, and then gains even more—plus, the dieter feels lethargic, unfocused, cold, and sometimes depressed.

And soy contains other anti-nutrients: phytic acid blocks mineral absorption, and enzyme inhibitors block the enzymes needed for protein digestion. Animal studies carried out in 1974 indicate that soy protein isolate, the major ingredient in modern soy foods, creates increased requirements for vitamins D, E, K, and B_{12} and deficiencies in many important minerals. Long-term consumption of high levels of soy foods can lead to serious nutritional deficiencies—definitely the wrong way to go if you're trying to lose weight. Yet, the U.S. government allows a health claim for foods containing soy protein, and many government agencies and health organizations encourage consumption of large amounts of soy foods.

Promoters of soy for weight loss point to the Asian diet, which they claim contains a lot of soy. In fact, soy consumption is relatively low in Asia, ranging from an average of two tablespoons per day in Japan to two teaspoons per day in China. Even so, thyroid problems are widespread in Asia, particularly in China. How much better to emulate the traditional practices of tropical peoples, who consume large amounts of thyroid-supporting coconut!

Since some people's motors burn faster and hotter than others, the point at which calorie restriction becomes excessive is different for everyone. Thus one woman who weighs 132 pounds may lose weight even if she eats 2500 calories, because she has a fast metabolism that burns calories efficiently; but someone of the same weight who has a slower metabolism may need to restrict her diet to 2000 calories to lose weight. By including coconut oil in our 2000-calorie plan, we ensure that you don't depress a slow metabolism even further.

In any diet, then, you don't want to restrict calories below the minimum number needed to support the basic functions, plus the amount needed for all your normal activities. Doing so will cause the body to lower its metabolism in order to prevent starvation. When that happens, *you cannot lose weight, no matter how little you eat.*

Quick and Easy Weight Loss Plan

Phase One: Moderate Weight Loss

Follow the 2500-calorie diet for two weeks. If you lose weight during this period (as many people do), continue this diet until your ideal weight is achieved. If you don't lose weight on Phase One, or need a more stringent diet for those last few pounds, move on to Phase Two.

Phase Two: Calorie Restriction

Follow the 2000-calorie diet until you achieve your desired weight, continuing to take your coconut oil before each meal and cod-liver oil before breakfast, as in Phase One.

Once you have achieved the weight that is right for you, you can move into Everyday Gourmet (see Chapter 8). However, you will probably need to limit desserts. If you gain weight on Everyday Gourmet, even when leaving out desserts entirely, first increase your intake of coconut by one tablespoon before each meal. If that doesn't stabilize your weight, follow Phase One indefinitely, or at least whenever you want to take off a few pounds.

Quick and Easy Beverages

Not only the foods in our meal plans but also the beverages you drink are important. Choosing the right beverage can provide essential nourishment, increase satiation, and help digestion. For weight loss, many people desperately need a replacement for sodas, including the sugar-free sodas made with aspartame.

One of the most satisfying, most digestible, and most nourishing beverages is whole raw milk. Since not everyone has access to it, we offer you an alternative in the form of our **Coconut Milk Tonic** (see recipe on page 220). Made

with coconut milk, a natural sweetener, and dolomite powder, this tonic is formulated to provide the same number of calories and the same amount of calcium as whole milk.

The Quick and Easy Weight Loss menu plans include raw whole milk or
Coconut Milk Tonic one or more times a day to provide adequate calcium and
medium-chain triglycerides for weight loss.

Here are some other beverages that you can use to accompany your meals:

Spritzer The easiest beverage to make. Simply add a small pinch of sea salt
and the juice of 1 lime, ½ lemon, or ¼ grapefruit to sparkling water. You'll
have a delicious, satisfying soft drink that goes well with food. The sea salt
provides important trace minerals, and the sour taste of the citrus fruit
helps digestion.

Kombucha A terrific sparkling fermented beverage from Russia, made by
fermenting sweetened tea with a culture from the kombucha mushroom.
You'll find a recipe for **Kombucha** on page 264, but you can also purchase
it at health food stores or by mail order (see Resources).

Coconut Fruit Shrub An easy, delicious, sweet-and-sour beverage (see
recipe on page 222) made with fresh fruit and coconut vinegar. The taste of
the vinegar disappears after a few days, leaving only complex fruit flavors.

Kefir Soda Chapter 10 includes several recipes for sparkling sodas made
with a culture of kefir powder or grains, including cream soda, ginger ale,
lemonade, and fruit sodas. The fermentation process provides enzymes
and beneficial bacteria. We recommend these beverages especially for anyone having trouble giving up the commercial soft drink habit. They're
wonderful and actually very easy (and a lot of fun) to make. You don't have
to deprive yourself—soft drinks actually can be good for you!

A Caution for Pregnant or Nursing Women

We do not recommend that women who are pregnant or nursing follow
Quick and Easy Weight Loss. You should not restrict calories at these times.
Instead, you can follow the Health Recovery or Everyday Gourmet plan, either of which will provide excellent nutrition for both you and your baby. (In
fact, nursing mothers should always include coconut oil in their diets because the lauric acid comes out in breast milk and helps protect the baby
against viruses and other pathogens.) Then, when your baby is weaned, you
can begin the weight-loss plan.

Start-Up Week for Quick and Easy Weight Loss

Here's a schedule for advance planning. During this week, you'll need to order and shop ahead for the necessary ingredients so everything is in place before you start.

Day One: Order Products by Mail, Scout Out Raw Milk

Scout out and order coconut and other products that you may or may not find in stores (see Resources for brand names and sources):

- Coconut milk and coconut oil (also available in many stores)
- Freeze-dried coconut (optional)
- High-vitamin cod-liver oil, liquid, or capsules
- Lacto-fermented condiments, such as sauerkraut and pickles. Be sure that what you buy has not been pasteurized or heated, but is made by the genuine process of lacto-fermentation. Several delicious brands are available.
- Dolomite powder (a calcium source if raw milk is unavailable). If you have access to raw milk, you won't need dolomite.
- Unrefined sea salt
- Kefir powder or kefir grains (if you want to try some kefir sodas; see recipes on pages 262–63).
- Raw milk. To find raw milk, visit realmilk.com or contact the nearest local chapter of the Weston A. Price Foundation (westonaprice.org). Raw milk is available in stores in several states and through direct farm purchase and cow-share programs in many other states.

Day Two: Cupboard Cleanout

Go on a tour of your kitchen cupboards and throw out all processed foods, especially products containing partially hydrogenated vegetable oil (crackers, cookies, pastries, doughnuts, chips, and snack foods), ready-to-eat breakfast cereals, and sauce mixes and other products likely to contain MSG. Remember that anything containing "spices," "spice mixes," "natural flavorings," and anything "autolyzed" or "hydrolyzed" is likely to contain MSG.

Day Three: Fridge and Freezer Free-Up

Get rid of all processed foods, prepared dinners, and low-fat dairy products in your fridge or freezer.

Day Four: Shop

Take a trip to the market or health food store to purchase ingredients for your first week of meals. Remember that you can use store-bought lacto-fermented condiments, recommended brands of whole-grain crackers, mayonnaise, and frozen broths if you don't want to make your own. Brand names are provided in the Resources section.

Whenever possible, purchase organic fruits and vegetables and organic or pasture-fed meats and eggs.

Shopping List for Quick and Easy Weight Loss

See Resources for recommended product brands and where to get them.

Coconut Products

These products generally are available at health food stores and specialty markets, which will soon be stocking more of them as demand grows.

- Coconut oil
- Whole canned coconut milk
- Unsweetened desiccated (dried) coconut

Fats and Oils

- Extra-virgin olive oil
- Cold-pressed sesame oil
- Cold-pressed flax oil
- Organic (ideally grass-fed) butter
- Ghee (optional)
- High-quality mayonnaise, preferably Delouis Fils brand (unless you make your own)

Dairy

- Organic whole-milk yogurt
- Organic whole-milk raw cheeses (the label should say the cheese is made from unpasteurized milk; available in most high-end markets and specialty stores or on the Internet)
- Organic cream cheese without additives
- Organic cream (preferably raw, but in any case not ultrapasteurized)

Sweeteners

A natural sweetener such as dehydrated cane sugar juice (sold as Rapadura or Sucanat), raw honey and/or maple syrup (Note: You'll use very few sweeteners on Quick and Easy Weight Loss.)

- Stevia powder

Breads, Cereals, and Legumes

- Rolled oats

- Sourdough and sprouted whole-grain bread
- Brown rice
- Whole-grain crackers
- Wheat berries or whole-wheat flour (if you want to make Coconut Crackers)

Animal Foods
- Eggs (preferably from pastured chickens)
- Fresh beef, lamb, and pork
- Organ meats, if you want to try them, such as calf's liver, beef heart, and turkey and chicken livers
- Organic chicken, duck, and turkey
- Nitrate-free, additive-free bacon, sausage, and salami
- Fresh paté or liverwurst without additives

Seafood
- Fresh wild fish
- Fresh and frozen shellfish
- Canned wild salmon, tuna without additives, and anchovies
- Salmon caviar (canned or fresh) or canned carp roe
- Smoked wild salmon

Fruits and Vegetables
- Fresh, seasonal produce, preferably organic
- Organic frozen produce

Nuts and Seeds
- Raw pecans, almonds, cashews, peanuts and/or walnuts (Note: You'll use very few nuts in Phase Two of Quick and Easy Weight Loss.)
- Pine nuts
- Organic natural peanut butter (be sure it does not contain partially hydrogenated vegetable oils)

Condiments
- Raw vinegar
- Organic spices (non-irradiated)
- Good-quality Dijon-style mustard
- Arrowroot powder (used as a thickener in stir-fries)
- Thai fish sauce
- Red and green curry paste
- Naturally fermented soy sauce
- Lacto-fermented condiments such as sauerkraut, kimchi, and pickles (brand names provided in the Resource section)

Canned and Frozen Foods
- Canned tomatoes, tomato paste
- Frozen meat stocks (chicken, fish, and beef)

Optional Miscellaneous Items
- Bonito flakes (if you want to make Quick Fish Stock, the base for several of our fish soup recipes)
- Ready-made kombucha
- Macaroons

To estimate quantities, look through the menu plans and recipes to decide which dishes you want to make, then consider how many meals you expect to cook over two weeks, and for how many people.

Day Five: Getting Started
Note: Bolded items are our own recipes, provided in Chapters 9 and 10.

- Make **Mary's Oil Blend** (page 188)
- Make **Coconut Sprinkles** (page 214)
- Begin a batch of **Crispy Nuts** (page 259)

Day Six: More Food Basics
- Make **Rich Chicken Stock** (page 224).
- Optional: Make a **Kefir Soda** (page 262) (especially recommended for anyone struggling to give up commercial sodas). You may also purchase ready-made kombucha, or simply make spritzers to go with your meals.
- Optional: Make a simple lacto-fermented condiment such as **Sauerkraut** (page 228) or **Bread and Butter Pickles** (page 231). You can also use purchased lacto-fermented condiments.

Day Seven: Final Prep (Optional)
These are all optional, since store-bought alternatives are available.

- Begin another **Kefir Soda** or lacto-fermented beverage (pages 261–64).
- Make another lacto-fermented condiment (pages 226–31).
- Make **Coconut Crackers** (page 209).
- Make **Mayonnaise** (page 238).

Phase One Menu Plans

During this phase, you will eat a regular, balanced diet containing plenty of fat but avoiding an excess of sugars and refined carbohydrates. In addition:

Keys to Weight-Loss Success

Be sure you always:

- Take 1 to 2 tablespoons of coconut oil in warm water or herb tea 20 minutes before each meal.
- Consume three servings of calcium-rich food, such as raw milk, raw cheese, bone broth (in soups, sauces, or gravies), or Coconut Milk Tonic, every day. If you work in an office and aren't able to eat a calcium-rich food for lunch, have an extra cup of raw milk or Coconut Milk Tonic, or 1½ ounces of cheese, in the evening. This amount of cheese provides the same amount of calcium as a glass of raw milk or Coconut Milk Tonic. It has about the same amount of calories as well, so there's no need for calorie adjustment.
- Check out the recipes and plan your cooking or buying in advance so that you have on hand key ingredients such as chicken broth, whole-grain crackers, lacto-fermented condiments, stock, mayonnaise, and healthy beverages.

- Take 1 to 2 tablespoons coconut oil in warm water or herb tea (such as mint or chamomile) 20 minutes before every meal.
- Take 1 teaspoon high-vitamin cod-liver oil (or the equivalent in capsules) before breakfast.

To determine how much coconut oil you need for each dose, use the formula given on page 110.

Although you will not be counting calories, the daily calorie level for the first week is about 2500. Be sure to avoid eating excess carbohydrates, though non-starchy vegetables are fine. Take coconut oil as directed to suppress appetite and boost metabolism. Many people report that this relatively liberal diet, with the addition of coconut oil, provides slow, steady weight loss. Phase One also helps you become familiar with a strict three-meal-per-day schedule and the satisfying tastes of traditional foods.

Bolded items indicate recipes provided in Chapters 9 and 10. Note that although the lunch menus do indicate that a spritzer is acceptable, the best option, should you be so inclined, would be to buy or make a Quick and Easy fermented beverage and take it to work.

Remember to take your dose of coconut oil before each meal (and cod-liver oil before breakfast)!

Tips for Streamlining the Menu Plans

The dishes in the Quick and Easy Weight Loss menus really are simple and easy. Moreover, they are available in restaurants if you don't have time to cook.

- If the only breakfast you have time to prepare during your work week is a coconut or yogurt smoothie (which can even be made the night before and consumed in the car on the way to work), then use your extra time on weekends to make eggs on Saturday and Sunday.
- If you work in an office, take your lunch to work (soup in a thermos, salads in covered containers, paté, cheese, Crispy Nuts, etc.). Or eat out, following our guidelines as much as possible.
- You may also want to make quantities large enough to provide leftovers to eat several days in a row.

Making Substitutions

The 14 days of menu plans for each phase are meant as guidelines—choose the ones that work for you and your lifestyle (and that you like to eat!). If there are any dishes we suggest that are not to your taste, or that you can't easily incorporate into your life, feel free to replace them with other selections you prefer from our wide range of recipes. (All recipes come with calorie counts.)

For example, if you prefer not to eat liver, you can substitute another recipe for a liver dish in the menu plans and take four desiccated liver tablets that day (see Resources for recommended brands).

If you are unable to buy raw milk, and don't have any prepared Coconut Milk Tonic (or don't have time to make it), you can substitute 1½ ounces of cheese to provide the same amount of calcium as a cup of the tonic.

DAY ONE

Breakfast: ½ grapefruit with 1 teaspoon **Coconut Sprinkles**
2 eggs fried in butter or coconut oil with 2 pieces nitrate-free bacon
1 slice whole-grain toast with coconut oil or butter
1 cup whole raw milk or warm **Coconut Milk Tonic**

Lunch: **Coconut Corn Soup**
Raw cheese or butter on whole-grain or **Coconut Crackers**
Spritzer or purchased kombucha

Dinner: **Mesclun Salad**
Baked Chicken with Coconut Peanut Sauce
Green Beans with Coconut
Kimchi (homemade or purchased)
Choice of **Quick and Easy Beverage**

DAY TWO

Breakfast: **Basic Oatmeal** with butter, natural sweetener, and **Coconut Sprinkles** or freeze-dried coconut
1 cup whole raw milk or warm **Coconut Milk Tonic**
Lunch: **Coconut Chicken Salad** (use leftover chicken from previous dinner)
Sliced tomatoes
Spritzer or purchased kombucha
Dinner: **Coconut Corn Soup**
Leg of Lamb with Root Vegetables
Sauerkraut (homemade or store-bought)
1 cup whole raw milk or warm **Coconut Milk Tonic**

DAY THREE

Breakfast: **Coconut Smoothie**
1 cup whole raw milk or warm **Coconut Milk Tonic**
Lunch: **Crispy Nuts** and raw cheese
Piece of fresh fruit
Spritzer or purchased kombucha
Dinner: **Watercress Salad**
Leftover **Red Meat Curry** (use leftover lamb from previous dinner)
Choice of **Quick and Easy Beverage**

DAY FOUR

Breakfast: **Super Scramble** with sausage or nitrate-free bacon
1 cup whole raw milk or warm **Coconut Milk Tonic**
Lunch: **Salmon–Cream Cheese Roll-Ups** (make your own or purchase at a specialty market)
Whole-grain or **Coconut Crackers** or bread with butter
Carrot and celery sticks
Spritzer or purchased kombucha

Dinner: **Caesar Salad**
Roast Beef
Slow-Bake Tomatoes
Steamed Spinach with butter
Sauerkraut (homemade or store-bought)
1 cup whole raw milk or 1 cup warm **Coconut Milk Tonic**

DAY FIVE

Breakfast: **English Breakfast**
1 cup whole raw milk or warm **Coconut Milk Tonic**
Lunch: Cold roast beef with shaved Parmesan cheese and sliced tomato
Bread and Butter Pickles or store-bought lacto-fermented pickle
Spritzer or purchased kombucha
Dinner: **Liver Stir-Fry**
Steamed Broccoli with butter
Sauerkraut (homemade or store-bought)
1 cup whole raw milk or warm **Coconut Milk Tonic**
Fresh fruit with **Coconut Sprinkles**

DAY SIX

Breakfast: Smoked salmon with cream cheese or butter on sourdough
whole-grain toast
Lunch: **Greek Salad** with Grilled Shrimp or Salami
Spritzer or purchased kombucha
Dinner: **Papaya Grapefruit Salad**
Indonesian Coconut Steak
Pineapple Chutney or store-bought lacto-fermented condiment
1 cup whole raw milk or warm **Coconut Milk Tonic**

DAY SEVEN

Breakfast: **Cheese Omelet**
Sourdough whole-grain toast with butter or coconut oil
1 cup whole raw milk or warm **Coconut Milk Tonic**
Lunch: **Chicken Liver Paté** or purchased paté (see Resources) with
whole-grain or **Coconut Crackers**
Bread and Butter Pickles or store-bought lacto-fermented pickles
Spritzer or purchased kombucha
Dinner: **Cream of Vegetable Soup**

Coconut-Crusted Salmon
Pineapple Chutney or purchased lacto-fermented condiment
Steamed Asparagus with butter
1 cup whole raw milk or warm **Coconut Milk Tonic**

DAY EIGHT

Breakfast: **Cream of Vegetable Soup**
Raw cheese with whole-grain or **Coconut Crackers**
Lunch: **Wild Salmon Salad** (make with leftover salmon from previous evening)
Bread and Butter Pickles or store-bought lacto-fermented pickle
½ cup sliced fresh pineapple
Spritzer or purchased kombucha
Dinner: Salad of baby greens with **Asian Dressing**
Green Thai Curry with Pork
Papaya Chutney or store-bought lacto-fermented condiment
1 cup whole raw milk or warm **Coconut Milk Tonic**

DAY NINE

Breakfast: **Ginger Oatmeal** with butter and **Coconut Sprinkles** or freeze-dried coconut
1 cup whole raw milk or warm **Coconut Milk Tonic**
Lunch: Leftover **Thai Curry with Pork**
Papaya Chutney or store-bought lacto-fermented condiment
Spritzer or purchased kombucha
Dinner: **Coconut Seviche**
Rib-Eye Steak with Mustard Cream Sauce
Green Beans with Coconut
Sauerkraut (homemade or store-bought)
1 cup whole raw milk or 1 cup warm **Coconut Milk Tonic**
Macaroon (homemade or store-bought)

DAY TEN

Breakfast: **Super Scramble** with bacon
1 cup whole raw milk or warm **Coconut Milk Tonic**
Lunch: Cold sliced steak with avocado and tomato
Bread and Butter Pickles or store-bought lacto-fermented pickles
Spritzer or purchased kombucha

Dinner: Salad of baby greens with **Asian Dressing**
Basic Baked Chicken
Sautéed Sweet Potato
Pineapple Chutney or store-bought lacto-fermented condiment
1 cup whole raw milk or warm **Coconut Milk Tonic**

DAY ELEVEN

Breakfast: **Basic Oatmeal** with butter or cream and **Coconut Sprinkles**
1 cup whole raw milk or warm **Coconut Milk Tonic**
Lunch: **Chicken Pesto Salad** made with leftover chicken from previous evening
Spritzer or purchased kombucha
Dinner: **Watercress Salad**
Sautéed Fillet of Sole
Stuffed Tomatoes
Steamed Spinach with butter
1 cup whole raw milk or warm **Coconut Milk Tonic**

DAY TWELVE

Breakfast: **Spanish Omelet**
1 cup whole raw milk or warm **Coconut Milk Tonic**
Lunch: Small steak or lamb chop topped with generous pat of butter
Steamed vegetables
Small green salad with olive oil and vinegar
Spritzer or purchased kombucha
Dinner: **Miso Soup with Cabbage**
Beef Stir-Fry with Pineapple
Coconut Rice
Kimchi (homemade or purchased)
1 cup whole raw milk or **Coconut Milk Tonic**

DAY THIRTEEN

Breakfast: Eggs fried in butter or coconut oil with Canadian bacon
1 cup whole raw milk or warm **Coconut Milk Tonic**
Lunch: **Salmon Roe on Toast**
Bread and Butter Pickles or store-bought lacto-fermented pickles
Spritzer or purchased kombucha

Dinner: Sliced tomatoes and feta cheese with olive oil and lemon juice
Coconut Shrimp Étouffée
Coconut Rice (can reheat from previous evening)
Sauerkraut (homemade or store-bought)
Baked Pears in Coconut Milk
Choice of **Quick and Easy Beverage**

DAY FOURTEEN

Breakfast: **Yogurt-Coconut Smoothie**
Lunch: Raw cheese with butter and whole-grain or **Coconut Crackers** or whole-grain toast
Bread and Butter Pickles or store-bought lacto-fermented pickle
Spritzer or purchased kombucha
Dinner: **Hawaiian Coconut Shrimp with Sweet-and-Sour Soy Sauce**
Barbequed Beef Ribs
Corn on the cob with butter
Sauerkraut (homemade or purchased)
Choice of **Quick and Easy Beverage**

Phase Two Menu Plans

On Phase Two, you'll be consuming about 2000 calories per day. Calorie counts are given for each menu item, for each meal as a whole, and for each day. As with Phase One, you can omit menus that you don't like and repeat those you do like, or to use up leftovers. Many of the lunch menus can be approximated with restaurant meals.

The Phase Two menus use special lower-calorie Quick and Easy Weight Loss versions of some of our recipes.

Note: The coconut oil you take before each meal and the cod-liver oil you take before breakfast are not listed in the menu plans but should be counted in the total calories for each meal. One tablespoon coconut oil contains 108 calories, and 1 teaspoon high-vitamin cod-liver oil contains 42 calories. If you use more than 1 tablespoon of coconut oil with each meal, add 108 calories per tablespoon to the totals listed.

DAY ONE

Breakfast: ½ grapefruit (50) with 1 teaspoon **Coconut Sprinkles** (18)
1 fried egg (101) with 2 pieces nitrate-free bacon (100)
1 cup whole raw milk or warm **Coconut Milk Tonic** (189)
Total calories: 608

Lunch: **Easy Coconut Fish Soup** (253)
2 ounces raw hard cheese (such as cheddar) (200) with 3 whole-grain or **Coconut Crackers** (60)
Spritzer (20)

Total calories: 641

Dinner: 2 cups baby greens (24) with 1 tablespoon **Basic Dressing** (87)
Easy Baked Chicken (312)
¼ cup **Sauerkraut** (homemade or store-bought) (8)
1 cup whole raw milk or warm **Coconut Milk Tonic** (189)

Total calories: 728
Total daily calories: 1978

DAY TWO

Breakfast: **Yogurt-Coconut Smoothie** (Quick and Easy Weight Loss version) (444)

Total calories: 594

Lunch: **Coconut Chicken Salad** (made with leftover chicken from previous dinner) (495)
1 sliced tomato (22)
Spritzer (20)

Total calories: 645

Dinner: **Miso Soup with Cabbage** (56)
Rib-Eye Steak with Mustard Cream Sauce (362)
¼ cup **Sauerkraut** (8)
Steamed Asparagus (75)
1 cup raw whole milk or warm **Coconut Milk Tonic** (189)

Total calories: 797
Total daily calories: 2036

DAY THREE

Breakfast: **Ginger Oatmeal** (144) with 2 tablespoons cream (62) and 1 tablespoon sweetener (50)
1 cup whole raw milk or warm **Coconut Milk Tonic** (189)

Total calories: 595

Lunch: **Asian Chef's Salad** (Quick and Easy Weight Loss version) (406)
Spritzer (20)

Total calories: 534

Dinner: Sliced tomatoes with juice of ½ lemon (10) and ½ ounce feta cheese (50)
Baked Lamb Chop with Red Peppers and Onion (353)
Steamed Spinach (69)

¼ cup **Sauerkraut** (28)
1 cup whole raw milk or warm **Coconut Milk Tonic** (189)
Total calories: 797
Total daily calories: 1926

DAY FOUR

Breakfast: **Yogurt-Coconut Smoothie** (Quick and Easy Weight Loss version) (444)
Total calories: 594
   Lunch: **Fish Roe Spread** (or 2 ounces store-bought paté) (245) with 3 whole-grain or **Coconut Crackers** (60) and 1 tablespoon butter (108)
Spritzer (20)
Total calories: 666
  Dinner: **Miso Soup** (56)
3 ounces roast beef, ¼" fat (326)
Steamed Brussels Sprouts (81)
¼ cup **Sauerkraut** (8)
1 cup whole raw milk or warm **Coconut Milk Tonic** (189)
Total calories: 768
Total daily calories: 2028

DAY FIVE

Breakfast: 1 medium sliced orange (65) with 1 teaspoon **Coconut Sprinkles** (18)
Cheese Omelet (305)
Total calories: 538
   Lunch: 2 ounces cold roast beef (217) with 1 tablespoon **Mayonnaise** (100)
1 sliced tomato (22)
1 ounce shaved Parmesan cheese (100)
¼ cup **Bread and Butter Pickles** or store-bought lacto-fermented pickles (20)
Spritzer (20)
Total calories: 587
  Dinner: **Coconut-Crusted Salmon** (401)
Steamed Spinach (69)
¼ cup **Kimchi** (homemade or store-bought) (10)
1 cup whole raw milk or warm **Coconut Milk Tonic** (189)
Total calories: 777
Total calories: 1902

DAY SIX

Breakfast: **Basic Oatmeal** (100) with 2 tablespoons cream (62) and 1 tablespoon sweetener (50)
1 cup whole raw milk or warm **Coconut Milk Tonic** (189)
Total calories: 551
Lunch: **Coconut Fish Spread** (made with leftover salmon from previous
evening (320) with 3 whole-grain or **Coconut Crackers** (60)
1 sliced tomato (22)
¼ cup **Bread and Butter Pickles** or store-bought lacto-fermented
pickles (20)
Spritzer (20)
Total calories: 442
Dinner: **Watercress Salad** (242)
Liver Stir-Fry (Quick and Easy Weight Loss version) (388)
¼ cup **Sauerkraut** (homemade or store-bought) (8)
1 cup whole raw milk or warm **Coconut Milk Tonic** (189)
Total calories: 935
Total daily calories: 1928

DAY SEVEN

Breakfast: 2 ounces smoked salmon (90) with 1 ounce cream cheese (100)
on 1 slice toasted whole-grain bread (60)
1 cup whole raw milk or warm **Coconut Milk Tonic** (189)
Total calories: 589
Lunch: **Fish Roe Spread** (370)
3 whole-grain or **Coconut Crackers** (60)
Spritzer (20)
Total calories: 558
Dinner: **Papaya Grapefruit Salad** (242)
Cheese Omelet (305)
Steamed Broccoli (74)
1 cup choice of **Quick and Easy Beverage** (70)
Total calories: 799
Total daily calories: 1946

DAY EIGHT

Breakfast: ½ grapefruit (50) with 1 teaspoon **Coconut Sprinkles** (18)
1 egg fried in butter or coconut oil (101) with 2 pieces nitrate-free
bacon (100)

1 cup whole raw milk or 1 cup warm **Coconut Milk Tonic** (189)
Total calories: 608
   Lunch: 3 ounces steak or lamb chop (200) topped with 1 tablespoon
              butter (108)
              1 cup steamed vegetables (50)
              Spritzer (20)
Total calories: 486
   Dinner: **Spicy Coconut Broth** (216)
              Cajun Swordfish with Corn (344)
              ¼ cup **Kimchi** (10) (homemade or store-bought)
              1 cup whole raw milk or warm **Coconut Milk Tonic** (189)
Total calories: 867
Total daily calories: 1961

DAY NINE

Breakfast: **Ginger Oatmeal** (144) with 2 tablespoons cream (62) and 1 table-
              spoon sweetener (50)
              1 cup whole raw milk or warm **Coconut Milk Tonic** (189)
Total calories: 595
   Lunch: **Salmon Roe on Toast** (186)
              1 ounce raw hard cheese (100), such as cheddar
              1 ripe pear (100)
              Spritzer (20)
Total calories: 514
   Dinner: **Miso Soup** (56)
              Chicken with Sweet-and-Sour Sauce (345)
              Steamed Cabbage (69)
              ¼ cup **Pineapple Chutney** (20) or purchased lacto-fermented
              condiment
              1 cup choice of **Quick and Easy Beverage** (70)
              1 cup fresh berries (60) with 2 tablespoons cream (62)
Total calories: 734
Total daily calories: 1843

DAY TEN

Breakfast: 1 medium sliced orange (65) with 1 teaspoon **Coconut
              Sprinkles** (18)
              Cheese Omelet (305)
Total calories: 538
   Lunch: **Chicken Caesar Salad** (558)

Spritzer (20)
Total calories: 686
Dinner: **Easy Coconut Chicken Soup** (299)
Hearty Hamburger with Sautéed Onion (304)
¼ cup **Bread and Butter Pickles** or store-bought lacto-fermented pickles (10)
1 cup choice of **Quick and Easy Beverage** (70)
Total calories: 791
Total daily calories: 2015

DAY ELEVEN

Breakfast: **Yogurt-Coconut Smoothie** (Quick and Easy Weight-Loss version) (444)
Total calories: 594
Lunch: **Steak Tartare** (209) (or 2 ounces purchased paté) with 3 whole-grain or **Coconut Crackers** (60) and 1 tablespoon butter (108)
Spritzer (20)
Total calories: 505
Dinner: **Coconut Seviche** (194)
Chicken Liver Supreme (370)
Steamed Asparagus (75)
¼ cup **Sauerkraut** (homemade or store-bought) (8)
1 cup raw whole milk or warm **Coconut Milk Tonic** (189)
Total calories: 944
Total daily calories: 2043

DAY TWELVE

Breakfast: **Coconut Smoothie** (Quick and Easy Weight Loss version) (462)
1 cup whole raw milk or warm **Coconut Milk Tonic** (189)
Total calories: 801
Lunch: **Salmon–Cream Cheese Rolls** (homemade or store-bought) (247)
3 whole-grain or **Coconut Crackers** (60) plus 1 tablespoon butter (108)
¼ cup **Sauerkraut** (homemade or store-bought) (10)
Spritzer (20)
Total calories: 553
Dinner: **Vegetable Beef Soup** (315)
Watercress Salad (262)
1 cup choice of **Quick and Easy Beverage** (70)
Total calories: 755
Total daily calories: 2109

DAY THIRTEEN

Breakfast: **Super Scramble** (209) with 1 slice toasted whole-grain bread (60)
1 cup whole raw milk or warm **Coconut Milk Tonic** (189)
Total calories: 608

  Lunch: **Vegetable Beef Soup** (315)
2 whole-grain or **Coconut Crackers** (40) with 1 tablespoon butter
(108)
Spritzer (20)
Total calories: 591

  Dinner: 2 cups baby greens (24) with 2 tablespoons **Basic Dressing** (156)
Indian-Style Coconut Curry (392)
¼ cup **Papaya Chutney** (20) or purchased lacto-fermented condiment
1 cup choice of **Quick and Easy Beverage** (70)
Total calories: 662
Total daily calories: 1861

DAY FOURTEEN

Breakfast: **Basic Oatmeal** (100) with 2 tablespoons cream (62) and 1 tablespoon sweetener (50)
1 cup whole raw milk or warm **Coconut Milk Tonic** (189)
Total calories: 551

  Lunch: **Greek Salad** with Grilled Shrimp or Salami (464)
1 fresh orange (65)
Spritzer (20)
Total calories: 657

  Dinner: 2 cups baby greens (24) with 1 tablespoon **Asian Dressing** (74)
Pork-Broccoli Stir-Fry (349)
1 cup whole raw milk or 1 cup warm **Coconut Milk Tonic** (189)
Total calories: 744
Total daily calories: 1952

Now it's time to turn to Chapter 9, for luscious coconut recipes, and Chapter 10, for savory recipes using traditional foods, to get started on a diet plan that won't feel like dieting!

Chapter Seven

Health Recovery

This chapter presents Health Recovery, a plan that enhances recovery from a wide range of health problems by emphasizing digestibility and concentration of nutrients. All the Eat Fat, Lose Fat plans will gradually upgrade your immune system, stabilize your blood sugar, help prevent illness, and increase your energy long term. However, if you have a more serious (or chronic) illness, or are recovering from any of the serious health issues outlined below, you should follow Health Recovery, an intensive version of our program.

Health Recovery focuses on relatively simple meals. Homemade bone broths are critical, as are lacto-fermented foods and beverages. The plan also emphasizes raw animal foods. If necessary, you can consume four to six smaller meals a day instead of three larger meals.

Continue on Health Recovery until you gain more strength and appetite. Once your health has improved, move on to Quick and Easy Weight Loss if you need to lose weight, or to Everyday Gourmet if you want to maintain or increase your weight.

The Eat Fat, Lose Fat principles can have a profound impact on turning around serious and chronic illnesses. You should consider Health Recovery if you have any of the following conditions:

Adrenal weakness: reduced libido, low energy, fatigue, difficulty handling stress

Allergies and hay fever

Asthma

Attention-deficit disorder

Chronic fatigue syndrome, anemia

Colds and flu

Constipation

Diabetes and insulin resistance

Emotional problems: anxiety, depression, mood swings	Immune system/autoimmune disorders
Food cravings	Irritable bowel syndrome, gas, Crohn's disease
Fungal infections: candida	Skin problems: eczema, dry skin, wrinkles, scaly patches, hair loss
Gallbladder ailments	
Hormonal imbalance/women's diseases	Thyroid imbalance
	Viral infections: Epstein-Barr, herpes, HIV/AIDS
Hypoglycemia	

Note: For any of these conditions, you should be under the care of a quali-fied health practitioner. The advice below is not intended as a substitute for medical counsel. Be sure to consult with your health-care provider before be-ginning the plan.

You'll find step-by-step instructions on how to follow Health Recovery (and two weeks' worth of menu plans) in this chapter. Recipes are provided in Chapters 9 and 10. Because some of the foods, preparation techniques, and supplements we'll recommend in Health Recovery may be new to you, be sure you've read Chapter 4, on our nutritional approach to weight loss, and Chap-ter 5, on traditional foods and superfoods, to understand our reasons for in-cluding these items in the diet. While some may seem foreign to a Western diet, they actually are time-honored traditional nutritional strategies used suc-cessfully in many cultures throughout the world for health recovery. It's defi-nitely worth the effort to learn about these new foods and techniques if you've been struggling with your health.

Core Elements of Health Recovery

The core elements of this plan build on the principles of Quick and Easy Weight Loss, but with several differences. Let's see first how they resemble our weight-loss program. As on Quick and Easy Weight Loss, you will:

1. **Correct metabolic fat disturbances through upgrading your fat intake by**

   - consuming coconut oil and coconut products;
   - supplementing with cod-liver oil to obtain vitamins A and D, as well as the omega-3 fatty acids EPA and DHA; and
   - eliminating harmful trans fats and commercial vegetable oils.

2. **Emphasize nutrient-dense foods.**

The difference is that for Health Recovery, there is much more emphasis on the following:

- **Homemade bone broths** For Health Recovery, you need the nutrient-dense, gelatin-rich goodness of real stock or bone broth. The gelatin in such broths is key to relieving digestive disorders, fatigue, diabetes, asthma, and allergies.

- **Increased dosage of vitamins A and D** by taking cod-liver oil along with high-vitamin butter oil (described on page 102). See page 101 for tips on taking cod-liver oil painlessly, either as a liquid or in capsules.

- **Lacto-fermented beverages** Providing nutrients and beneficial enzymes, these are key to relieving digestive disorders, kidney problems, skin disorders, allergies and asthma, and alleviating food and alcohol cravings.

- **Raw animal foods** to provide vitamins B_6 and B_{12}. Raw dairy products and/or raw and marinated meat and fish are a key part of the Health Recovery strategy.

- **More superfoods** Increased amounts of liver, fish eggs, and other nutrient-dense foods that nourished healthy traditional peoples.

- **A supplement of desiccated liver** (in addition to cod-liver oil) to increase strength, stamina, and energy as you recover from illness.

- **Soaked grains** Many digestive disorders stem from the inability to digest grains and legumes. In Health Recovery, we allow only grains that have been thoroughly soaked or breads that are genuine sourdough. It is particularly important to avoid cold breakfast cereals, granola, and any other grain products that are likely to irritate the digestive tract. If your health problems stem from an allergy to wheat, even soaked whole-grain products should be eliminated, at least until you recover completely. Use rice crackers instead of whole-wheat crackers.

- **More frequent meals,** particularly for people who have difficulty taking in high levels of calories at one meal.

If You Need to Lose Weight

In Health Recovery, calorie restriction takes a backseat. This is because, in order to maximize the diet's health benefits, you'll more intensively incorporate a variety of traditional foods like those in the list above. For most people with health problems, it is more important to nourish the cells with these healthful foods than to worry about calorie counting.

If you need to lose weight, *and* your weight is connected to your health challenge (for example, if you have diabetes, food cravings, or chronic fatigue), we advise you to follow Quick and Easy Weight Loss, eating three meals per day (that is, avoiding the between-meal snacks in Health Recovery) but adding in the following features of Health Recovery:

- Bone broths
- Increased coconut dosage
- Increased dosage of cod-liver oil accompanied by high-vitamin butter oil
- More raw animal foods
- Supplement of desiccated liver
- Increased use of lacto-fermented beverages

Major Health Challenge or Convalescence

If you are struggling with any of the following, whatever your weight, do not attempt caloric restriction until you are stronger:

- Recovery from surgery
- Life-threatening illness
- Debilitated, weak condition
- Chemotherapy
- Serious digestive disorder
- Malnutrition

Obviously, this is not a license to eat indiscriminately. Instead, you should carefully follow the recommended diet in order to rebuild your health.

Adrenal Weakness: Reduced Libido, Low Energy, Fatigue, Chronic Fatigue Syndrome, Difficulty Handling Stress

If you are experiencing low energy or any of the above conditions, lowered adrenal function is probably the culprit. Your adrenal glands produce a variety of hormones that regulate various bodily functions, such as mineral metabolism, glucose balance, and response to injury and healing. In addition, your adrenal glands produce the stress hormones, which means that difficulty dealing with stress often accompanies adrenal weakness.

What Your Adrenals Need

The special fatty acids in coconut oil give quick energy and prevent low blood sugar. And the nutrients in cod-liver oil are vital for hormone production, along with vitamin and mineral absorption.

Vitamin A To do their job, your adrenal glands (and the entire hormone production pathway) need the nutritional building-block cholesterol along with plentiful vitamin A, obtained through the foods on our diet.

In a 2001 study reported in *Prostaglandins, Leukotrienes, and Essential Fatty Acids,* researchers found that people with adrenal disorders that respond to corticosteroids (synthetic adrenal hormones) also respond to EPA and DHA, which are amply present in cod-liver oil, as well as in the other traditional foods we recommend. The efficient absorption and use of these fat components is guaranteed by the saturated fat in this diet.

Vitamin D According to a 1996 study published in *Brain Research: Molecular Brain Research,* activated vitamin D in the adrenal glands regulates an enzyme needed to produce dopamine, epinephrine, and norepinephrine, substances in the brain that help us feel good and help provide energy.

That's how, acting in synergy with other foods, cod-liver oil, by supplying vitamin D and vitamin A , will boost you out of a low-energy state.

Vitamin C To maintain optimal function, our adrenals need the vitamin C complex, provided in this diet by fresh fruits and vegetables, particularly those that have been lacto-fermented. When cabbage is fermented to make sauerkraut, its vitamin C levels increase tremendously. You'll learn how to prepare fermented foods in Chapter 10. We also recommend acerola powder or amla tablets, described on page 100, as a natural vitamin C supplement.

Salt Since the adrenal glands need salt to function properly, people with adrenal fatigue need more salt in their diet. You can use unrefined salt liberally, even drinking beverages with a pinch of added salt (quite helpful for insomnia in people with adrenal problems).

What to Avoid

Trans fats Key to healthy adrenal function is avoiding all trans fatty acids in processed foods, for these interfere with the enzyme systems that the body uses to make adrenal hormones.

Sugar and caffeine It's also crucial that people with adrenal problems avoid sugar and caffeine. These substances are stimulants that activate the body's stress response, causing the adrenal gland to produce adrenaline. The result is an outpouring of adrenal hormones. The body develops a cycle of adrenaline energy surges followed by exhaustion, forcing the adrenals to produce compensating hormones to recover from the adrenaline surges.

Over time, this cycle leads to adrenal exhaustion. Remember: Your body

---

Elaine's Story: Weight Loss and Sweet Cravings

Weight loss was Elaine's goal in following the Eat Fat, Lose Fat plan, but she discovered other benefits even before the pounds began to come off. She had been feeling generally fatigued and was subject to mood swings. She usually gave in to her sweet cravings, even though she knew this would prevent her from losing weight.

One Monday morning, only three days after beginning to take coconut oil, she felt a tremendous energy rush. It kept her going well past the midmorning "blahs" when she would normally have gone for a doughnut or muffin. Her mind stayed clear and focused on her work, and she couldn't believe how much she got done that day.

As the days passed, Elaine found her mood swings leveling out, even with the onset of PMS. And within two weeks she lost three pounds.

---

was not designed to produce adrenaline all the time, so don't hype your energy with caffeine or sugar. These stimulants may buy you fast energy cheaply in the short term, but you'll pay dearly for it over the long term.

For most of us, the main energy "drain" is actually the digestion of our food. Processed foods, pasteurized milk products, and excess carbohydrates (even whole grains) exhaust our reserves, so that when we assimilate foods more easily (as we do when they are properly prepared), we suddenly have a huge reserve available for tasks such as muscular function, thinking, exercise, and other more creative pursuits.

Using raw milk, eating lacto-fermented foods, soaking grains, and consuming gelatin-rich bone broths greatly improve digestion and thus help combat low energy.

Anemia

If anemia is contributing to your fatigue, the vitamin A in cod-liver oil will help this condition. We actually cannot absorb iron from our food without vitamin A. In third-world countries, anemia is very common, even though the foods eaten contain adequate iron. Public health officials have discovered that the best way to treat the anemia is not by giving iron, but by giving vitamin A, preferably in the form of cod-liver oil.

Allergies and Hay Fever

You may not realize that allergies and hay fever are closely related to adrenal function. In fact, adrenal hormones (like cortisol) control your body's response to allergens. An overactive response will produce inflammation, which can manifest as asthma, rashes, or hay fever.

Since the adrenal cortex is very sensitive to blood sugar levels, eating refined carbohydrates (like bread, pasta, doughnuts, soda, and chips) can cause allergies, with allergic reactions triggered by low blood sugar.

Therefore, the best treatment for allergies is not the conventional therapy, cortisone, a drug that suppresses and eventually weakens your adrenal glands, but a natural program of nutrition and supplements that rebuild and rebalance your adrenal cortex.

If you are prone to allergies, we recommend that you do the following to rebuild your adrenal strength:

- Absolutely avoid all refined carbohydrates—bread, pasta, and sugar—as well as fruit juices and most sweet foods, even natural sweeteners such as maple syrup and honey, if you have any allergic symptoms.
- Use coconut oil, along with other traditional fats, to provide satiety and keep your blood sugar stable and within the normal range.
- Take your coconut and cod-liver oils: many studies have shown that the omega-3 fats in cod-liver oil relieve allergy symptoms. Remember that your body uses omega-3 fatty acids much more efficiently when you are also eating saturated fats.

Asthma

The lungs secrete a fluid called a surfactant that enables them to function properly. This fluid is made of two fatty acids, *both* of which are saturated. In fact, the lungs cannot function without saturated fats!

A study published in the journal *Thorax* in 2003 indicates that children brought up on butter and whole milk have much less asthma than those fed vegetable oils and reduced-fat milks. What's more, European researchers have found evidence that trans fatty acids in the diet actually *promote* asthma.

Furthermore, numerous studies have shown that EPA and DHA, the very long-chain omega-3 fatty acids found in cod-liver oil, help relieve asthma. Once again, these fatty acids are used more efficiently when you eat ample saturated fats.

Based on this evidence, our diet effectively treats asthma in three ways:

- by including plenty of saturated fats
- by providing synergy between coconut oil, other saturated fats, and omega-3 fatty acids
- by eliminating trans fats

Attention-Deficit Disorder

How can children sit still in school and concentrate when their diet does not provide the nutrients that their brains need to function properly? The typical American breakfast of cold cereals, bread, jam, pastries, and sweet juice is a recipe for ADD—not only for children but also for adults. Such foods provide few nutrients and rapidly flood the bloodstream with sugar, resulting in a letdown an hour or two later. More than any other organ, the brain needs sugar, in the form of glucose, so when our blood sugar drops after the morning rush brought on by low-fat, high-sugar foods, distraction and fuzzy thinking inevitably result.

Instead, assure a steady supply of glucose, by eating not sugar but fats, which slow down the absorption of glucose into the bloodstream. A good high-fat breakfast, like eggs (a brain food) or soaked grains consumed with butter or cream, ensures even energy throughout the morning—whereas a high-sugar breakfast puts you on a roller coaster of sugar surges and lows.

Many studies have found that the omega-3 fatty acids in cod-liver oil can improve brain function, memory, learning, and behavioral disorders. Scientists have also learned that vitamin D and calcium—or both taken together—combined with a good diet that includes trace minerals can improve disorders such as ADD. In our diet, cod-liver oil provides vitamins A and D to ensure that the minerals in your food, especially calcium, are absorbed.

That's why we so strongly emphasize the importance of eating a healthy breakfast.

Finally, anyone with ADD must avoid all trans fats. University research has demonstrated that trans fats promote ADD/ADHD (attention-deficit/hyperactivity disorder) in children.

Ricky's Story: No More Colds

Ricky and his wife, Marjorie, use coconut oil primarily for cooking, but they also take therapeutic doses to prevent illness by boosting their immune systems. Since they started using coconut oil, neither they nor their two young sons have ever had even a cold.

The moment they feel something coming on, they take 2 to 3 tablespoons of coconut oil a day in hot cereal, warm milk, or hot tea. Their sons get a tablespoon on toast with tahini spread, or mixed into hot cereal or warm milk. At 16 months, their younger son has never been sick—even though he's often exposed to germs at his day-care center.

Colds and Flu

Sally personally attributes her own escape from the flu the last few years to the addition of coconut oil to her diet. Flu is caused by a virus that has a lipid coating, and coconut oil makes this type of pathogenic virus disintegrate. (Good bacteria have a coating made of sugar molecules and are impervious to the effects of coconut oil; in fact, coconut oil encourages the growth of beneficial bacteria.)

Many studies have shown that adequate vitamin A is critical for fighting infection, so the coconut oil/cod-liver oil combination is ideal for preventing bacterial infections. Bone broths also help protect against infection, while lacto-fermented foods provide good bacteria that, along with plentiful vitamin C, fight the pathogenic ones.

Constipation

It's well known that dietary fiber is important for colon health. In our diet, desiccated coconut, vegetables, and whole grains provide fiber.

However, consuming fiber is not a panacea. While fiber does speed elimination time, high-fiber foods that have not been prepared correctly can irritate and even damage the villi (tiny structures that absorb nutrients) in the small intestine, leading to poor absorption. (This is why adding Metamucil, a source of insoluble fiber, to the normal American diet will not heal constipation in the long term.)

A better strategy is to encourage the growth of beneficial bacteria in the bowel by consuming coconut oil and lacto-fermented foods and beverages. In fact, although they eat no fiber at all, the Eskimos maintain bowel health by eating fermented foods.

Denis Burkett, a British physician who lived and worked in Africa during the 1950s, 1960s, and 1970s, noted that Africans eating their traditional diet high in grains and tubers had between one and three substantial bowel movements every day, and that the time between ingestion and excretion was 24 hours or less. He saw a connection between this ease of elimination and the Africans' very low incidence of bowel diseases such as hemorrhoids, appendicitis, colitis, Crohn's disease, ulcerative colitis, gallbladder disease, and colon cancer. Dr. Burkett attributed this robust bowel health to the large amount of fiber in the native African diet.

While fiber consumption is helpful, there are many other traditional foods in the African diet that support intestinal health. Africans eat ample fermented foods, use bitter vegetables and herbs (which stimulate the bile and therefore help digest fats), and consume many foods rich in vitamin D, such as insects and dried shrimp (vitamin D is also important for colon health).

Burkett did not realize that Africans traditionally prepared grains and other high-fiber foods like cassava by soaking and fermenting them. Proper elimination depends not only on high-fiber food, but on your diet as a whole, and how you prepare your foods.

Diabetes and Insulin Resistance

A high-fat diet that includes coconut oil helps regulate blood sugar levels. Before the discovery of insulin, the *only* treatment for diabetes was a diet consisting largely of fat. Since trans fats interfere with insulin receptors in the cells, replacing trans fats with coconut oil and other healthy fats is the number one measure for preventing and reversing the insulin resistance so characteristic of type II diabetes. As for type I diabetes (the autoimmune type), eating the traditional foods recommended in Health Recovery will not necessarily heal a defective pancreas, but it will go a long way toward preventing the side effects of diabetes, such as kidney and retinal problems and impaired tissue repair.

Beyond that, our three-pronged approach to healthy fat nutrition will also help those with Syndrome X (also known as pre-diabetes), a combination of health problems associated with type II diabetes, including obesity and hypertension, insulin resistance, and stroke. Here's why:

- Replacing trans fats with good traditional fats will prevent trans fats from interfering with insulin receptors.
- Without vitamin D, your body cannot adequately use insulin, and thus may release excess amounts of it, leading to glucose intolerance, the inability to properly metabolize glucose. Research has found that low

---

Stewart's Story

Stewart was a retired software engineer in his late 60s who had had type II diabetes for several years. He was overweight, had high blood pressure, felt tired all the time, and—especially distressing—his eyesight was fading. His physician discovered protein in his urine, a sign that the diabetes was at an advanced stage.

Stewart's life was made even more miserable by the drugs he took to lower his blood sugar and blood pressure—not to mention his boring low-cal, low-fat diet. Yet none of these measures successfully controlled the disease.

Stewart consulted a holistic practitioner, who put him on a diet rich in healthy fats and low in carbohydrates. Along with other traditional remedies, he began taking cod-liver oil and eating lots of egg yolks.

Within six months, Stewart lost over 25 pounds. All his previous indicators of diabetes returned to normal—even his eyesight got better—and he was able to reduce and eventually stop his drug intake.

levels of vitamin D in the blood are associated with high levels of insulin. This means that the more vitamin D you have circulating in your blood, the less insulin your body releases and the better your blood sugar balance will be. And since in some people vitamin D deficiency inhibits insulin production, vitamin D may protect against type I as well as type II diabetes.

A number of studies have tested vitamin D–rich cod-liver oil with both insulin-dependent (type I) and non-insulin-dependent (type II) diabetes. For both conditions, cod-liver oil helped balance blood sugar and improved markers of the disease. Vitamin A in cod-liver oil also promotes wound healing and protects the retina, both problem areas for diabetics.

The traditional foods in our diet are especially important since those suffering from diabetes cannot make any vitamin A from carotenes (vitamin A precursors found in vegetables) and therefore need more animal-source vitamin A from cod-liver oil and the other animal foods.

Emotional Problems: Anxiety, Depression, Mood Swings

You may be surprised to learn how profoundly your diet can influence your moods—both for better and for worse. That's why it's important to know not only which foods can help, but also which ones to avoid.

Anxiety

Anxiety is also related to adrenal imbalance. On this diet, the coconut oil/ cod-liver oil synergy protects you from the energy dives caused by low blood sugar and also helps your body make the adrenal hormones needed to deal with stress.

Here's how it works: As you know, to produce key adrenal hormones, your body needs cholesterol (found in animal foods) and vitamin A (found in cod-liver oil). This combination builds stress hormones while soothing your nerves (since cod-liver oil's EPA and DHA support nerve function). And as we've said, the saturated fats you'll enjoy on this diet (including those in dairy products and meats as well as in coconut oil) promote optimal utilization of these omega-3 fatty acids.

Many people have noticed that a sense of calmness ensues from adopting a diet that includes plenty of good-quality saturated fat at every meal. That's because these fats help stabilize the blood sugar; when you eat too many carbohydrates and not enough fat, your blood sugar may drop too low between meals, contributing to a feeling of anxiety.

Again, preparation methods are important. The various B vitamins protect us from mental disorders, depression, and anxiety. By soaking whole grains, we greatly increase the amount of B vitamins they contain. In addition, taking nutritional yeast, rich in B vitamins, can help with all conditions of anxiety, depression, and mood swings.

What to Avoid Avoiding harmful substances in your diet is just as critical as eating the right foods.

- **Trans fats:** Trans fats *inhibit* the production of stress hormones from cholesterol, so removing these from the diet is another big step toward calmness.

- **Additives:** Once you eliminate processed foods from your diet, you'll no longer be consuming the many additives they contain. Additives like MSG, aspartame, and artificial flavors actually are nerve toxins that can contribute to nervous disorders and stress.

Depression

The nutrients in cod-liver oil have a proven record against depression. In fact, some studies indicate that cod-liver oil works better than drugs like Prozac in warding off the blues! This effect is enhanced by its synergy with coconut oil.

When your blood sugar drops too low, you're more vulnerable to depression. Eating plenty of fat, including coconut oil, with each meal helps prevent this perilous dip from occurring between meals. So coconut oil's ability to boost your metabolism and prevent hunger between meals also helps relieve depression.

Seasonal Affective Disorder Vitamin D–rich cod-liver oil, together with coconut oil, can also help this condition. In one study, subjects treated with vitamin

---

Marian's Story

Marian loved her job writing advertising copy. But although she was only in her early 40s, she felt tired all the time and had a growing sense that nothing seemed worth doing anymore. She found it particularly hard to get through the winter in the northern city where she lived. Marian was a vegetarian and liked to discover and prepare interesting recipes, but nothing she ate tasted good anymore.

Then she learned from friends who belonged to the Weston A. Price Foundation that a local farm was delivering raw milk, cream, and butter to the city. They persuaded her to substitute these dairy products for the low-fat versions she had been using and to start taking cod-liver oil and coconut oil. She also began eating organic foods.

The first thing Marian discovered was that these new foods were *delicious*. Putting raw cream on her strawberries in the morning gave her a sense of pleasure she hadn't felt for a long time. Soon she noticed that she had a lot more energy. Gradually, her outlook improved—and six weeks later, she realized she hadn't felt depressed in days.

D recovered completely from depression, while a second group treated only with exposure to light for two hours a day did not.

Mood Swings

Plentiful fat in this diet minimizes mood swings by helping stabilize blood sugar ups and downs. And many studies have found that the omega-3 fatty acids in cod-liver oil can relieve symptoms of bipolar disorder (manic depression) by providing the brain with the nutrients it needs to function properly.

Food Cravings

Cravings arise when you don't get vital nutrients from food. On our program, you'll find that when your body is well fed, you won't crave excessive unhealthy food.

The elements of Health Recovery—satisfying coconut oil, vitamin A– and D–rich cod-liver oil, and our traditional food preparation techniques—combine to enable you to fully assimilate your food's nutrients. That's why, on this diet, food cravings will fade away.

Fungal Infections: Candida

Either taken internally or used topically (on the skin), coconut oil has strong antifungal properties. Research indicates that the lauric acid in coconut oil, as well as the monolaurin that the body makes from coconut oil, kills fungus on the skin and in the gut.

Both antibiotic use and consumption of hard-to-digest foods (particularly unsoaked whole grains) can cause candida to proliferate. The candida fungus also feeds on simple carbohydrates (sugar and white flour). That's why the best approach to candida is to remove sugar, refined grains, and improperly prepared whole grains from your diet.

At the same time, you need to include coconut oil with its antifungal properties. On Health Recovery, you'll do just that.

Gallbladder Ailments

Coconut oil is the ideal fat for those suffering from gallbladder ailments because most of the fatty acids in coconut oil do not require bile for digestion.

Conventional medical thinking says that if you have stones in your gallbladder, it is diseased and needs to come out. But does the presence of gallstones really mean that the gallbladder is diseased?

Let's take a closer look. When we eat fat, the gallbladder releases bile into the digestive tract to break the fat down into absorbable fatty acids. The gallbladder acts as a holding tank for the bile, which is secreted by the liver and is made out of cholesterol.

In our view, the presence of gallstones means that your body has increased its reservoir of cholesterol. If you have low cholesterol, your body needs such a reservoir on hand because it cannot be assured of getting adequate cholesterol from the bloodstream. Thus, it's actually counterproductive to reduce the fat in your diet, for this would only increase the body's tendency to store fat and hence to form gallstones. Instead, the best way to eliminate gallstones is to give your gallbladder the cholesterol it needs by eating adequate amounts of animal fats.

But it's crucial to eat the *right* fats. When people eat a lot of vegetable oils and trans fats, the gallbladder can become inflamed easily. That's yet another reason why eliminating those fats is so important. And when someone misguidedly follows a low-fat diet, the gallbladder stops working, still another harmful effect of the low-fat diets we've all been told are so healthy.

If Your Gallbladder Has Been Removed

What should you eat if you've had your gallbladder removed? While the conventional advice is to go on an extreme low-fat diet, we don't recommend that. Your body still needs good fats and still produces bile to digest them. Even without your gallbladder, you should eat healthy animal fats and avoid processed vegetable oils.

The liver is a rhythmical organ that secretes bile at certain times of the day, ideally at mealtimes. If you still have your gallbladder, you always have bile stored and so do not necessarily have to eat at set times of the day. If your gallbladder has been removed, you should eat meals rhythmically: three meals a day at approximately the same time each day, with no snacks in between.

To enhance the sense of rhythm and supplement the supply of bile, we recommend a supplement of ox bile at each meal, taken according to the manufacturer's directions (see Resources). Swedish bitters, ½ teaspoon mixed with a little water, taken just before each meal, may also be helpful.

A survey published in *The Lancet* in 1981 indicates that people whose gallbladders have been removed have an increased risk of colon cancer. In order to provide ample protection for your colon, be sure to take cod-liver oil and other foods rich in vitamin D. And avoid all processed and grilled meats and any foods containing carcinogenic substances.

Hormonal Imbalance/Women's Diseases

The combination of ample vitamins A and D from cod-liver oil with other features of our diet helps keep your hormones balanced and your reproductive system healthy. Here's how: vitamin D supports hormone production in both men and women. According to a study published in the *Journal of Nutri-*

Alice's Story: Menorrhagia

For nearly four years, Alice, a San Diego caterer, suffered from menorrhagia, a debilitating condition characterized by extremely heavy menstrual bleeding along with severe abdominal, back, and/or leg cramping. She described it as "having a never-ending period."

Since Alice knew that this spectrum of disorders is often caused by excess estrogen, and can be ameliorated by vitamin A, she began taking a small amount of cod-liver oil (supplying about 12,000 IU of vitamin A per day).

Although her symptoms improved a bit, they worsened whenever she was subject to stress. Once she had to cater a special dinner and got so stressed out that the menorraghia hit her full force, making it hard even to walk.

Then Alice joined the Weston A. Price Foundation and read our website and magazine. She discovered that much higher doses of cod-liver oil might help—as high as 90,000 IU. "I don't know if I can get that down!" she told a fellow member. However, she decided to try it, and took two full tablespoons of high-vitamin cod-liver oil a day (providing 60,000 IU of vitamin A) for three days. After the first day, the bleeding was 50 percent less! By the third day, it was gone—and has not returned. A condition that had lasted over four years cleared up after just three days on high-dosage cod-liver oil. Alice also found that her sleep was more restful.

Alice now takes a daily maintenance dose of 30,000 IU of vitamin A, in the form of a liquid mixed with water, since after some experimentation she discovered that this method is actually more pleasant and easier on her digestion than taking a lot of capsules. Today she can fulfill her catering duties and is even thinking of training with renowned chef Jacques Pépin!

---

tion, 1992, and confirmed in subsequent research, infertility is associated with low vitamin D.

If you suffer from PMS, the cod-liver oil, mineral-rich tonics, and other foods on our diet will ease your symptoms, for studies show that additional dietary calcium, magnesium, and vitamin D can completely reverse PMS. These same foods will also help eliminate menstrual migraines, which are associated with low levels of vitamin D and calcium.

Even more serious reproductive disorders, such as PCOS (Polycystic Ovarian Syndrome), have been corrected by supplementation with vitamin D and calcium, according to a study published in *Steroids*, 1999. And that's not all. In a study reported in the *Mayo Clinic Proceedings*, 2003, women with PCOS also lost weight when they ate a diet with ample medium-chain saturated fats. And this weight loss lasted for at least one year.

Your body needs vitamin A, another key nutrient supplied by cod-liver oil, for every step of hormone production, from cholesterol to estrogen and progesterone. Fibroid tumors caused by hormonal imbalance have been completely eliminated with doses of vitamin A as high as 90,000 IU per day. As well as consuming nutrients key to reproductive health, you'll need to eliminate trans fatty acids from your diet. These harmful fats actually interfere with the enzymes necessary to make sex hormones from cholesterol.

Hypoglycemia

The drops in blood sugar that bring on the symptoms of hypoglycemia—sweating, trembling, dizziness, anxiety, and so on—can be prevented by eating plenty of healthy fats at each meal. Coconut oil combined with the other traditional fats in our diet is a delicious way to do just that. It's also important to keep sweet foods to a minimum, but with plenty of satisfying fats in the diet your craving for sweets will be much less.

Some people have found that eating properly soaked grains also helps minimize drops in blood sugar levels, a phenomenon that scientists have yet to explain.

Immune System/Autoimmune Disorders

The nutrients in coconut and cod-liver oil play an important role in bolstering the immune system. While saturated fats in general are immune system enhancers, the fatty acids in coconut oil do this best of all. The omega-3 fatty acids—particularly the EPA and DHA in cod-liver oil—are important for an effective immune response to injury or illness. And the fatty acids from coconut oil enhance their effect.

Monolaurin In 1996, researchers at the University of Minnesota looked at the disease-fighting action of monolaurin, a compound the body makes from the lauric acid in coconut oil. Aware that it inhibits a variety of toxins produced by

---

Susie's Story: Soaked Oatmeal Better Than Eggs and Bacon

Susie loved her morning oatmeal but had to give it up because it always led to a sudden plunge in her blood sugar at midmorning. By 10 A.M. she would be ravenously hungry, with a headache, nausea, and trembling hands.

Susie concluded that she was allergic to oats, and sorrowfully gave up this delicious food. Then she learned about soaking grains and decided to give oatmeal another try. She soaked the oats overnight in warm water with a little vinegar added, and in the morning cooked them and ate them with maple syrup and plenty of butter.

This time, there was no midmorning letdown—in fact, at 1 P.M. Susie was still going strong, without a hunger pang, even though she had put plenty of maple syrup on her porridge. Now she eats oatmeal frequently—in fact, she finds that it sticks to her ribs longer than a breakfast of bacon and eggs.

the pathogenic bacteria *streptococci* and *staphylococci,* they also found that monolaurin stimulates production of disease-fighting T cells.

Vitamin D Research published in 1994 in the *Journal of Cellular Biochemistry*
suggests that vitamin D also contributes to a healthy immune system by regulating both the components of the immune system that fight infection and those
that counter inflammation. Further research published in 2000 indicates that
low levels of vitamin D are associated with several autoimmune diseases, including multiple sclerosis, Sjögren's syndrome, rheumatoid arthritis, thyroidi-
tis, and Crohn's disease.

Vitamin A is essential for the production of T cells, so cod-liver oil boosts the
immune system in this way as well.

Supporting Liver Health

A healthy liver is essential for a healthy immune system. Thus, nutrients
that support liver function are vital for combating immune system disorders.

Decades ago, researchers suggested that gelatin assists liver function. The
liver uses the amino acid glycine—a major component of gelatin—for detoxi-
fication, and its ability to detoxify depends on the amount of glycine available.

Fructose in fruit juices and anything sweetened with high-fructose corn syrup
are very damaging to the liver because all fructose must be processed in the liver.
Animal studies carried out during the 1990s at the U.S. Department of Agriculture revealed that animals fed diets high in fructose suffered damage to their
livers similar to that produced by diets high in alcohol. Anyone with an autoimmune disease (or any condition associated with poor liver function) should
avoid these substances. (By contrast, saturated fats support liver function.)

Jenny's Story: Breast Cancer

When Jenny was diagnosed with stage-4 breast cancer, her doctors gave her a 50-50 chance
of surviving. She had a mastectomy, then chemotherapy, but her cancer kept spreading. Finally,
she was told it was inoperable.

Then she read some articles by Mary Enig and others, describing the use of virgin coconut oil
to treat HIV/AIDS by improving immune functioning. She decided to try boosting her own immune
system with coconut oil, to make it strong enough to fight the cancer.

She followed our program, eating traditional foods, taking cod-liver oil, and using coconut oil
for cooking, as salad oil, mixed in hot drinks, and on her skin. For six months she took no other
medication. When she finally went back to her doctors, they discovered she was in remission, as
she still is today.

Ronnie's Story

Ronnie, a delivery-service driver, was friendly with Eleanor, who worked for a company where he made daily deliveries. One day, as he was leaving, Ronnie remarked that he was going on his lunch break but knew he wouldn't enjoy it, since he had gastritis, which gave him stomach pain after every meal.

Eleanor suggested he try coconut oil and even ordered some for him. He began cooking with it—for example, gently frying chicken in coconut oil instead of the vegetable oils he had been using. His gas and other discomfort cleared up completely—until one evening when he had dinner out at a restaurant that proudly advertised its use of vegetable oils for cooking. That night, Ronnie's symptoms returned with a vengeance—and he realized that vegetable oils really were not as healthy as proclaimed.

Irritable Bowel Syndrome, Colitis, and Crohn's Disease

Our synergistic combination of coconut oil, cod-liver oil, gelatin-rich bone broths, and soaked and fermented traditional foods will help heal all the diseases of the gut.

IBS

In 2003, the *New England Journal of Medicine* published a major article on the causes and treatment of irritable bowel syndrome (IBS). The authors pointed out that as many as 15 percent of American adults suffer from symptoms associated with this uncomfortable disease, including abdominal pain, cramping, bloating, gas, diarrhea, and constipation.

Since intestinal health is central to overall bodily health, it's important to understand the properties of a healthy gut. So let's take a closer look at what goes on in the digestive tract.

The intestines are populated by many different organisms, all of which interact with each other and with your gut walls. Like all living things, these organisms need to consume and to excrete. When the bowel system shifts toward disease, both the population of organisms inside the bowel and the characteristics of the bowel wall itself undergo certain changes. The numbers of beneficial bacteria decline, while the amount of undigested or partially digested foodstuff increases. Pathogenic bacteria and fungi multiply, along with the toxic by-products that these abnormal microorganisms produce. In the small intestine, the villi are disturbed and deformed. The function of nerves in the intestinal walls becomes abnormal, and the absorption of food is compromised. These changes result in the distressing symptoms so familiar to the many sufferers of IBS.

By supporting the growth of beneficial bacteria, coconut oil can enormously benefit people with IBS. Cod-liver oil is also extremely helpful because it encourages the production of prostaglandins that the body uses to fight inflammation.

Colitis

Colitis, characterized by inflammation in the colon leading to diarrhea and bloody stools, actually responds better to the type of omega-3 fatty acids in cod-liver oil than to medication, according to studies carried out in Spain and published in 1990 and 1992. Thus, cod-liver oil should be the first thing you reach for to treat this condition.

A recent animal study carried out in Germany found that omega-3 fatty acids promoted the presence of beneficial lactobacilli in the gut. These fatty acids were especially effective when taken with probiotics (protective microorganisms), which are provided by fermented foods.

Consuming coconut oil strengthens the beneficial effect of omega-3 fatty acids. In fact, coconut oil provides the perfect fuel—medium-chain triglycerides—for beneficial microorganisms in the colon. Furthermore, coconut oil's medium-chain fatty acids work with the vitamin A in cod-liver oil to enhance the immune system.

Crohn's Disease

As doctors seek to find the causes of Crohn's disease, one popular theory is that the body's immune system reacts to a virus or a bacterium, causing ongoing inflammation of the intestine. People with Crohn's disease tend to have immune system abnormalities, but clinicians don't know whether these abnormalities are a cause or a result of the disease. Several studies have identified low-level measles virus as a major cause of chronic Crohn's disease. The measles virus is a lipid-coated virus, a type known to be vulnerable to monolaurin, the antiviral substance derived from coconut oil.

Gas and Bloating

Even if you only have relatively mild intestinal problems, like gas and bloating, the antimicrobial properties of coconut oil will help you by fighting gas-producing bacteria in your intestines.

Making grains and legumes more digestible through proper preparation and eating gut-soothing, gelatin-rich broths will go still further to prevent gas and bloating.

How Our Diet Heals Intestinal Disorders

If you have intestinal problems, it's important not only to take coconut oil and cod-liver oil, but also to modify your diet with the right food preparation techniques. In Chapter 10, you'll learn to soak grains and legumes, prepare fermented foods, and make bone broths.

Norman's Story

Norman considered himself something of a health-and-fitness expert. He worked out regularly and paid particular attention to his diet, which included eating granola and soymilk for breakfast every day. So he couldn't understand why he had constant gas and bloating.

Then he heard about the work of the Weston A. Price Foundation and consulted Mary Enig, who suggested he change his breakfast to soaked, fermented whole-grain cereal with yogurt and eliminate soymilk. Suddenly, his gas and bloating were gone. He also found that he had more energy throughout the day.

Soaking and fermenting Unless grains and legumes are soaked and fermented as we recommend, the tannins (astringent, bitter-tasting substances in plants), enzyme inhibitors, mineral blockers, and difficult-to-digest proteins and carbohydrates in these foods can block nutrient absorption and irritate the gut lining.

If you have any intestinal disorders, avoid all cold breakfast cereals, granola, and other heavy whole-grain products. Instead, use our methods to soak and cook your grains for better absorption. You'll then be able to consume grains and beans with much less strain on your digestive tract and fully benefit from the nutrients and fiber they contain.

Bone broths Another feature of our traditional foods program that's especially helpful for IBS and Crohn's disease is gelatin-rich bone broths.

Broths help you digest food while also calming an inflamed digestive tract. Traditionally, gelatin (which is extracted by boiling bones) has a reputation as a health restorer that soothes the digestive tract and aids digestion. Furthermore, gelatin is rich in the amino acid glycine, which helps digestion by enhancing gastric acid secretion. A study published in 1982 in the *American Journal of Physiology* found that gelatin promoted digestion by boosting the secretion of gastric juices, bringing the amount of hydrochloric acid in the stomach to normal levels.

The amino acids in broth also act as a tonic for the bowel wall. So anyone who suffers from IBS should drink lots of broth made from bones, and use it in nourishing soups, stews, sauces, and gravies.

Skin Problems: Eczema, Dry Skin, Wrinkles, Scaly Patches, Hair Loss

Topically applied, coconut oil helps wounds heal faster and improves skin quality. Take it orally to help keep skin soft, minimize wrinkles, and help heal eczema and similar skin problems.

The synergistic combination of saturated fatty acids in coconut oil and long-chain super unsaturated fatty acids in cod-liver oil contributes to beautiful skin by helping keep the right fatty acids in the cell membranes. Vitamins A and D in cod-liver oil are also important for healthy skin. Many people have reported that their skin tone improves when they consume coconut oil and also use it on their skin.

Coconut oil also helps prevent hair loss by supporting thyroid function. Hair loss is one of the first symptoms of low thyroid function. When thyroid function is restored, hair usually grows back.

Unsaturated Fats Make Wrinkles

While saturated fats help prevent wrinkles, unsaturated fats actually contribute to wrinkles. That's because unsaturated fats are usually rancid and contain free radicals that do a lot of damage inside the body—including promoting wrinkles. Studies performed by several plastic surgeons during the 1980s found that women who consumed lots of vegetable oil had far more wrinkles and looked much older than women who consumed saturated fats.

Drinking Water Won't Help

Many researchers tell people with dry skin to drink lots of water. Unfortunately, this doesn't help much. That's because the water in our cells actually comes from metabolizing fats. (The water we drink mostly goes into the bloodstream, rather than the cells, and then out via the kidneys.) So dry skin means there is a relative imbalance or deficiency of fats—especially in relation to the amount of carbohydrates in the diet. People with dry skin are often hypoglycemic and crave sugar because they are eating a diet that's high in carbohydrates but deficient in good-quality fat.

Once you change this ratio—so that more calories come from fats than from carbohydrates—the body produces more water for the cells. What's more, it will now have more fatty acids available for the oil-producing glands, which are our natural moisturizers.

Good fats for properly moist skin include butter, lard, coconut oil, olive oil, and small amounts of flax oil.

Thyroid Imbalance

All by itself, coconut oil improves thyroid function. When people with hypothyroidism (insufficient production of thyroid hormone) start taking coconut oil, they frequently report higher body temperature and increased energy due to improved thyroid function. Many thyroid sufferers are able to eliminate thyroid medication completely when they start taking coconut oil. (Of course, you should never go off thyroid medication without consulting your healthcare practitioner.)

Diane's Story: Hypothyroidism

Diane suffered from hypothyroidism. Her symptoms included weight gain, hair loss, dry skin, and intolerance to cold. Diane was distressed that she couldn't keep her weight down, even when she ate very little. But when she went on Health Recovery, increasing her consumption of coconut oil to four tablespoons daily and using butter and unrefined sea salt, she lost weight for the first time in years—more than 15 pounds. And after she had been taking the oil about two weeks, her below-normal body temperature began to increase.

Best of all, Diane was thrilled to discover that her previously thinning gray hair was growing in darker and thicker. Her skin lost its wrinkles and grew soft; even some freckled patches began to fade.

The combination of coconut oil with the vitamin A in cod-liver oil (which the thyroid gland needs in high amounts) can have even more dramatic effects on thyroid health because this combination gives the thyroid the basic components it needs to function properly. Unrefined salt and seafoods (particularly fish broth) also support thyroid function by providing iodine. Butter from grass-fed cows is an excellent source of both iodine and vitamin A.

You'll also be eliminating soy foods, which inhibit thyroid function.

High thyroid Coconut oil will also normalize thyroid function if you have an overactive thyroid.

Viral Infections: Epstein-Barr, Herpes, HIV/AIDS

The medium-chain fatty acids in coconut oil kill the pathogenic lipid-coated viruses in the digestive tract that cause these viral infections. As for vitamin A, a 1994 *Washington Post* article hailed it as "cheap and effective, with wonders still being (re)discovered," noting that vitamin A supplements help prevent infant mortality in third-world countries caused by viruses and other pathogens, protect victims of measles (caused by a virus) from severe complications, and prevent mother-to-child transmission of HIV virus. Consuming coconut oil along with cod-liver oil will give the body a double defense against these pathogenic viruses. In fact, monolaurin made from the lauric acid in coconut oil has been shown to knock out the measles virus and is the strongest anti-HIV substance ever studied.

The remarkable benefits of the coconut/cod-liver oil synergy in helping address health challenges are greatly enhanced by the use of time-honored foods, preparation methods, and natural supplements that have nurtured many traditional populations. So let's get started on the Health Recovery Plan!

Christine's Story: Beet Kvass Relieved Fatigue and Fungi

Christine suffered from candida for years, with gas, bloating, and fatigue. She tried every anti-candida diet, but nothing worked. Then she learned about beet kvass from the Weston A. Price Foundation website. It sounded strange, but she decided to give it a try. She made up a batch and drank one cup before each meal. The results were magical. Her candida symptoms cleared up immediately, and she was thrilled to find that her fatigue was banished.

Health Recovery Plan

Lacto-Fermented Beverages for Health Recovery

Key to the success of the Health Recovery diet plan are lacto-fermented beverages. These beverages supply beneficial lactic acid and healthy flora for the digestive tract, as well as mineral ions that the body can readily use.

On this plan, you'll be consuming lacto-fermented beverages at least three times a day. Use beet kvass, coconut kefir, ginger ale, and kombucha interchangeably, according to your preferences (for descriptions of these drinks, see pages 261–64).

Start-Up Week for Health Recovery

Day One: Order Products by Mail, Scout Out Raw Milk

Scout out and order coconut and other products that you are unlikely to find in stores.

- Coconut milk and coconut oil (although these usually are available in stores)
- Powdered kefir culture or grains to make fermented beverages
- Ready-made kombucha (if you don't want to make your own)
- Basic supplements such as high-vitamin cod-liver oil, high-vitamin butter oil, desiccated liver, and amla-C or acerola powder
- Lacto-fermented condiments, such as sauerkraut, kimchi, and pickles, if not available locally in stores
- Dolomite powder (a calcium source if raw milk is unavailable)
- Unrefined sea salt
- Scout out a source of raw milk in your area. Raw milk is particularly important on Health Recovery, so if you want optimal results, do your best to procure it. For sources, visit realmilk.com or contact your nearest Weston A. Price Foundation chapter leader. Chapter leader contact information is posted at westonaprice.org.

Day Two: Cupboard Cleanout

Go on a tour of your kitchen cupboards and throw out all processed foods, especially products containing partially hydrogenated vegetable oil (crackers, cookies, pastries, doughnuts, chips, snack foods, etc.), extruded breakfast cereals, and sauce mixes and other products likely to contain MSG. Remember that anything containing "spices," "spice mixes," "natural flavorings," and anything "autolyzed" or "hydrolyzed" is likely to contain MSG.

Day Three: Fridge and Freezer Free-Up

Get rid of all processed foods, prepared dinners, and low-fat dairy products in your fridge or freezer.

Day Four: Shop

Take a trip to the market/health food store to purchase ingredients for your first week of meals. Consult the Resources section for our recommendations of optimal products and where to obtain them.

Whenever possible, purchase organic fruits and vegetables and organic or pasture-fed meats and eggs.

Note: You can use store-bought lacto-fermented condiments, whole-grain crackers, good oils, and mayonnaise. In a pinch, you can also use frozen broths, but we really encourage you to make your own.

Shopping List for Health Recovery

See Resources for recommended product brands and where to get them.

Coconut Products
- Coconut oil
- Whole canned coconut milk

These products generally are available at health food stores and specialty markets, which will soon be stocking more items as the demand grows.

Fats and Oils
- Extra-virgin olive oil
- Cold-pressed sesame oil
- Cold-pressed flax oil
- Good-quality butter (preferably pasture-fed)
- Good-quality mayonnaise, preferably Delouis Fils brand

Dairy
- Organic whole-milk yogurt
- Organic whole-milk raw cheeses (check labels to be sure the cheeses are

made from unpasteurized milk; they are available in most high-end markets and specialty stores or on the Internet)
- Good-quality cream (not ultrapasteurized)

Sweeteners
- Natural sweeteners, such as dehydrated cane sugar juice (sold as Rapadura or Sucanat), raw honey, maple syrup, and maple sugar
- Organic molasses (any kind)
- Stevia powder

Breads, Cereals, and Legumes
- Rolled oats
- Sourdough and sprouted whole-grain bread
- Whole-grain crackers or rice crackers (if you cannot tolerate wheat)

Nuts and Seeds
- Raw pecans, almonds, cashews, peanuts and/or walnuts, and flax seeds

Animal Foods
- Eggs (preferably from pastured chickens)
- Fresh beef and lamb, liver and heart
- Beef bones (if you want to make beef stock)
- Organic chicken, duck, and turkey, and chicken livers

Seafood
- Fresh wild fish and fish carcasses (for making stock)
- Fresh and frozen shellfish
- Canned wild salmon and canned cod's liver (which actually tastes like tuna!)
- Salmon caviar (canned or fresh) or canned carp roe
- Smoked wild salmon

Fruits and Vegetables
- Fresh, seasonal produce, preferably organic
- Organic frozen produce, particularly berries

Condiments
- Raw vinegar
- Naturally fermented soy sauce
- Organic spices (non-irradiated)
- Good-quality Dijon-style mustard
- Lacto-fermented condiments such as sauerkraut, kimchi, and pickles
- Thai fish sauce

Daily Supplements for Health Recovery

We recommend the following daily supplements for everyone on Health Recovery:

- 1 to 2 tablespoons coconut oil in warm water or herb tea before each meal
- ½ teaspoon high-vitamin butter oil
- At least 2 teaspoons high-vitamin cod-liver oil, 4 teaspoons regular cod-liver oil, or capsules totaling 20,000 IU of vitamin A
- 4 capsules desiccated liver
- 2 tablets amla-C or ¼ teaspoon acerola powder
- ½ teaspoon Swedish bitters or apple cider vinegar mixed with water before every meal provides liver support in case you have difficulty digesting the increased amount of fats in this diet, or have digestive problems that manifest as stomach cramps, gas, or diarrhea

Miscellaneous
- Swedish bitters and/or raw apple cider vinegar
- Ready-made kombucha (if you do not make other lacto-fermented beverages) or kombucha culture
- Bonito flakes (if you want to make **Quick Fish Stock**, see page 226)

Day Five: Getting Started
- Make **Rich Chicken Stock** (page 224)
- Make **Homemade Whey** (page 227)

Day Six: More Food Basics
- Make **Coconut Kefir** (page 222)
- Make **Beet Kvass** (page 263)
- Make **Sauerkraut** (page 228) if you do not use purchased sauerkraut

Day Seven: Final Prep (Optional)
- Make **Beef Stock** (page 225)
- Make **Kombucha** (page 264) or **Kefir Ginger Ale** (page 262)
- Make **Coconut Crackers** (page 209)

If You're Gluten Intolerant
If your health problems derive from gluten intolerance, eliminate all gluten-containing grains (such as oats, wheat, and rye). For breakfast, replace oatmeal with eggs or smoothies and use rice crackers instead of crackers or bread based on wheat.

How to Use This Menu Plan

The Health Recovery menu plan can be tailored to your individual needs. If you have a very serious digestive disorder, for example, you may do best on a diet that features mostly liquid foods—such as tonics and soups. If you have chronic fatigue, you may be drawn to mostly raw animal foods or organ meats like liver. We also encourage you to repeat various menus in order to use up leftovers, and, of course, to omit items you don't like. (*Note:* If you don't like liver, don't worry—taking four desiccated liver capsules a day as noted in our supplement list will supply the needed nutrients from liver.)

Becoming accustomed to new ingredients and food preparation techniques may take some time, so feel free to substitute ingredients or use shortcuts when you need to. If you don't have time to prepare mayonnaise, for example, find a good-quality health food store product. You'll find listings of the best brands in our Resources section. Use organic ingredients wherever possible.

Here are some tips on integrating our diet into a busy life:

- If the only breakfast you have time to prepare during your work week is a coconut or yogurt smoothie (which can even be made the night before and consumed in the car on the way to work), then use your extra time on weekends to make eggs on Saturday and Sunday.
- If you work in an office, take your lunch to work (soup in a thermos, salads in covered containers, paté, cheese, Crispy Nuts, etc.). Or eat out, following our guidelines as much as possible.

You may find that after a period of avoiding gluten-containing grains as you follow Health Recovery, you'll become able to include properly prepared glutinous grains in your diet again.

Health Recovery Menu Plans

Bolded items indicate recipes provided in Chapters 9 and 10.
Note: Recipes for lacto-fermented beverages appear on pages 262–64.

DAY ONE

Breakfast: ½ to 1 cup lacto-fermented beverage
Ginger Oatmeal with butter and natural sweetener or **Coconut Smoothie**
Snack: **Raw Milk Tonic** or **Coconut Milk Tonic**
Lunch: ½ to 1 cup lacto-fermented beverage
Coconut Chicken Soup

A Note for Pregnant and Nursing Women

It's fine to follow Health Recovery if you are pregnant or nursing. In fact, this plan will provide excellent nutrition for both you and your baby. Nursing mothers should always include coconut oil in their diets because the lauric acid in the oil comes out in breast milk and helps protect the baby against viruses and other pathogens.

Whole-grain, rice, or **Coconut Crackers** with raw cheese and butter

Snack: **Raw Milk Tonic** or **Coconut Milk Tonic**

Dinner: ½ to 1 cup lacto-fermented beverage
Coconut Beef Soup with Vegetables
Whole-grain, rice, or **Coconut Crackers** with butter

DAY TWO

Breakfast: ½ to 1 cup lacto-fermented beverage
Super Scramble with sourdough whole-grain toast and butter or coconut oil and/or nitrate-free bacon

Snack: **Coconut Chicken Broth**

Lunch: ½ to 1 cup lacto-fermented beverage
Coconut Beef Soup with Vegetables

Snack: ½ to 1 cup lacto-fermented beverage
Raw Milk Tonic or **Coconut Milk Tonic**

Dinner: ½ to 1 cup lacto-fermented beverage
Coconut Marinated Fish
Liver Stir-Fry
Lacto-fermented condiment (homemade or store-bought)

DAY THREE

Breakfast: ½ to 1 cup lacto-fermented beverage
Coconut Smoothie

Snack: **Raw Milk Tonic** or **Coconut Milk Tonic**

Lunch: ½ to 1 cup lacto-fermented beverage
Coconut Fish Soup

Snack: **Raw Milk Tonic** or **Coconut Milk Tonic**

Dinner: ½ to 1 cup lacto-fermented beverage

Coconut Fish Soup
Steak Tartare (or purchased paté) on whole-grain, rice, or
Coconut Crackers
Lacto-fermented condiment (homemade or store-bought)

DAY FOUR

Breakfast: ½ to 1 cup lacto-fermented beverage
Basic Oatmeal with butter and natural sweetener
Snack: **Raw Milk Tonic** or **Coconut Milk Tonic**
Lunch: ½ to 1 cup lacto-fermented beverage
Cod's Liver Spread (or store-bought paté) with whole-grain,
rice, or **Coconut Crackers**
Snack: **Raw Milk Tonic** or **Coconut Milk Tonic**
Dinner: ½ to 1 cup lacto-fermented beverage
Cream of Vegetable soup
Easy Baked Salmon
Steamed Spinach with butter

DAY FIVE

Breakfast: ½ to 1 cup lacto-fermented beverage
Yogurt Smoothie
Snack: **Raw Milk Tonic** or **Coconut Milk Tonic**
Lunch: ½ to 1 cup lacto-fermented beverage
Wild Salmon Salad
Lacto-fermented condiment (homemade or store-bought)
Snack: **Coconut Orange Julius**
Dinner: ½ to 1 cup lacto-fermented beverage
Creamy Onion Soup
Baked Lamb Chop with Red Peppers and Onions
Steamed Broccoli with butter
Lacto-fermented condiment (homemade or store-bought)

DAY SIX

Breakfast: ½ to 1 cup lacto-fermented beverage
Coconut Smoothie
Snack: **Raw Milk Tonic** or **Coconut Milk Tonic**
Lunch: ½ to 1 cup lacto-fermented beverage

Creamy Onion Soup
Salmon Roe on toast
Snack: **Coconut Broth**
Dinner: ½ to 1 cup lacto-fermented beverage
Chicken Liver Paté (or store-bought paté) on whole-grain, rice,
or **Coconut Crackers**

DAY SEVEN

Breakfast: ½ to 1 cup lacto-fermented beverage
Basic Oatmeal with butter and **Coconut Sprinkles**
Snack: **Raw Milk Tonic** or **Coconut Milk Tonic**
Lunch: ½ to 1 cup lacto-fermented beverage
Smoked wild salmon with butter and whole-grain, rice, or
Coconut Crackers
Snack: **Raw Milk Tonic** or **Coconut Milk Tonic**
Dinner: ½ to 1 cup lacto-fermented beverage
Miso Soup with Cabbage
Hearty Hamburger with Sautéed Onions
Steamed Asparagus
Lacto-fermented condiment (homemade or store-bought)

DAY EIGHT

Breakfast: ½ to 1 cup lacto-fermented beverage
Ginger Oatmeal with butter and natural sweetener
Snack: **Coconut Broth**
Lunch: ½ to 1 cup lacto-fermented beverage
Roe Spread on whole-grain toast with butter
Snack: **Raw Milk Tonic** or **Coconut Milk Tonic**
Dinner: ½ to 1 cup lacto-fermented beverage
Easy Baked Chicken
Steamed Broccoli with butter

DAY NINE

Breakfast: ½ to 1 cup lacto-fermented beverage
Super Scramble with sourdough whole-grain toast and butter or
coconut oil and/or nitrate-free bacon
Snack: **Raw Milk Tonic** or **Coconut Milk Tonic**

Lunch: ½ to 1 cup lacto-fermented beverage
     Coconut Chicken Salad
Snack: **Coconut Broth**
Dinner: ½ to 1 cup lacto-fermented beverage
     Coconut Broth
     Simple Baked Salmon
     Steamed Cabbage

DAY TEN

Breakfast: ½ to 1 cup lacto-fermented beverage
     Coconut Smoothie
Snack: **Raw Milk Tonic** or **Coconut Milk Tonic**
Lunch: ½ to 1 cup lacto-fermented beverage
     Easy Coconut Chicken Soup
     Toasted whole-grain sourdough bread with butter or coconut oil
Snack: **Raw Milk Tonic** or **Coconut Milk Tonic**
Dinner: ½ to 1 cup lacto-fermented beverage
     Miso Soup with Cabbage
     Hearty Hamburger with Sautéed Onions
     Coconut Green Beans
     Lacto-fermented condiment (homemade or store-bought)

DAY ELEVEN

Breakfast: ½ to 1 cup lacto-fermented beverage
     Ginger Oatmeal with butter and natural sweetener
Snack: **Raw Milk Tonic** or **Coconut Milk Tonic**
Lunch: ½ to 1 cup lacto-fermented beverage
     Asian Chef's Salad with Noodles
Snack: **Raw Milk Tonic** or **Coconut Milk Tonic**
Dinner: ½ to 1 cup lacto-fermented beverage
     Salad of baby greens with **Asian Salad Dressing**
     Fish and Shrimp Stew

DAY TWELVE

Breakfast: ½ to 1 cup lacto-fermented beverage
     Yogurt Smoothie
Snack: **Coconut Broth**
Lunch: ½ to 1 cup lacto-fermented beverage

Fish and Shrimp Stew
Snack: **Coconut Broth**
Dinner: ½ to 1 cup lacto-fermented beverage
Coconut Mushroom Soup
Omelet or **Super Scramble** with whole-grain toast and butter
Steamed Broccoli

DAY THIRTEEN

Breakfast: ½ to 1 cup lacto-fermented beverage
Coconut Smoothie
Snack: **Raw Milk Tonic** or **Coconut Milk Tonic**
Lunch: ½ to 1 cup lacto-fermented beverage
Coconut Mushroom Soup
Raw cheese with **Crispy Nuts** and whole-grain, rice, or **Coconut Crackers**
Snack: **Raw Milk Tonic** or **Coconut Milk Tonic**
Dinner: ½ to 1 cup lacto-fermented beverage
Cream of Vegetable Soup
Sautéed Fillet of Sole
Steamed Spinach
Coconut Mashed Potatoes

DAY FOURTEEN

Breakfast: ½ to 1 cup lacto-fermented beverage
Basic Oatmeal with butter and **Coconut Sprinkles**
Snack: **Coconut Broth**
Lunch: ½ to 1 cup lacto-fermented beverage
Cream of Vegetable Soup
Raw cheese with whole-grain, rice, or **Coconut Crackers**
Snack: **Raw Milk Tonic** or **Coconut Milk Tonic**
Dinner: ½ to 1 cup lacto-fermented beverage
Papaya Grapefruit Salad
Kosher Pot Roast
Sauerkraut (homemade or store-bought)

Turn now to Chapter 9, for coconut-based recipes, and Chapter 10, for recipes based on healing, nourishing traditional foods, to begin your own recovery of health.

Chapter Eight

Everyday Gourmet

Congratulations! You've reached your ideal weight with Quick and Easy Weight Loss or experienced improved health with Health Recovery. Now you can enjoy even more variety and culinary delights with Everyday Gourmet, a diet plan that not only helps you maintain your weight and your health, but will also delight the other members of your family and keep them in top shape as well. Everyday Gourmet is a lifelong, delicious, and satisfying diet based on healthy fats, whole foods, and traditional preparation techniques.

All the foods listed in this menu plan are homemade, but, as with the other plans, you can substitute purchased lacto-fermented condiments, kombucha, commercial (healthful) mayonnaise, frozen stock, crackers, bread, and many other items as necessary. The menus are meant to provide guidelines for healthy eating and can be adjusted to suit your schedule and individual tastes. There are plenty of recipes to appeal to those who like to cook, and many simple ones for those with limited time.

We don't list supplements for this diet, but we do highly recommend taking cod-liver oil daily in liquid or capsule form to supply about 10,000 IU of vitamin A, along with some of the superfoods described in Chapter 5. Choose them according to your individual needs, as Chapter 5 explains.

If you need to watch your weight, remember to leave out the desserts (or eat them only occasionally), go easy on carbohydrate foods like bread and rice, and include one to two tablespoons coconut oil in warm water or herb tea before every meal.

This plan uses a larger variety of coconut products, including freeze-dried coconut, coconut cream, coconut vinegar, and even—as a flavoring for desserts—coconut rum! We've also provided recipes for more grain products (including ready-to-eat breakfast cereals) for active people who tolerate grains well and don't need to lose weight. Many of the techniques and guidelines you'll

How to Use This Menu Plan

Becoming accustomed to new ingredients and food preparation techniques may take some time, so feel free to substitute ingredients or use shortcuts when you need to. If you don't have time to prepare mayonnaise, for example, find a good-quality health food store product. You'll find listings of the best brands in our Resources section. Use organic ingredients wherever possible.

Here are some tips on integrating our diet into a busy life:

- If the only breakfast you have time to prepare during your work week is a coconut or yogurt smoothie (which can even be made the night before and consumed in the car on the way to work), then use your extra time on weekends to have eggs on Saturday and Sunday.
- If you work in an office, take your lunch to work (soup in a thermos, salads in covered containers, paté, cheese, Crispy Nuts, etc.). Or eat out, following our guidelines as much as possible.
- You may also want to make quantities large enough to provide leftovers to eat several days in a row.

Substitutions

The 14 days of menu plans are meant as guidelines—choose the ones that work for you and your lifestyle (and that you like to eat!). If there are any dishes we suggest that are not to your taste, or that you can't easily incorporate into your life, feel free to replace them with other selections you prefer from our wide range of recipes.

For example, if you prefer not to eat liver, you can substitute another recipe for a liver dish in the menu plans and, if you wish, take four desiccated liver tablets that day to supply the nutrients the liver would have provided (consult Resources for recommended brands).

follow are similar to those of Health Recovery, but here the emphasis is on high-quality, enjoyable, life-promoting cuisine.

Start-Up Week for Everyday Gourmet

Day One: Order Products by Mail, Scout Out Raw Milk
Scout out and order coconut and other products that you are unlikely to find in stores.

Dining Away from Home

How do you follow our program at a restaurant, at friends' or relatives' houses, or when you travel? You won't be able to follow it to the letter, but here are a few tips:

Restaurants

- It's easier to follow the plan at upscale restaurants than at low-cost ones. Try to eat out less frequently, but when you do, go to a restaurant where the food is made on the premises by trained chefs. Avoid fast-food places like the plague.
- Take your coconut oil just before going out.
- Don't eat the bread.
- For a beverage, order sparkling water with pieces of lemon.
- Avoid soups unless you're sure they're made from scratch. Ask whether the soup is made from a "base." If the answer is yes, don't order the soup—it will be loaded with MSG.
- Ask for olive oil and vinegar on your salad.
- In general, order simple foods, without sauces, unless you are sure the sauces have been made from bone broths. Instead of a sauce, put butter on your meat and fish.
- Don't order anything fried.
- Skip the dessert.

Dinner Parties

You don't want to be so strict about your diet that you can't eat at other people's homes. If the hosts are relatives or people you know well, you can offer to bring a dish yourself and eat that, choosing wisely from the other dishes available. At business dinners or more formal dinner parties, you sometimes just have to eat what's served.

On the Road

Take along a substantial snack that won't need refrigeration. A good choice is a container of Crispy Nuts and good-quality Parmesan cheese, which doesn't spoil easily. You can make a meal from this combination alone if you can't find suitable restaurant food. You can also make sandwiches using whole-grain sourdough bread, butter or mayonnaise, and good-quality cheese and/or cold cuts. Take a bottle of kombucha or lacto-fermented beverage along and enjoy a wonderful lunch!

A Note for Pregnant and Nursing Women

It's fine to follow Everyday Gourmet if you are pregnant or nursing. In fact, this plan will provide excellent nutrition for both you and your baby. Nursing mothers should always include coconut oil in their diets because the lauric acid in the oil comes out in breast milk and helps protect the baby against viruses and other pathogens.

- Coconut milk (also available in many stores)
- Coconut oil (also available in many stores)
- Coconut cream
- Freeze-dried coconut
- Lacto-fermented condiments, such as sauerkraut, kimchi, and pickles, if you do not want to make your own and if not available locally. You'll find names of several delicious brands in the Resource section. Be sure that what you buy has not been pasteurized or heated, but is made by the genuine process of lacto-fermentation.
- Lard
- Unrefined sea salt
- Kefir powder or kefir grains (if you want to try some of the kefir sodas; recipes on pages 262–63)
- Raw milk: scout out a source of raw milk products (and other farm products) in your area. To find raw milk, visit realmilk.com or contact the nearest local chapter of the Weston A. Price Foundation, posted at westonaprice.org. Raw milk is available in stores in several states and through direct farm purchase and cow-share programs in many other states.

Day Two: Cupboard Cleanout

Go on a tour of your kitchen cupboards and throw out all processed foods, especially products containing partially hydrogenated vegetable oils (crackers, cookies, pastries, doughnuts, chips, snack foods, etc.), extruded breakfast cereals, and sauce mixes and other products likely to contain MSG. Remember that anything containing "spices," "spice mixes," "natural flavorings," and anything "autolyzed" or "hydrolyzed" is likely to contain MSG.

Day Three: Fridge and Freezer Free-Up

Get rid of all processed foods, prepared dinners, and low-fat dairy products in your fridge and freezer.

Day Four: Shop

Take a trip to the market/health food store to purchase ingredients for your first week of meals. Consult the Resources section for our recommendations of optimal products, and where to obtain them.

Whenever possible, purchase organic fruits and vegetables and organic or pasture-fed meats and eggs.

Shopping List for Everyday Gourmet

See Resources for recommended product brands and where to get them.

Coconut Products

These generally are available at health food stores and specialty markets, which will soon be stocking more items, as the demand for these foods grows.

- Coconut oil
- Whole canned coconut milk
- Unsweetened desiccated coconut

Fats and Oils

- Extra-virgin olive oil
- Cold-pressed sesame oil
- Cold-pressed flax oil
- Good-quality (ideally grass-fed) butter
- Ghee
- Good-quality mayonnaise (preferably Delouis Fils brand)

Dairy

- Organic whole-milk yogurt
- Whole-milk raw cheeses (check labels to be sure cheeses are made from unpasteurized milk; available in most high-end markets and specialty stores or on the Internet)
- Cream cheese without additives
- Cream (preferably raw, but at least not ultrapasteurized)

Sweeteners

- Dehydrated cane sugar juice (sold as Rapadura or Sucanat)
- Raw honey
- Maple syrup and maple sugar
- Molasses

Breads, Cereals, and Legumes

- Rolled oats
- Sourdough and sprouted whole-grain bread

- Brown rice
- Dry beans
- Whole-grain crackers
- Wheat berries or whole-wheat flour

Animal Foods
- Eggs (preferably from pastured chickens)
- Fresh beef, lamb, and pork
- Organ meats if you want to try them, such as calf's liver, beef heart, and chicken livers
- Organic chicken, duck, and turkey
- Nitrate-free, additive-free bacon, sausage, and salami
- Fresh paté or liverwurst without additives

Seafood
- Fresh wild fish
- Fresh and frozen shellfish
- Canned wild salmon, tuna without additives, anchovies, and cod's liver (which actually tastes like tuna!)
- Smoked wild salmon
- Salmon caviar (canned or fresh) or canned carp roe

Fruits and Vegetables
- Fresh, seasonal produce, preferably organic
- Organic frozen produce

Nuts and Seeds
- Raw pecans, almonds, cashews, peanuts, and/or walnuts
- Pine nuts
- Natural peanut butter (be sure it does not contain partially hydrogenated vegetable oils)

Condiments
- Raw vinegar
- Organic spices (non-irradiated)
- Good-quality Dijon-style mustard
- Arrowroot powder (used in stir-fries and cookies)
- Thai fish sauce
- Red and green curry paste
- Naturally fermented soy sauce
- Lacto-fermented condiments, such as sauerkraut, kimchi, and pickles, if you do not want to make your own (brand names provided in the Resources section)

Canned Goods
- Canned tomatoes and tomato paste
- Frozen meat stocks (chicken, fish, and beef)

Miscellaneous
- Macaroons
- Ready-made kombucha
- Unsweetened cocoa powder
- Bonito flakes (if you want to make **Quick Fish Stock,** the base for several of our fish soup recipes)
- Coconut Rum (for several of the desserts)

Specialty Asian Products
Several of our recipes call for specialty products, available at Asian markets.
- Coconut sugar
- Kaffir lime leaves
- Galangal (Thai ginger)
- Lemongrass
- Coconut vinegar
- Tamarind paste
- Jasmine essence

Day Five: Getting Started
- Make **Mary's Oil Blend** (page 188)
- Make **Coconut Sprinkles** (page 214)
- Begin a batch of **Crispy Nuts** (page 259)
- Make **Homemade Whey** (page 227)

Day Six: More Food Basics
- Make **Rich Chicken Stock** (page 224)
- Make one lacto-fermented beverage (pages 261–64)
- Make one lacto-fermented condiment (pages 226–31)

Day Seven: Final Prep
- Make **Beef Stock** (page 225)
- Make **Coconut Granola** (page 209) or **Breakfast Cereal** (page 258)
- Make **Coconut Crackers** (page 209)

Everyday Gourmet Menu Plans

Bolded items indicate recipes provided in Chapters 9 and 10.

DAY ONE

Breakfast: 2 fried eggs with bacon
Whole-grain toast with **Coconutty Butter**
Whole raw milk or **Coconut Milk Tonic**

Lunch: **Coconut Chicken Soup**
Coconut Crackers with raw cheese and butter
Kombucha

Dinner: Salad of baby greens with **Asian Salad Dressing**
Baked Chicken with Coconut Peanut Sauce
Green Beans with Coconut
Papaya Chutney
Kefir Cream Soda
Coconut Custard

DAY TWO

Breakfast: **Basic Oatmeal** with butter, natural sweetener, and **Coconut Sprinkles**

Lunch: **Coconut Chicken Salad**
Spritzer

Dinner: **Coconut Corn Soup**
Leg of Lamb with Root Vegetables
Sauerkraut
Ginger Ale
Coconut Ice Cream

DAY THREE (A DAY ON THE GO—QUICK MEALS)

Breakfast: **Coconut Smoothie**

Lunch: **Crispy Nuts** and raw cheese
Kombucha
Coconut Macaroons

Dinner: **Watercress Salad**
Leftover Leg of Lamb Curry
Coconut Rice
Kefir Ginger Ale

DAY FOUR

Breakfast: **Super Scramble** with sausage or bacon
          Coconut Muffins
Lunch: **Coconut Shrimp Cakes**
          Salad of baby greens with **Asian Salad Dressing**
          Pineapple Chutney
          Kefir Cream Soda
Dinner: **Caesar Salad**
          Roast Beef
          Coconut Eggplant Fritters
          Sauerkraut
          Coconut Mousse Pie
          Kefir Ginger Ale

DAY FIVE

Breakfast: **Coconut Granola** with cream and fresh fruit
Lunch: **Cold Roast Beef** with **Mayonnaise** and sliced tomatoes
          Bread and Butter Pickles
          Kombucha
Dinner: **Coconut Waldorf Salad**
          Liver Stir-Fry
          Coconut Mashed Potatoes
          Sauerkraut
          Kefir Cream Soda
          Fresh fruit with **Coconut Sprinkles** or freeze-dried coconut

DAY SIX

Breakfast: **Coconut Pancakes** with no-nitrate bacon or sausage
Lunch: **Salmon Roe on Toast**
          Whole raw milk or **Coconut Milk Tonic**
Dinner: **Watercress Salad**
          Indonesian Coconut Steak
          Steamed Asparagus
          Mango Chutney
          Kefir Ginger Ale
          Stewed Fruit with **Macaroons**

DAY SEVEN

Breakfast: Cheese Omelet
Sourdough whole-grain toast with butter
Lunch: **Chicken Liver Paté with Coconut Crackers**
Stewed Fruit with **Macaroons**
Dinner: **Miso Soup with Cabbage**
Coconut Crusted Salmon
Steamed Spinach with butter
Pineapple Chutney
Kombucha
Cocoa-Coconut Cake

DAY EIGHT

Breakfast: **English Breakfast**
Whole raw milk or **Coconut Milk Tonic**
Lunch: **Wild Salmon Salad** with avocado and tomato
Pineapple Chutney
Kefir Ginger Ale
Dinner: Salad of baby greens with **Asian Salad Dressing**
Thai Green Curry with Pork
Coconut Rice
Coconut Custard with fresh fruit
Kefir Cream Soda

DAY NINE

Breakfast: **Ginger Oatmeal** with butter and **Coconut Sprinkles**
Lunch: Leftover **Thai Green Curry with Pork**
Kombucha
Dinner: **Coconut Seviche**
Rib-Eye Steak with Mustard Cream Sauce
Steamed Spinach Sauerkraut
Kefir Ginger Ale
Coconut Peanut Cookies

DAY TEN

Breakfast: **Super Scramble** with no-nitrate bacon
Whole-grain toast with butter and **Coconutty Butter**

Lunch: **Cold sliced steak** with shaved Parmesan cheese, **Mayonnaise,** and tomato
Bread and Butter Pickles
Kefir Cream Soda
Dinner: Salad with **Basic Salad Dressing**
Mango Chicken
Steamed Asparagus
Kefir Cream Soda
Coconutty Tart

DAY ELEVEN

Breakfast: **Coconut Granola** with cream and fresh fruit
Coconut Cocoa
Lunch: **Asian Chef's Salad with Noodles**
Kombucha
Dinner: **Papaya Grapefruit Salad**
Salmon Eggplant Curry
Kombucha
Fresh Fruit with **Coconut Sprinkles** or freeze-dried coconut

---

DAY TWELVE

Breakfast: **Spanish Omelet**
Whole Raw Milk or **Coconut Milk Tonic**
Lunch: **Quesadilla**
Coconut Avocado Dip
Cilantro Salsa
Kefir Ginger Ale
Dinner: Mesclun salad with **Balsamic Salad Dressing**
Prawns in Almond and Coconut Cream
Basic Brown Rice
Kefir Cream Soda
Akwadu

DAY THIRTEEN

Breakfast: Fried eggs with **Hash Brown Potatoes**
Lunch: **Roe Spread** with whole-grain toast
Small green salad with **Basic Salad Dressing**
Kombucha

Dinner: Salad of baby greens with **Basic Salad Dressing**
    Mango Chicken
    Basic Brown Rice
    Pineapple Chutney
    Baked Pears in Coconut Milk
    Kefir Fruit Soda

DAY FOURTEEN

Breakfast: **Coconut Pancakes** with sausage
Lunch: **Greek Salad with Salami**
    Kombucha
Dinner: **Hawaiian Coconut Shrimp**
    Barbequed Beef Ribs
    Asian Coleslaw
    Pineapple Chutney
    Kefir Fruit Soda
    Coconut Carrot Cake

PARTY BUFFET MENU

Here's a buffet spread that will please everyone, no matter what they're used to eating!

Oyster Shooters
Fish Roe Spread with whole-grain toast or whole-grain or
Coconut Crackers
Chicken Liver Paté with whole-grain toast or whole-grain or
Coconut Crackers
Lamb Kofta with Coconut Sauce
Chicken Satay with Peanut Sauce
Asian Coleslaw
Fancy Coconut Rice
Fresh Fruit Platter
Macaroons
Coconut Kisses

Now you're ready to turn to Chapter 9, for fabulous coconut dishes, and Chapter 10, for savory dishes based on traditional foods, and find out what some of these intriguing-sounding recipes actually taste like!

Part Three

Recipes and Resources

Chapter Nine

Coconut Recipes

These luscious recipes, incorporating coconut in various forms, will help you get your daily coconut quota. We've provided Quick and Easy Weight Loss versions for some recipes that are included in the Quick and Easy menu plans.*

Note: Many recipes call for a "can" of coconut milk. Use the standard 13- to 14-ounce can.

COCONUT MILK
Makes about 1½ cups

Although most people will opt for canned coconut milk, if you'd like to make it from scratch, here's how to make fresh coconut milk.

2 coconuts

Using an ice pick, poke 2 holes in soft spots at the ends of the coconuts and allow the coconut water to drain out. Place in a preheated 350°F oven until the coconuts crack. Use a hammer to split them open. Separate coconut meat from the dark outer shell with a sharp knife. Dice white coconut meat into quarter-inch pieces. Place coconut meat in food processor and process until well broken up. Add 1 cup warm water and process until fluffy.

Line a strainer with a kitchen towel and place processed coconut meat in the strainer. Let the coconut milk drain into a glass container, squeezing out all liquid with the back of a wooden spoon or with your hands. Use immediately or refrigerate and use within 2 days.

---

*All recipes from other cookbooks are used with kind permission from the authors and publishers.

Soups

The easiest way to use coconut is to add whole coconut milk to soups. In fact, you can substitute coconut milk in any soup recipe that calls for milk or cream. The quality of the stock you use is critical to the richness, nourishment, and flavor of any soup. Use homemade stock (see pages 224–26) whenever possible, especially if you are following Health Recovery; or substitute frozen commercial stock (see Resources) or make **Quick Chicken Stock** (see pages 225).

COCONUT BROTH
Serves 4 • *216 calories per 1½ cup serving*

1 can whole coconut milk
4 cups chicken stock
1-inch piece ginger, peeled and chopped

1 teaspoon salt or 1 tablespoon Thai fish sauce
Juice of 1 lemon or 2 limes
½ teaspoon red or green curry paste

Place all ingredients in a medium pot over medium heat and simmer until flavors are blended, about 10 minutes.

EASY COCONUT CHICKEN SOUP
Serves 4 • *384 calories per 1½ cup serving*

This is a basic, easy coconut chicken soup recipe, an important component of both the Weight Loss and Health Recovery plans. The rice adds a bit of thickness, but it can be left out for the Weight Loss plan.

1 can whole coconut milk
3 cups chicken stock
½ cup brown rice (optional)
¼ teaspoon crushed red chiles
1-inch piece ginger, peeled and chopped
1 teaspoon salt or 1 tablespoon
Thai fish sauce

1 teaspoon Sucanat, Rapadura, or coconut
sugar
Juice of 1 lemon or 2 limes
1 tablespoon fresh basil leaves
1 cup chopped cooked chicken meat or
uncooked chicken meat cut into fine strips

Place all ingredients except chicken in a medium pot over high heat, bring to a boil, then reduce heat and simmer about 1½ hours, or until rice is thoroughly cooked. (If you are not using rice, simmer for about 30 minutes.) Add the chicken about 15 minutes before serving.

Quick and Easy Weight Loss version: Omit rice (299 calories per 1½ cup serving).

COCONUT CORN SOUP
Serves 6 • 229 calories per 1 cup serving

1 can whole coconut milk
4 cups chicken stock
28-ounce can fire-roasted chopped tomatoes
Kernels from 4 ears of corn

¼ teaspoon cayenne pepper
½ teaspoon dried thyme
Sea salt and freshly ground black pepper to taste

Place all ingredients in a large pot over medium heat, bring to a simmer, and cook 10 minutes.

EASY COCONUT SEAFOOD SOUP
Serves 6 • 253 calories per 1½ cup serving

1 can whole coconut milk
3 cups fish stock
1 pound fresh fish (any kind), cut into ½-inch pieces
¾ pound baby shrimp or crabmeat
1-inch piece ginger, peeled and chopped
1 tablespoon Thai fish sauce

2 jalapeño chiles, seeded and cut into fine strips
½ teaspoon red curry paste
1 teaspoon Sucanat, Rapadura, or coconut sugar
Juice of 1 lemon or 2 limes
1 tablespoon chopped fresh basil leaves

Place all ingredients in a large pot over medium heat. Bring to a simmer and cook until seafood is cooked through, about 15 minutes.

COCONUT BEEF SOUP WITH VEGETABLES
Serves 6 • 317 calories per 1½ cup serving

If you are using beef stock made from scratch, you can use the meat that comes with the meaty bones in the soup.

1 can whole coconut milk
4 cups beef stock
1 cup finely chopped leftover cooked beef
2 cups chopped organic fresh or frozen vegetables

¼ teaspoon cayenne pepper
Juice of 1 lemon or 2 limes
Sea salt and freshly ground black pepper to taste
1 tablespoon naturally fermented soy sauce or miso

Place all ingredients in a large pot over medium heat. Bring to a simmer and cook until vegetables are tender, about 15 minutes.

ASPARAGUS SOUP WITH COCONUT MILK
Serves 4   •   375 calories per 1½ cup serving

3 cups fresh asparagus,
   cut into ½-inch pieces
¼ cup butter or **Mary's Oil Blend** (page 188)
¼ cup unbleached white flour
1 can whole coconut milk

1½ cups chicken stock
1½ teaspoons grated fresh ginger
Juice of 1 lemon, or more to taste
Sea salt and freshly ground black pepper to
   taste

Blanch asparagus in a large pot of boiling water for 3 to 5 minutes. Drain and set aside. Melt butter in a large pot over medium heat. Slowly whisk in flour. Cook, stirring, for several minutes, until flour browns slightly. Slowly whisk in coconut milk and then stock. Add asparagus and ginger and simmer until asparagus is soft, about 10 minutes. Blend soup with a handheld blender. Add lemon juice and season with salt and pepper.

COCONUT MUSHROOM SOUP
Serves 6   •   287 calories per 1½ cup serving

4 tablespoons butter or **Mary's Oil Blend**
   (page 188)
2 medium onions, chopped
2 pounds fresh mushrooms,
   chopped coarsely
½ cup dry white wine or sherry
2 slices sourdough bread, broken into pieces

4 cups chicken stock
1 can whole coconut milk
Pinch of nutmeg
Sea salt and freshly ground black pepper to
   taste
1 tablespoon finely chopped fresh parsley,
   for garnish

Warm butter in a large pot over medium heat. Add onions and mushrooms and sauté for 10 minutes, or until softened. Add wine, bread, and chicken stock, raise heat to high, bring to a boil and skim. Reduce heat to medium, stir in coconut milk, and simmer about 15 minutes. Puree soup with a handheld blender. Add nutmeg and season with salt and pepper. Ladle into heated soup bowls and garnish with chopped parsley.

THAI COCONUT-CHICKEN SOUP
WITH GALANGAL AND OYSTER MUSHROOMS
Serves 6   •   296 calories per 1 cup serving

This recipe by Thai chef Kasma Loha-Unchit is posted at thaifoodandtravel.com. Galangal (a type of ginger that grows in Thailand), lemongrass, and kaffir lime leaves are unique to Thai cooking and give this delicious soup its distinctive taste. They are available, along with the coconut sugar, in Asian markets. You can use fresh or frozen galangal. Use a brand of coconut milk that does not contain emulsifiers (see Resources), so the coconut cream can separate and rise to the top.

Quantities of the fish sauce, lime juice, coconut sugar, and white pepper are to taste. Add each slowly, tasting between additions, to achieve a balance among salty, sour, hot, and sweet flavors.

2- to 3-inch piece fresh or frozen galangal,
  or 6 to 8 dried pieces
2 stalks lemongrass
1 can whole coconut milk
4 cups homemade chicken stock
1 pound boneless, skinless chicken thighs,
  cut into bite-sized pieces
4 small shallots, crushed
4 serrano chiles, seeded and thinly sliced

4 fresh kaffir lime leaves, thinly slivered
½ pound fresh oyster mushrooms, cut in half
  if stems are large
4 to 6 tablespoons Thai fish sauce
½ teaspoon freshly ground white pepper
Juice of 2 or more limes
1 to 2 tablespoons coconut sugar
¼ cup fresh cilantro leaves, for garnish

Using a sharp knife, thinly slice galangal root; it is not necessary to peel it unless the outside is old and has turned brown. Cut off and discard bottom tip of lemongrass and remove loose outer leaf or leaves. Slice at a long slanted angle, into 1-inch pieces, all the way up the stalk close to where the grass blade starts. Smash and bruise with the flat side of a cleaver to release the aromatic oils and flavor.

Place galangal and lemongrass in a soup pot. Spoon off as much of the coconut cream as possible and reserve. Add the watery coconut milk or stock to the pot, bring to a boil over high heat, then lower heat and simmer, covered, over low heat for about 20 minutes.

Bring stock back to a rolling boil. Stir in chicken and shallots. Return to a boil, then lower heat and simmer until chicken has lost its raw pink color. Add chiles and lime leaves. Cook another 1 to 2 minutes, then stir in mushrooms and reserved coconut cream. Add white pepper, lime juice, and enough coconut sugar to balance the sour taste of the lime juice. Ladle into serving bowls and garnish with cilantro.

Appetizers

COCONUT SEVICHE
Serves 4 • 191 calories per serving

---

1 teaspoon sea salt
½ cup fresh lime juice
1 pound whitefish or tuna, cut into ¼-inch cubes
1½ cups coconut cream
1 teaspoon grated fresh ginger
1 bunch scallions, chopped

1 tablespoon chopped fresh cilantro
1 medium tomato, peeled, seeded, and
  chopped
1 clove garlic, crushed
Boston lettuce leaves, for serving

Place salt and lime juice in a medium bowl, toss with fish, and marinate at least 4 hours in the refrigerator. Drain fish and pat dry with paper towels. Place fish in a medium bowl, add coconut cream, ginger, scallions, cilantro, tomato, and garlic, and mix well. Serve on Boston lettuce leaves.

CRUDITÉS WITH DIP
Serves about 10 as an hors d'oeuvre • *20 calories per serving of vegetables; 80–100 calories per tablespoon of dip*

1 pound carrots, peeled and cut into strips
2 green peppers, seeded and cut into strips
2 red peppers, seeded and cut into strips
2 bunches green onions, trimmed
1 large jicama, peeled and cut into strips

2 cups sauce or dip such as
Coconut Red Pepper Sauce (page 189),
Cilantro-Coconut Pesto (page 190),
Coconut Avocado Dip (page 190),
Coconut Peanut Sauce (page 189), or
Curried Mayonnaise (page 239)

Arrange vegetables on a platter and serve with a bowl of sauce or dip.

HAWAIIAN COCONUT SHRIMP WITH SWEET-AND-SOUR SOY SAUCE
Serves 8 • *470 calories per serving*

24 large shrimp, peeled
½ cup unbleached white flour
Sea salt and freshly ground pepper, to taste
2 egg whites

3 cups desiccated coconut
6 tablespoons lard, goose fat, or **Mary's Oil Blend** (page 188)
1 cup **Sweet-and-Sour Soy Sauce** (page 239)

You may prepare the shrimp whole or split lengthwise and folded out in butterfly fashion. Mix flour with salt and pepper on a large plate. Lightly beat egg whites in a medium bowl. Spread coconut on a large plate. Dip shrimp in flour mixture, then in egg whites. Roll each shrimp in shredded coconut until well covered. Heat lard in a large cast-iron skillet over medium-high heat and fry shrimp until browned and crispy, about 5 minutes on each side. Serve with Sweet-and-Sour Soy Sauce.

COCONUT SHRIMP CAKES
Makes 12 cakes (3 servings) • *379 calories per 4 cake serving*

1 pound small peeled and cooked shrimp
2 scallions, minced very fine
⅓ cup desiccated coconut, plus more for dredging
1 tablespoon finely chopped fresh cilantro

½ teaspoon grated fresh ginger
4 tablespoons **Mary's Oil Blend** (page 188) or coconut oil
1 cup **Sweet-and-Sour Soy Sauce** (page 239), for serving

Pat shrimp dry, place in a blender, and pulse until a paste is formed. Add scallions, coconut, cilantro, and ginger and pulse until blended. Form shrimp mixture into 12 small cakes. Spread coconut for dredging on a large plate. Warm oil blend in a large skillet over medium heat. Dredge shrimp mixture in coconut and fry gently until golden brown, about 5 minutes on each side. Serve with Sweet-and-Sour Soy Sauce.

COCONUT FISH SPREAD
Makes about 1½ cups • 40 calories per tablespoon

1 cup leftover cooked fish
1 tablespoon fresh lime juice
2 cloves garlic, crushed
¾ cup sour cream or crème fraîche

Sea salt and freshly ground pepper to taste
½ cup grated fresh coconut or 2 tablespoons
    freeze-dried fine-cut coconut

Place fish, lime juice, garlic, and sour cream in a food processor and blend until almost smooth. Season with salt and pepper. Add coconut and blend in with a few quick pulses. Place in a large bowl and refrigerate for 2 hours before serving. Serve as a spread on coconut or whole-grain crackers or whole-grain bread.

BEEF KOFTA IN COCONUT SAUCE
Serves about 32 as an hors d'oeuvre • 105 calories each

Kofta are little meatballs, said to have originated in Europe and then been carried to India by early travelers. Frequently served in northern Indian cuisine, kofta can be made with beef, lamb, fish, crab, shrimp, or lobster. Garam masala is a traditional spice mix from India, usually sold with other spices in Indian and upscale markets.

1 pound ground beef (or lamb)
1 medium onion, finely chopped
1 clove garlic, crushed
½ teaspoon finely grated fresh ginger
1 small green or red chile,
    seeded and finely chopped

1½ teaspoons sea salt
1 teaspoon garam masala
1 egg
½ cup **Mary's Oil Blend** (page 188) or ghee
Kofta Sauce (recipe follows)

Mix all ingredients except oil in a large bowl and form into small balls. Heat oil blend in a large skillet over medium-high heat. Fry kofta until golden brown, about 5 minutes on each side. Drain on paper towels and simmer in Kofta Sauce for 10 minutes.

KOFTA SAUCE
Makes 16 servings • *65 calories per serving*

2 tablespoons **Mary's Oil Blend**
(see below) or ghee
2 medium onions, chopped
2 cloves garlic, finely chopped
1 teaspoon turmeric
1 teaspoon chili powder

1 teaspoon garam masala
2 tomatoes, chopped
1 tablespoon fresh lemon juice
1 teaspoon sea salt
1 can whole coconut milk

Place oil blend in a large sauté pan over medium heat. Add onions and garlic and sauté until golden, about 10 minutes. Add turmeric, chili powder, and garam masala and cook, stirring, about 1 minute. Add tomatoes, lemon juice, and salt. Stir in coconut milk. Add meatballs to the sauce, cover, and simmer 10 minutes.

FISH KOFTA
Serves about 32 as an hors d'oeuvre • *95 calories each*

¾ cup sourdough whole-grain breadcrumbs
½ cup plain whole yogurt
1½ pounds cooked, flaked fish
Sea salt to taste
⅛ teaspoon turmeric
⅛ teaspoon cayenne pepper

⅛ teaspoon ground cardamom
¼ teaspoon ground cumin
¼ teaspoon ground coriander
½ teaspoon ground ginger
1 teaspoon garam masala
½ cup **Mary's Oil Blend** (see below) or ghee

Place breadcrumbs and yogurt in a large bowl, stir, and let sit for 5 to 10 minutes, until moisture is absorbed. Stir in the rest of the ingredients (except oil) and form into small balls. Heat oil blend in a large skillet over medium-high heat. Fry kofta until golden, about 5 minutes on each side. Drain on paper towels and simmer in Kofta Sauce (recipe above), covered, for 10 minutes.

Salad Dressings and Sauces

MARY'S OIL BLEND
Makes 3 cups • *119 calories per tablespoon*

This wonderful blend of three oils can be used in salad dressings or as a cooking oil. When used for cooking, flavors come through beautifully, and the blend does not burn as easily as pure coconut oil. In salads, it provides all the benefits of coconut oil and does not have the strong taste of olive oil. In mayonnaise, it provides firmness when chilled. Be sure that the sesame oil you purchase is truly expeller expressed or cold pressed, since the very high temperatures used during processing destroy the unique protective antioxidants in sesame oil. Since we use this blend in many recipes, we suggest you make enough to have on hand whenever you need it.

1 cup coconut oil, gently melted
1 cup expeller-expressed or cold-pressed
  sesame oil

1 cup extra-virgin olive oil

Mix all ingredients together in a glass jar, cover tightly, and store at room temperature.

COCONUT PEANUT SAUCE
Makes 2 cups   •   43 calories per tablespoon

6 garlic cloves, coarsely chopped
2-inch piece fresh ginger, peeled and chopped
1 large bunch fresh cilantro, chopped
1 tablespoon extra-virgin olive oil
1 teaspoon Asian hot chili oil

¾ cup natural peanut butter
⅜ cup naturally fermented soy sauce
3 tablespoons rice or coconut vinegar
½ can whole coconut milk

Place garlic, ginger, and cilantro in a food processor and pulse until finely chopped. Add all remaining ingredients and pulse until well blended. To warm sauce, place in a medium bowl set in a pan of hot water over very low heat.

COCONUT RED PEPPER SAUCE
Makes 1½ cups   •   17 calories per tablespoon

This is delicious as a dip for raw vegetables, with crab cakes, or with simple baked chicken. Use canned or fresh roasted and peeled red peppers (available in upscale markets).

¾ pound roasted red peppers, drained
2 cloves garlic, coarsely chopped
Juice of 1 lemon

⅓ cup sun-dried tomatoes packed in olive oil
½ cup whole coconut milk
Pinch of sea salt

Place all ingredients in a food processor and process until smooth.

HOT COCONUT SAUCE
Makes about 1 cup   •   48 calories per tablespoon

Use this versatile sauce on vegetables, fish, and meat.

½ cup grated fresh coconut or
 ¼ cup dessicated coconut meat
1 small onion, finely chopped

½ cup whole coconut milk
½ teaspoon chili powder
Juice of ½ lemon

Place all ingredients in a small saucepan over low heat and simmer until onion is softened, about 10 minutes.

COCONUT AVOCADO DIP
Makes about ¾ cup   •   35 calories per tablespoon

1 ripe avocado
3 tablespoons coconut cream

Sea salt and freshly ground black pepper
Juice of ½ lemon

Mash avocado until smooth, mix in coconut cream and lemon juice and add seasoning to taste.

CILANTRO-COCONUT PESTO
Makes about 1½ cups   •   69 calories per tablespoon

This pesto can be used as a dip or as a sauce for fish or meat.

1 bunch fresh cilantro, stems removed
5 cloves garlic, peeled
2 teaspoons sea salt
½ cup **Crispy Macadamia Nuts** or **Walnuts**
 (page 259)

Juice of 1 lemon
1 teaspoon grated fresh ginger
½ cup **Mary's Oil Blend** (page 180)
½ cup whole coconut milk

Place cilantro, garlic, salt, and nuts in a food processor and pulse to form a coarse paste. Add lemon juice and ginger and pulse a few more times. While the machine is running, add the oil blend drop by drop, forming a thick emulsion. Finally, pulse in the coconut milk. Check seasoning; you may wish to add more salt.

Salads

COCONUT CHICKEN SALAD
Serves 4 • *495 calories per serving*

2 cups cooked diced chicken meat
6 stalks celery, finely chopped
6 green onions, finely chopped
1 red pepper, seeded and finely chopped
1 cup **Curried Mayonnaise** (page 239)
½ cup **Crispy Slivered Almonds** (page 259)

2 tomatoes, cut into wedges
1 tablespoon chopped cilantro, for garnish
4 tablespoons freeze-dried coarse-cut
 coconut or **Coconut Sprinkles** (page 214),
 for garnish

Mix chicken, celery, peppers, and onions with curried mayonnaise. Mix in the almonds. Divide among four plates. Decorate with tomato wedges and garnish with cilantro and coconut.

CHICKEN PESTO SALAD
Serves 4 • *313 calories per serving*

½ cup **Cilantro-Coconut Pesto** (page 190)
 or **Pesto** (page 240)
2 cups cooked chopped chicken meat
1 small onion, chopped

1 red pepper, seeded and sliced into thin strips
1 green pepper, seeded and sliced into thin
 strips
Sea salt to taste

Mix all ingredients together in a large bowl.

COCONUT WALDORF SALAD
Serves 6 • *294 calories per serving*

4 large apples
Juice of 1 lemon
4 stalks celery, chopped
1 cup **Crispy Walnuts** (page 259), chopped
1 tablespoon chopped fresh cilantro
½ cup **Mayonnaise** (page 238)

Lettuce leaves, for serving
4 tablespoons freeze-dried coarse-cut
 coconut or **Coconut Sprinkles** (page 214)
 for garnish
Sliced cherry tomatoes, for garnish

Peel apples and cut into ½-inch chunks. Immediately place in a large bowl and toss with lemon juice. Stir in celery, walnuts, cilantro, and mayonnaise. Place lettuce leaves on six plates and and divide salad among the plates. Garnish with coconut and sliced cherry tomatoes.

Seafood Entrées

THAI MARINATED FISH IN COCONUT CREAM
Serves 4 • 287 calories per serving

---

1 pound whitefish, or other mild fish,
   cut into ½-inch cubes
½ cup fresh lime juice
1 teaspoon sea salt
1 cup green beans
2 tablespoons **Mary's Oil Blend** (page 188)
   or lard

1 bunch scallions, chopped
1 red pepper, seeded and sliced
1 clove garlic, finely minced
¾ cup coconut cream
Cilantro sprigs, for garnish

Place fish in a large bowl and stir in lime juice and salt. Cover and place in refrigerator to marinate for 4 hours. Drain. Remove strings from beans, cut lengthwise and then into 1-inch pieces. Heat oil blend in a medium sauté pan over medium heat. Add scallions, red pepper, garlic, and green beans and sauté for several minutes, until tender. Add fish and coconut milk and simmer, stirring frequently, for about 10 minutes, until vegetables are tender and fish is cooked through. Garnish with cilantro sprigs.

BRAZILIAN SHRIMP STEW
Serves 4 • 470 calories per serving

1½ pounds fresh large shrimp,
   shelled and deveined
Juice of 2 lemons
1 onion, finely chopped
1 clove garlic, minced
2 tablespoons white wine vinegar

½ teaspoon sea salt, plus more to taste
1 tablespoon chopped fresh cilantro
1 can whole coconut milk
1 cup **Crispy Cashews** (page 259),
   processed into a coarse meal
Freshly ground black pepper to taste

Place shrimp in a mixture of lemon juice, onion, garlic, vinegar, and salt and marinate for 30 minutes. Place in a medium saucepan over medium heat. Add cilantro, coconut milk, cashews, salt and pepper to taste. Simmer, covered, for about 15 minutes, until shrimp are cooked through. Serve with **Coconut Rice** (page 206).

Quick and Easy Weight Loss version: Omit cashews (370 calories per serving).

FISH AND SHRIMP STEW
Serves 6 • *383 calories per serving*

This is a traditional recipe from Mozambique. Serve with **Coconut Rice** (page 206).

1 pound uncooked medium shrimp
(about 21 to 25 to the pound)
Eight 4-ounce sea bass or red snapper steaks,
about 1 inch thick
1 tablespoon sea salt
3 tablespoons **Mary's Oil Blend** (page 188)
1 cup finely chopped onions

2 medium bell peppers, seeded and finely
chopped
2 medium firm-ripe tomatoes, peeled, seeded
and finely chopped
1 tablespoon finely chopped fresh cilantro
½ teaspoon red chile flakes
1 can whole coconut milk

Shell and devein shrimp, wash under cold running water, and pat dry with paper towels. Pat fish steaks dry and sprinkle them with 1 teaspoon salt on each side. Set shrimp and fish aside.

Warm oil blend in a large heavy skillet over medium heat. Add onions and peppers and sauté for about 5 minutes, stirring frequently, until soft but not brown. Add tomatoes and cook, stirring frequently, until most of the liquid in the pan evaporates and the mixture thickens. Remove the pan from the heat, then stir in cilantro, chile flakes, and remaining teaspoon salt, and taste for seasoning.

Arrange 4 of the fish steaks in a heavy saucepan large enough to hold them in one layer. Scatter half of the shrimp over and around the fish, and spoon half the vegetable mixture over them. Add the remaining fish steaks and shrimp and cover them with the rest of the vegetables.

Pour in coconut milk and bring to a simmer over medium heat. Reduce heat to its lowest point. Cook, partially covered, for about 20 minutes, or until shrimp are firm and pink and the fish flakes easily when prodded with a fork.

COCONUT SHRIMP ÉTOUFFÉE
Serves 6 • *581 calories per serving*

36 large shrimp with shells, fresh or frozen
¼ cup vinegar (any kind)
4 tablespoons **Mary's Oil Blend** (page 188)
or lard
2 large onions, chopped
1 green pepper, seeded and chopped
2 ripe plum tomatoes, seeded and chopped
4 cloves garlic, mashed

½ cup butter
½ cup unbleached white flour
1 can whole coconut milk
¼ teaspoon cayenne pepper
½ teaspoon dried thyme
Sea salt to taste

Shell and devein shrimp, wash well, and reserve in refrigerator. Place shells in a large pot, cover with water, and add vinegar. Let sit about 15 minutes, then bring to a boil over high heat. Skim any scum that comes to the surface, reduce heat, and simmer, uncovered, for 1 hour. Remove shrimp shells and reserve stock for the étouffée.

Heat oil blend in a large sauté pan over medium heat. Add onions and green pepper and sauté until soft, about 5 minutes. Add tomatoes, raise heat to high, and sauté, stirring constantly, until liquid has evaporated. Remove pan from heat and stir in garlic.

Melt butter in a large heavy pot over medium heat. Stir in flour and cook, stirring constantly with a wooden spoon, for about 5 minutes, or until flour turns light brown. Slowly add 2 cups of shrimp stock and coconut milk, stirring constantly with a whisk, until sauce thickens, about 5 minutes. Add sautéed vegetables, cayenne, thyme, and salt. Add shrimp, reduce heat to low, and simmer, stirring frequently until shrimp are cooked through, thinning with a little shrimp stock or water if necessary. Serve in soup bowls with **Coconut Rice** (page 206).

COCONUT-CRUSTED SALMON
Serves 4 • *408 calories per serving*

4 tablespoons melted butter	½ cup desiccated coconut
1 teaspoon sea salt	1⅓ pounds wild salmon fillet
⅛ teaspoon paprika	

Preheat oven to 350°F. Mix melted butter with salt, paprika, and coconut in a small bowl. Spread over salmon. Place salmon in a buttered Pyrex pan and bake for about 10 minutes, or until salmon is cooked through and crust is lightly browned.

LEAF-WRAPPED SALMON WITH CILANTRO-COCONUT STUFFING
Serves 8 • *334 calories per serving*

3 heads butter lettuce or other soft-leaf lettuce	8 small hot or 4 medium mild fresh green chiles
1 bunch fresh cilantro	1 tablespoon grated fresh ginger
⅓ cup fresh mint leaves	Sea salt and freshly ground black pepper to taste
1 cup desiccated coconut	
⅓ cup fresh lemon juice	2 wild salmon fillets, about 1½ pounds each, skin removed
8 cloves garlic, peeled	

Preheat oven to 350°F.

Prepare lettuce leaves by dipping whole heads into a pot of boiling filtered water for about 10 seconds each. Remove immediately. Drain, separate leaves, and spread out on kitchen towels. Meanwhile, prepare stuffing by placing cilantro, mint, coconut, lemon juice, garlic, chiles, and ginger in a food processor. Process into a thick paste and season with salt and pepper.

Butter an oblong Pyrex dish and line it with one layer of overlapping lettuce leaves. Place 1 salmon fillet on the lettuce leaves skinned side down. Spread stuffing over the fillet and set other fillet on top, skinned side up. Fold lettuce leaves up to cover sides and a portion of the top of the fish. Cover top with one layer of overlapping leaves and tuck under. Bake for 45 minutes. To serve, cut fish with lettuce wrapping crosswise into slices about 1 inch thick.

SALMON AND EGGPLANT CURRY
Serves 4   •   432 calories per serving

1 pound Japanese eggplant
Sea salt
2 tablespoons **Mary's Oil Blend**
  (page 188) or lard
1 can whole coconut milk
1 cup fish stock
2 to 3 teaspoons green curry paste

1 tablespoon Thai fish sauce
Juice of 1 lemon or 2 limes
2 teaspoons coconut sugar
2 kaffir lime leaves
¼ cup coarsely chopped fresh basil
1 pound wild salmon, cut into 1-inch cubes

Peel eggplant and cut into ½-inch cubes. Place in a colander and toss with sea salt; let stand about 1 hour. Rinse and squeeze dry in a kitchen towel. Warm oil blend in a large sauté pan. Add eggplant and sauté until lightly browned, about 8 minutes. Add coconut milk and fish stock, bring to a boil, then reduce to a simmer. Add curry paste, fish sauce, lemon juice, and coconut sugar. Add salmon, lime leaves, and basil and simmer about 10 minutes, or until salmon is cooked through.

PRAWNS IN ALMOND AND COCONUT CREAM
Serves 6   •   438 calories per serving

3 tablespoons **Mary's Oil Blend** (page 188)
  or ghee
2 bay leaves
1-inch piece cinnamon stick
5 whole cardamom pods
1½ pounds (about 24) fresh prawns, shelled
3 cloves garlic, chopped
1 teaspoon grated fresh ginger
1 large onion, chopped
1 tablespoon unbleached white flour

3 tablespoons ground **Crispy Almonds**
  (page 259)
2¼ cups coconut cream
⅛ teaspoon cayenne pepper
1 teaspoon coconut or maple sugar
1 teaspoon sea salt
1 tablespoon fresh lemon juice
2 tablespoons chopped fresh cilantro
2 tablespoons **Crispy Almond Slivers**,
  for garnish

Heat oil blend in a large frying pan over medium heat. Add bay leaves, cinnamon stick, and cardamom pods and sauté for about 2 minutes, or until flavors are released. Add prawns and cook on both sides, about 3 minutes total. Remove prawns and set aside. Add garlic, ginger, and onions and sauté until onions are clear, about 8 minutes. Add flour and ground almonds. Cook 2 minutes, sitrring constantly. Add coconut cream, cayenne, and sugar, bring to a boil, and simmer for 10 minutes, or until flavors amalgamate.

Return prawns to the pan and add salt. Simmer about 8 minutes, or until cooked through. Add lemon juice and cilantro. Remove bay leaves, cinnamon stick, and cardamom pods. Garnish with almond slivers.

Poultry Entrées

Whenever possible, use grass-fed, farm-raised chicken (see Resources).

BAKED CHICKEN WITH COCONUT PEANUT SAUCE
Serves 6 • *400 calories per serving*

1 whole chicken, including head and feet
   if possible
1 tablespoon melted butter

Salt and freshly ground black pepper to taste
1¾ cups **Coconut Peanut Sauce** (page 189)

Preheat oven to 350°F.

Cut up chicken, reserving backs, wings, neck, head, and feet (neck, head, and feet are optional if not desired or not provided by your local market) for making chicken stock. Place breasts, thighs, and drumsticks, skin side up, in a stainless-steel baking pan. Brush with butter and sprinkle with salt and pepper.

Note: Chicken may be prepared the day ahead to this point and reserved, covered, in the refrigerator while you make stock.

Place chicken in oven and bake about 2 hours, or until golden brown. Remove to a heated platter and serve with Coconut Peanut Sauce.

INDIAN-STYLE CHICKEN CURRY
Serves 6 • *385 calories per serving*

1½ pounds skinless chicken meat,
   cut into ½-inch pieces
4 tablespoons ghee or **Mary's Oil Blend**
   (page 188)
2 medium onions, finely chopped
2 tablespoons turmeric
1 tablespoon ground fenugreek
1 teaspoon ground cumin
¼ teaspoon cayenne pepper

½ teaspoon ground cloves
1 teaspoon ground coriander
1 teaspoon ground cardamom
2 cups chicken stock
Juice of 1 to 2 lemons
2 cloves garlic, peeled and mashed
1 can whole coconut milk
Sea salt to taste

Pat chicken pieces dry with paper towels. Heat ghee in a large skillet over medium-high heat. Add chicken pieces and sauté in batches. Remove each batch with a slotted spoon and set aside. Add onions and sauté until soft. Add spices and sauté, stirring, for several minutes, or until flavors are released. Add chicken stock and lemon juice and bring to a boil. Stir in garlic, chicken, and coconut milk.

Lower heat and simmer, uncovered, for about 15 minutes, stirring frequently, until sauce is reduced and thickened. Season with salt. Serve with traditional curry garnishes such as chopped green onions, **Chopped Crispy Peanuts** (page 259), raisins, and **Coconut Sprinkles** (page 214) or freeze-dried coconut meat. This dish is excellent with **Cucumber Raita** (page 244).

THAI CHICKEN CURRY
Serves 4 • *475 calories per serving*

This recipe is adapted from *It Rains Fishes: Legends, Traditions and the Joys of Thai Cooking* by Kasma Loha-Unchit. Tamarind paste is available in Asian markets. Use a brand of coconut milk that does not contain emulsifiers and will separate, so you can skim off the cream (see Resources).

1 can whole coconut milk
2 tablespoons red curry paste
3 tablespoons finely ground **Crispy Peanuts**
  (page 259)
Thai fish sauce to taste
1 tablespoon coconut sugar
1 pound boneless chicken thigh meat,
  cut into bite-sized chunks

1 medium potato, cut in ½-inch cubes
2 tablespoons whole **Crispy Peanuts**
8 to 10 baby pearl onions, peeled
1 jalapeño chile, seeds removed
  and cut into slivers
2 teaspoons tamarind paste dissolved
  in 1 tablespoon hot water

Spoon about ⅔ cup thick coconut cream from top of the can of coconut milk into a medium saucepan. Heat over medium-high heat. Reduce until bubbly and oils begin to separate, 3 to 5 minutes. Add the curry paste, mashing it to mix with the cream. Fry paste in cream for a few minutes, until it is aromatic. Add ground peanuts and some of remaining coconut milk, enough to make a smooth, thick sauce. Season with fish sauce and coconut sugar.

Add chicken to sauce and cook over medium heat until the pieces change color and are no longer pink and raw on the outside. At this point the chicken will start to let out the juices inside. The mixture should appear wet, but if it is still dry and there is not enough sauce, add more coconut milk. Add potatoes and whole peanuts, cover, and lower heat.

Simmer for about 10 minutes, stirring occasionally to check consistency. The chicken should be in a rich sauce. If sauce is too thick, add more coconut milk. Stir in baby pearl onions and jalapeños. Cover and simmer another 5 to 10 minutes, or until potatoes and onions are tender.

Taste the curry sauce. Sprinkle in more fish sauce and coconut sugar as needed to adjust the flavors to your liking and stir in the tamarind. The curry should taste slightly sweet.

VIETNAMESE CHICKEN CURRY
Serves 4 • *496 calories per serving*

This curry recipe comes from Vietnam and contains sweet potato. It is adapted from *The Vietnamese Cookbook* by Diana My Tran.

2 teaspoons sea salt
½ teaspoon crushed red pepper
1 tablespoon coconut sugar
3 tablespoons curry powder
3 tablespoons tomato paste
1 pound boneless chicken breasts,
    cut into bite-sized pieces
2 tablespoons **Mary's Oil Blend**
    (page 188) or lard

3 garlic cloves, sliced
1 stalk lemongrass, peeled and cut
    into 1-inch pieces
1 cup chicken stock
1 can whole coconut milk
1 medium sweet potato,
    peeled and cut into large dice

In a large bowl, mash salt, red pepper, sugar, curry powder, and tomato paste together, using a fork. Coat chicken with this mixture and marinate for 10 minutes.

Heat oil blend in a deep pot or wok over medium-high heat. Add garlic and lemongrass and stir-fry until fragrant. Add chicken and stir-fry another 5 minutes, or until chicken browns slightly. Add stock and coconut milk. Stir in sweet potato and simmer for 20 minutes, or until sweet potato is tender.

MANGO CHICKEN
Serves 6 • *366 calories per serving*

This unusual dish from Western Samoa combines the tastes of coconut milk and mango.

1 large onion, thinly sliced
2 mangos, peeled and sliced
1 whole chicken, cut into pieces
2 tablespoons melted coconut oil or butter
1 teaspoon sea salt
½ teaspoon freshly ground pepper

¼ teaspoon paprika
Pinch of nutmeg
Grated rind of 1 lemon
1 cup chicken stock
Juice of 1 lemon
1 can whole coconut milk

Preheat oven to 350°F.

Strew onion slices in a large stainless-steel baking dish. Arrange mango slices in a layer on top of onions and place chicken pieces (breasts, legs, and thighs), skin side up, over mango. (Use the chicken backs and neck to make chicken stock unless you'd prefer not to, or are having trouble finding these at your local market.) Mix together coconut oil, salt, pepper, paprika, nutmeg, and lemon rind in a small bowl and brush on chicken pieces. Bake for about 1½ hours, or until chicken is nicely browned.

Remove chicken and mango slices to a heated platter. Pour chicken stock into the dish and bring to a boil over high heat, scraping up coagulated juices. Reduce heat and simmer, stirring in lemon juice and coconut milk. Strain into a small saucepan and continue to simmer to allow the liquid to reduce and thicken slightly.

BAKED COCONUT CHICKEN
Serves 6 • 421 calories per serving

1 cup sourdough breadcrumbs	1 egg
1 tablespoon curry powder	6 chicken thighs
1 teaspoon sea salt	¼ cup butter
1 cup desiccated coconut	¼ cup coconut oil
½ cup fresh orange juice	

Preheat oven to 350°F.

Mix together breadcrumbs, curry powder, salt, and coconut on a large plate. Pour orange juice into a small bowl and beat egg in another small bowl. Dip chicken thighs in orange juice, then in beaten egg, and then in breadcrumb mixture. Place prepared thighs in a buttered Pyrex pan just large enough to hold them. Melt butter and coconut oil together in a small saucepan over medium heat and pour over chicken. Bake for at least 1 hour, or until chicken is cooked through and nicely browned.

CHICKEN SATAY WITH PEANUT SAUCE
Serves 6 • 457 calories per serving

1½ pounds boneless chicken breasts, cut into pieces	1 clove garlic, crushed
½ cup coconut cream	1 small onion, finely chopped
1 tablespoon naturally fermented soy sauce	1 teaspoon sea salt
1 tablespoon fresh lemon juice	**Peanut Satay Sauce** (recipe follows)

Combine coconut cream, soy sauce, lemon juice, garlic, onion, and salt in a large bowl. Add chicken, cover, and place in refrigerator to marinate for several hours. Thread onto skewers and grill over a fire, on a barbecue, or under a grill, about 10 minutes per side, or until chicken is well-cooked but not dry. Serve with Peanut Satay Sauce.

PEANUT SATAY SAUCE

1 tablespoon coconut oil
1 onion, finely chopped
1 teaspoon grated fresh ginger
2 cloves garlic, crushed
½ cup natural peanut butter
1 cup coconut cream

2 tablespoons naturally fermented soy sauce
2 teaspoons coconut or maple sugar
1 jalapeño chile, seeded and finely chopped
2 tablespoons fresh lemon juice
Sea salt to taste

Warm coconut oil in a medium sauté pan over medium heat. Add onion, ginger, and garlic and sauté gently until onion is clear and golden. Add peanut butter and coconut cream and stir well. Add soy sauce, sugar, jalapeño, and lemon juice and season with salt. Lower heat and simmer for 10 minutes, or until sauce is thoroughly warmed.

Red Meat Entrées

Whenever possible, use grass-fed, farm-raised meats (see Resources).

LEFTOVER RED MEAT CURRY
Serves 4   •   436 calories per serving

2 tablespoons lard or **Mary's Oil Blend**
    (page 188)
2 cups leftover beef or lamb,
    cut into ¼-inch pieces
1 can whole coconut milk
2 cups beef stock
1 teaspoon red curry paste
1-inch piece ginger, peeled and chopped

Juice of 1 lemon or 2 limes
1 teaspoon coconut or maple sugar
1 teaspoon sea salt
2 tablespoons chopped fresh basil leaves
1 red pepper, seeded and cut into strips
1 cup Chinese peas, ends removed and cut on
    an angle into ½-inch pieces

Warm lard in a large pot over medium heat. Add meat and sauté, stirring frequently, for 10 minutes, or until meat has browned. Add remaining ingredients and simmer until vegetables are tender.

KOSHER POT ROAST WITH COCONUT GRAVY AND ROOT VEGETABLES
Serves 8 • 678 calories per serving

2 pounds chuck roast or skirt steak
¼ cup red wine vinegar or fresh lemon juice
About ½ cup unbleached white flour
Sea salt and freshly ground black pepper
   to taste
4 tablespoons **Mary's Oil Blend** (page 188)
1 cup red wine
2 to 3 cups beef stock

1 teaspoon tamarind paste (optional) or several
   slivers orange peel
1 pound carrots, peeled and cut into sticks
1 pound parsnips, peeled, cored, and cut into
   sticks
1½ pounds small red potatoes, washed but not
   peeled
1 can whole coconut milk

Tenderize the roast with a home tenderizer (available in hardware or kitchen stores). Rub red wine into roast. Place roast, along with remaining marinating liquid, in a shallow dish. Cover and keep in refrigerator several days, turning occasionally, or at room temperature for several hours. Preheat oven to 300°F. Mix flour, salt, and pepper together on a large plate. Discard marinade from roast, dry roast well with paper towels, and dredge in flour mixture. Heat oil blend in a large, ovenproof casserole over medium-high heat and brown roast on all sides. Remove to a plate. Add remaining flour mixture to oil and stir until well blended and browned. Add 1 cup red wine to pot and bring to a boil over high heat. Add stock, tamarind, and roast, bring back to a boil, cover, and place in oven for about 2 hours. Add carrots, parsnips, and potatoes, and cook another 2 hours, or until vegetables are very tender.

To serve, remove roast and vegetables to a platter. Add coconut milk to sauce and bring to a boil, reduce to desired thickness, and season with salt and pepper. Serve sauce separately in a gravy boat.

INDONESIAN COCONUT STEAK
Serves 4 • 546 calories per serving

3 tablespoons lard or **Mary's Oil Blend**
   (page 188)
1 large onion, sliced
1 garlic clove, crushed
1½ pound boneless sirloin or skirt steak,
   sliced into ½-inch strips
1 teaspoon ground ginger
1 teaspoon ground cumin
1 teaspoon ground coriander
1 teaspoon chili powder

⅔ cup desiccated coconut
2 teaspoons coconut or maple sugar
1 tablespoon fresh lemon juice
1¼ cups beef stock
1 red pepper, seeded and sliced thin,
   for garnish
2 to 3 small green chiles, seeded and sliced
   thin, for garnish
Small onion slices, for garnish

Heat lard in a large sauté pan over medium-high heat. Add onion slices and garlic and sauté 5 minutes, or until soft. Add beef and sauté, stirring, until browned, about 10 minutes. Stir in spices and cook 2 minutes. Stir in coconut, sugar, lemon juice, and beef stock. Lower heat and simmer, uncovered, 20 to 25 minutes, stirring occasionally, until sauce is reduced and meat is well coated. Garnish with slivers of bell pepper, green chiles, and small onion slices.

CURRIED LAMB CHOPS
Serves 4 • 635 calories per serving

2 tablespoons **Mary's Oil Blend** (page 188)
1 small onion, finely diced
2 cloves garlic, crushed
1 jalapeño chile, seeded and chopped
4 **Crispy Macadamia Nuts** (page 259)
½ teaspoon turmeric
½ teaspoon ground ginger
1 teaspoon grated lemon rind

Four 6-ounce lamb chops
Juice of 1 lemon
1 teaspoon coconut or maple sugar
1 teaspoon ground coriander
1 can whole coconut milk
1 cup beef or lamb stock
Sea salt and freshly ground black pepper to
  taste

Place oil blend, onion, garlic, jalapeño, macadamia nuts, turmeric, ground ginger, and lemon rind in a blender or food processor and process into a paste. Fry paste in a heavy frying pan over medium-high heat, stirring constantly, for 2 minutes. Dry off chops, add to pan and fry on both sides until brown, about 5 minutes each side. Add lemon juice, sugar, coriander, coconut milk, and stock and stir well. Reduce heat, cover, and simmer until chops are almost tender, about 20 minutes. Season with salt and pepper.

THAI COCONUT PORK CURRY
Serves 4 • 568 calories per serving

1 pound lean pork, cut into bite-sized strips
½ cup coconut or rice vinegar
1 pound Japanese eggplant,
  peeled and cut into bite-sized chunks
Sea salt
¼ cup lard or **Mary's Oil Blend** (page 188)
1 can whole coconut milk

2 to 3 teaspoons green curry paste
2 kaffir lime leaves
1 tablespoon Thai fish sauce
Juice of 1 lemon or 2 limes
2 teaspoons coconut sugar
¼ cup coarsely chopped fresh basil
1 jalapeño chile, seeded and finely chopped

Place pork in a large bowl, cover with vinegar, and marinate for several hours at room temperature. Place eggplant in a colander, toss with salt, and let sit for 1 hour. Rinse and drain eggplant, wrap in a kitchen towel, and squeeze out moisture. Drain pork from vinegar and pat dry. Warm lard in a large sauté pan over medium-high heat. Add pork and sauté until moisture evaporates and pork browns, about 10 minutes. Remove pork with a slotted spoon. Add eggplant and sauté in remaining lard. Return pork to pan, add remaining ingredients, and bring to a simmer. Simmer, covered, about 10 minutes, or until eggplant is tender.

INDONESIAN PORK IN COCONUT MILK
Serves 4 • 500 calories per serving

---

1 pound pork, cut into small cubes
¼ cup rice or coconut vinegar
2 small red chiles, seeded and finely chopped
2 small jalapeño chiles,
   seeded and finely chopped
3 cloves garlic, finely chopped
1-inch piece fresh ginger,
   peeled and finely chopped

2 teaspoons coconut or maple sugar
1 teaspoon salt
2 tablespoons lard or **Mary's Oil Blend**
   (page 188)
1 medium onion, diced
1 teaspoon grated lemon peel
Juice of 1 lemon
1 can whole coconut milk

Place pork in a large bowl, cover with vinegar, and marinate at room temperature for several hours. Drain and pat dry with paper towels. Put pork in a large bowl and stir in chiles, garlic, ginger, sugar, and salt. Marinate in this mixture at room temperature for 30 minutes.

Heat lard in a large sauté pan over medium heat. Add onion and sauté until softened, about 10 minutes. Add pork and marinade. Stir-fry mixture for 3 minutes. Add lemon peel, lemon juice, and coconut milk. Stir well and bring to a simmer. Simmer, uncovered, until pork is tender and sauce has thickened, about 40 minutes.

Vegetables

COCONUT MASHED POTATOES
Serves 6 • About 200 calories per serving

---

4 large baking potatoes
½ cup whole coconut milk
4 tablespoons butter or **Mary's Oil Blend**
   (page 188)

Sea salt to taste
1 tablespoon chopped fresh parsley
   or cilantro, for garnish

Peel potatoes, place in a large pot, and cover with water. Bring to a boil over high heat, then lower heat and simmer until potatoes are soft. Pour water out of pan and mash potatoes coarsely with a potato masher. Add coconut milk and butter and beat until smooth with a handheld electric beater. Season with salt. Transfer to a serving dish and garnish with parsley or cilantro.

COCONUT CARROTS
Serves 4 • *343 calories per serving*

1 pound carrots, peeled and cut into
　½-inch rounds
¼ cup ghee
¼ cup filtered water

2 tablespoons honey
½ cup **Coconut Sprinkles** (page 214) or freeze-
　dried fine-cut coconut

Blanch carrots in a large pot of boiling water until just tender. Drain and pat dry. Place in a large pan with ghee, water, and honey. Boil vigorously to reduce the liquid to a glaze, stirring frequently. Transfer to a serving dish and toss with Coconut Sprinkles or freeze-dried coconut.

COCONUT EGGPLANT FRITTERS
Serves 6 • *571 calories per serving*

2 large eggplants
Sea salt
½ cup lard or **Mary's Oil Blend**
　(page 188)

½ cup unbleached white flour
Sea salt and freshly ground black pepper to taste
½ recipe batter for **Coconut Pancakes**
　(page 208)

Peel eggplants and cut into ¼-inch slices. Rub each side with salt, place in a bowl, cover loosely with a kitchen towel, and leave for about 1 hour. Rinse eggplant slices in a colander and pat dry with paper towels. Heat lard in a large skillet over medium-high heat. Mix together flour, salt, and pepper on a large plate. Place pancake batter in a medium bowl. Dredge eggplant slices in flour mixture, then dip into batter. Fry on both sides until golden, about 5 minutes each side. Remove to paper towels and drain.

COCONUT CORN
Serves 6 • *287 calories per serving*

2 tablespoons ghee or **Mary's Oil Blend**
　(page 188)
1 green pepper, seeded and diced
1 red pepper, seeded and diced
1 red onion, peeled and chopped

2 tablespoons curry powder
Kernels from 8 ears of corn
1 can whole coconut milk
1 tablespoon chopped fresh cilantro
Sea salt to taste

Warm ghee in a large sauté pan over medium heat. Add peppers and onion and sauté until soft, about 5 minutes. Stir in curry powder. Add corn and coconut milk and bring to a simmer. Simmer, uncovered, until sauce thickens, about 5 minutes. Stir in cilantro and season with salt.

STRING BEANS WITH COCONUT
Serves 4 • 125 calories per serving

4 cups string beans, ends removed
2 tablespoons butter

2 tablespoons desiccated coconut

Cut string beans lengthwise with a knife, or use a food processor to make a French cut. Place in top of a two-part vegetable steamer and steam about 10 minutes, until bright green and just tender. Meanwhile, warm butter in a small skillet over medium heat. Add coconut and sauté until golden, about 3 minutes. Transfer beans to a serving dish and toss with the coconut-butter mixture.

INDIAN VEGETABLE MEDLEY WITH COCONUT
Serves 6 • 247 calories per serving

1 medium eggplant, peeled, cubed,
  and salted
3 medium zucchini, seeded,
  sliced into sticks, and salted
¼ cup **Mary's Oil Blend** (page 188) or ghee
2 cloves garlic, crushed
2 teaspoons black mustard seeds
2 teaspoons yellow mustard seeds
2 teaspoons cumin seeds

1 red pepper, seeded and sliced
1 green pepper, seeded and sliced
3 medium carrots, peeled and cut into
  sticks
1 cup chopped raw spinach
1 cup sweet potato, peeled and cut into
  sticks
1 cup coconut cream
1 cup plain whole yogurt

Let salted eggplant and zucchini sit for about 1 hour. Rinse in a colander and drain. Wrap in a kitchen towel and squeeze out excess moisture. Heat oil blend in large sauté pan over medium heat. Add garlic, mustard seeds, and cumin seeds; cover and cook for 1 minute. Add vegetables and cook, stirring occasionally, until vegetables are tender, about 10 minutes. Add coconut cream and yogurt and cook uncovered, stirring frequently, about 10 minutes, or until the sauce thickens.

Smoothies

YOGURT-COCONUT SMOOTHIE
Serves 1 • 544 calories

½ cup fresh or frozen berries
1 cup plain whole yogurt (or **Kefir**; page 261)
2 tablespoons maple syrup

2 egg yolks
1 tablespoon melted coconut oil

Place berries in a food processor and process to a puree. Add yogurt or kefir, maple syrup, and egg yolks and process until smooth. With the motor running, slowly add the coconut oil.

Quick and Easy Weight Loss version: Use a pinch of stevia powder in place of maple syrup (444 calories).

COCONUT SMOOTHIE
Serves 1   •   662 calories

1 ripe banana   2 egg yolks
½ cup whole coconut milk   1 teaspoon pure vanilla extract
2 tablespoons maple syrup

Place banana in food processor and process to a puree. Add remaining ingredients and process to a puree. Add enough water to obtain desired consistency.

Quick and Easy Weight Loss version: Use a pinch of stevia powder in place of maple syrup (562 calories).

Grains

Most of our grain recipes call for soaking to make the grains more digestible and neutralize phytic acid and enzyme inhibitors. The one exception is brown rice, which we cook for a long time in mineral-rich stock. Rice contains lower amounts of phytic acid and enzyme inhibitors than other grains, and these inhibitors are more easily neutralized in rice than in other grains.

Several recipes call for freshly ground whole-grain flour. Ideally, you would grind your own flour from whole-wheat berries at home, using a grain grinder, to be sure that the flour is fresh. If you buy whole-grain flour in a store, be sure to store it in the refrigerator or freezer.

COCONUT RICE
Serves 8   •   332 calories per serving

4 tablespoons butter, ghee, or   1 can whole coconut milk
   Mary's Oil Blend (page 188)   2½ cups chicken stock
3 cardamom pods   ½ teaspoon sea salt
2 cups long-grain brown rice   Pinch of saffron (optional)

Warm butter in a heavy, flameproof casserole over medium heat. Open cardamom pods and add to the casserole. Add rice to casserole and sauté, stirring constantly, until rice begins to turn whitish or milky, about 5 minutes. Pour in coconut milk and chicken stock, add salt and saffron, and bring to a rolling boil. Boil, uncovered, for about 10 minutes, or until water has reduced to level of the rice. Reduce heat to lowest setting, cover pot tightly, and cook for at least 1½ hours, or as long as 3 hours, if possible. Do not remove lid during cooking.

FANCY COCONUT RICE
Serves 8 • 531 calories per serving

This is a delicious party dish served with pork or chicken.

¼ cup ghee or clarified butter
½ cup chopped **Crispy Cashews** (page 259)
½ cup raisins
Pinch of nutmeg
½ teaspoon ground cardamom

¼ cup Sucanat, Rapadura, or maple sugar
1 cup **Coconut Sprinkles** (page 214) or freeze-dried fine-cut coconut
4 cups cooked **Coconut Rice** (previous recipe), prepared with saffron

Warm ghee in a medium skillet over medium heat. Add cashews and raisins and sauté about 5 minutes. Stir in nutmeg, cardamom, and sweetener and sauté, stirring, until sweetener dissolves. Fold cashew mixture and coconut into hot rice.

COCONUT RICE SALAD
Serves 8 • 396 calories per serving

4 cups cooked **Coconut Rice** (page 206), omitting saffron
1 red pepper, seeded and diced
1 green pepper, seeded and diced

1 bunch green onions, chopped
1 cup finely chopped fresh pineapple
½ cup raisins
¾ cup **Basic Salad Dressing** (page 237)

Mix all ingredients together in a large bowl. The rice can be pressed into a ring mold and inverted for serving.

COCONUT-LIME RICE
Serves 8 • 434 calories per serving

4 tablespoons butter, ghee, or **Mary's Oil Blend** (page 188)
2 cups long-grain brown rice
1 can whole coconut milk
2½ cups chicken stock
½ teaspoon sea salt
3 tablespoons clarified butter or ghee
1 tablespoon mustard seeds

½ cup chopped **Crispy Cashews** or **Almonds** (page 259)
½ teaspoon turmeric
2 jalapeño chiles, seeded and finely chopped
½ cup chopped fresh cilantro
½ cup fresh lime juice

Melt butter in a heavy, flameproof casserole over medium heat. Add rice and sauté, stirring constantly, until rice begins to turn whitish or milky, about 5 minutes. Pour in coconut milk and chicken stock, add salt, and bring to a rolling boil. Boil, uncovered, for about 10 minutes, or until water has reduced to the level of the rice. Reduce heat to lowest setting, cover tightly, and cook for at least 1½ hours, or as long as 3 hours. Do not remove lid during cooking.

While rice is cooking, warm clarified butter in a small skillet. Add mustard seeds, cashews, turmeric, and jalapeños and cook for 5 minutes, or until soft. Fold into cooked rice, along with cilantro and lime juice. Cook rice another 5 to 10 minutes and serve.

COCONUT PANCAKES
Makes about 20 • 125 calories per pancake

These pancakes cook more slowly than unsoaked whole-grain flour or white flour pancakes. The texture will be chewy but light and the taste pleasantly sour. Serve with melted butter and maple syrup or raw honey. Leftover pancakes can be put in an oven set at 200°F and allowed to dry out to make crispy pancakes, which are delicious with **Coconutty Butter** (page 212).

2 cups freshly ground spelt, kamut, or
  whole-wheat flour
2 cups **Kefir** (page 261) or yogurt
2 eggs, lightly beaten
½ teaspoon sea salt

1 teaspoon baking soda
2 tablespoons melted butter
1 cup **Coconut Sprinkles** (page 214) or
  freeze-dried coconut

Soak flour in kefir in a warm place for 12 to 24 hours. Stir in remaining ingredients and thin with water to desired consistency. Brush a griddle or cast-iron skillet with a little butter, heat, and cook pancakes about 5 minutes on each side or until nicely browned.

COCONUT MUFFINS
Makes about 15 • 207 calories per muffin

For best results, use stoneware muffin tins. The muffins will rise nicely but sink back down as they cool. The result is a dense, chewy muffin.

3 cups freshly ground spelt, kamut, or
  whole-wheat flour
2 cups whole yogurt or **Kefir** (page 261)
2 eggs, lightly beaten
1 teaspoon sea salt
¼ cup maple syrup

2 teaspoons baking soda
1 teaspoon pure vanilla extract
3 tablespoons melted butter
1 cup **Coconut Sprinkles** (page 214) or
  freeze-dried fine-cut coconut

Soak flour in yogurt in a warm place for 12 to 24 hours. Muffins will rise better if soaked for 24 hours. Preheat oven to 325°F. Blend in remaining ingredients. Pour into well-buttered and floured muffin tins (preferably stoneware), filling about three-quarters full. Bake for about 45 minutes, or until a toothpick inserted in center of muffin comes out clean. Cool on a wire rack before removing muffins.

COCONUT CRACKERS
Makes about 40 crackers • about 20 calories per cracker

If you have the time to make your own crackers, these will be superior to any-thing you can buy in the store. Unfortunately, as of this writing, there is no brand of commercial crackers made with coconut oil.

2½ cups freshly ground spelt, kamut,
   whole-wheat, or rye flour, or a mixture
1 cup plain yogurt
1 teaspoon sea salt

1½ teaspoon baking powder
½ cup melted coconut oil
Unbleached white flour

Mix flour with yogurt and leave in a warm place for 12 to 24 hours. Preheat oven to 200°F. Place soaked flour, salt, baking powder, and ¼ cup coconut oil in a food processor and process until well blended. Roll out to about ¹⁄₁₆ inch on a pas-try cloth dusted with white flour to prevent sticking. Cut into 2-inch squares with a knife. Place on an oiled cookie sheet, brush with remaining ¼ cup coconut oil, and bake in oven (or a dehydrator) for several hours, or until completely dry and crisp. Store in an airtight container in the refrigerator.

POPCORN
Makes 8 cups • 94 calories per cup

---

2 tablespoons **Mary's Oil Blend**
   (page 188)
¼ cup popcorn

Sea salt to taste
¼ cup melted coconut oil or butter,
   or a mixture

Warm oil blend in a large, heavy skillet over medium heat. Add popcorn, cover tightly, and cook, shaking constantly until popping starts. Lower heat slightly and cook, shaking, until popping dies away. (If using a popper, place oil blend and corn in the popper and proceed according to instructions.) Transfer popcorn to a large bowl. Dribble on melted coconut oil and shake on salt. Mix well and serve.

COCONUT GRANOLA
Makes 12 cups • 748 calories per ½-cup serving

This ingenious granola recipe is the invention of Sonja Kepford, a Weston A. Price Foundation chapter leader. The oats are soaked in a yogurt mixture and then slow-baked in a warm oven or a dehydrator. Granola is very caloric and should be avoided by those trying to lose weight, as well as by those who have a poor toler-ance of grains.

8 cups rolled oats
½ cup melted butter
½ cup melted coconut oil
1½ cups whole yogurt
2 cups water
½ cup raw honey

1 teaspoon sea salt
1 teaspoon ground cinnamon
1 cup **Coconut Sprinkles** (page 214) or freeze-
    dried fine-cut coconut
2 cups chopped **Crispy Nuts** (page 259)
1 cup raisins

Mix oats, butter, coconut oil, yogurt, and water together in a large bowl. Pat down, cover with a plate, and leave on the kitchen counter for 2 days. Preheat oven to 200°F. Place honey, salt, and cinnamon in a small bowl and set in a small pot of simmering water until honey warms and becomes thin. Mix honey with oat mixture. Place on 2 parchment-lined cookie sheets and bake for several hours, until completely dry and crisp. Mix with Coconut Sprinkles, chopped nuts, and raisins. Store in airtight container in refrigerator. Serve with whole raw milk or cream diluted with a little water.

Legumes

JAMAICAN-STYLE BEANS AND RICE
Serves 8   •   257 calories per serving

1 cup red kidney beans
1 tablespoon **Homemade Whey** (page 227),
    vinegar, or fresh lemon juice
1 can whole coconut milk
1 bunch green onions, chopped
3 jalapeño chiles, seeded and chopped

3 cloves garlic, mashed
2 teaspoons dried thyme
2 teaspoons sea salt
1 teaspoon dried green peppercorns, crushed
1 cup brown rice, soaked at least 7 hours

Place beans in a large bowl and cover with warm water. Stir in whey and leave overnight in a warm place. In the morning, drain and rinse beans and place in a pot. Add enough water to cover beans, bring to a boil, and skim. Add remaining ingredients except rice. Lower heat, cover, and simmer for 6 to 8 hours, or until beans are very tender. Drain rice and add to the pot along with enough filtered water to cover the rice and beans by about ½ inch. Bring to a boil and cook, uncovered, until liquid has reduced to level of rice and beans. Lower heat, cover, and cook on lowest heat for about 30 minutes, or until rice is tender.

COCONUT BLACK-EYED PEAS
Serves 8 • 286 calories per serving

This recipe comes from Tanzania.

1 cup black-eyed peas	1 tablespoon ground coriander
2 tablespoons **Homemade Whey** (page 227),	2 teaspoons turmeric
vinegar, or fresh lemon juice	1 tablespoon chopped fresh cilantro
2 tablespoons ghee or	1 cup desiccated coconut
Mary's Oil Blend (page 188)	2 cups diced cooked potatoes
3 cloves garlic, crushed	Juice of 1 lemon or 2 limes
1 teaspoon chili powder	Sea salt to taste
1 tablespoon ground cumin	

Place black-eyed peas in a large bowl and cover with warm water. Stir in whey and leave overnight in a warm place. In the morning, drain and rinse black-eyed peas and place in a large pot. Add enough water to cover peas, bring to a boil, and skim. Cook for about 3 hours and drain.

Heat ghee in a large sauté pan over medium heat. Add garlic and chili powder and sauté for half a minute. Add cumin, coriander, turmeric, and cilantro. Cook for another minute or two, stirring often to blend. Add coconut and mix well. Add cooked beans and potatoes. Add lemon juice and season with salt. Cook for another 10 minutes or so, until thoroughly warmed.

NUTS

Our coconut-nut recipes use **Crispy Nuts** (page 259). Although very nutritious, nuts are highly caloric and should be avoided if you are trying to lose weight.

COCONUT WALNUTS OR PECANS
Makes 2 cups • 350 calories per ¼-cup serving

2 tablespoons butter	½ teaspoon plus a pinch of sea salt
2 tablespoons Rapadura, Sucanat,	2 cups **Crispy Walnuts** or Pecans (page 259)
or maple sugar	1 egg white
½ cup freeze-dried fine-cut coconut	

Preheat oven to 300°F. Melt butter with Rapadura, coconut, and ½ teaspoon salt and toss with nuts. In a clean bowl, beat egg white with a pinch of salt until soft peaks form. Fold in nuts. Spread on cookie sheets and bake for about 30 minutes, turning occasionally, until egg white is thoroughly dried. Store in an airtight container in the refrigerator.

COCONUTTY BUTTER
Makes 2½ cups • *320 calories per ¼-cup serving*

This nut butter is so delicious that it's hard to stop eating it. So if you are on the Quick and Easy Weight Loss plan, do not make Coconutty Butter! (However, it's great for those who need to gain weight.)

2 cups **Crispy Nuts** (page 259),
   such as peanuts, almonds, or cashews
1 teaspoon sea salt

2 tablespoons raw honey
¾ cup coconut oil, softened

Place nuts and salt in a food processor and grind to a fine powder. Add honey and coconut oil and process until "butter" becomes smooth. It will be somewhat liquid but will harden when chilled. Store in an airtight container in the refrigerator. Serve at room temperature.

COCONUTTY FUDGE
Makes about 2 dozen small squares • *188 calories per square*

---

2 cups **Crispy Almonds** (page 259)
1 cup coconut oil, softened
1 cup raw honey
1 cup carob or cocoa powder

2 teaspoons chocolate extract
   (if using carob powder)
1 teaspoon pure vanilla extract
½ teaspoon sea salt

Place all ingredients in a food processor and process until well blended. Line a large loaf pan with parchment paper and spread mixture about ½ inch thick. Wrap up in parchment paper and refrigerate several hours. Cut into small squares and store in an airtight container in the refrigerator.

COCONUT ALMOND COOKIES
Makes about 20 • *185 calories per cookie*

1½ cups **Crispy Almonds** (page 259),
   plus 20 to top cookies
½ cup coconut oil or butter, softened
1 cup arrowroot powder
½ cup Rapadura, Sucanat, or maple sugar
½ teaspoon sea salt

Grated rind of 1 lemon
1 teaspoon pure vanilla extract
1 teaspoon pure coconut extract
½ cup desiccated or freeze-dried fine-cut
   coconut

Preheat oven to 300°F. Place almonds in a food processor and process to a fine meal. Add remaining ingredients, except 20 almonds, and process until well blended. Form dough into walnut-sized balls and place on buttered cookie sheets. Press an almond into each. Bake for about 5 minutes, then press cookies down lightly with a fork. Bake another 15 minutes, or until lightly browned. Let cool completely before removing to an airtight container. Store in refrigerator.

COCONUTTY CANDIES
Makes about 32 • 146 calories per candy

Children love these!

½ cup **Crispy Almonds** (page 259)
1½ cups coconut oil, softened
⅔ cup freeze-dried fine-cut coconut
5 tablespoons cocoa powder

¼ cup raw honey
3 tablespoons butter, softened
½ cup natural peanut butter or hazelnut butter

Grind almonds in a food processor. Add remaining ingredients and process until well blended. Pour into ice cube trays and refrigerate or freeze.

COCONUT-ALMOND KISSES
Makes about 12 • 53 calories per kiss

2 egg whites
Pinch of sea salt
¼ cup Rapadura, Sucanat, or maple sugar
⅛ cup cocoa powder

¼ teaspoon pure almond extract
½ cup **Crispy Almonds** (page 259) ground up in a food processor
1 cup desiccated coconut

Preheat oven to 375°F. Line a cookie sheet with parchment paper and rub with butter or coconut oil. Beat egg whites with a pinch of salt in a very clean bowl until stiff. Beat in sweetener, cocoa powder, and almond extract. Fold in almonds and coconut. Drop by rounded teaspoonfuls onto cookie sheet. Bake for 12 to 15 minutes, or until nicely colored. Remove from oven, let stand a minute or two, then remove with a spatula and cool completely on a rack.

Desserts

Coconut is an absolutely delicious ingredient in desserts. Occasional desserts like these, made with coconut and other whole foods such as fruit, butter, cream, nuts, and eggs, are fine in moderation for most people. If you're struggling with weight gain, though, you must curtail your consumption of sweets, even healthy sweets. When you do eat sweets, choose those containing coconut products, which will minimize the tendency to gain weight.

And if you're on Phase Two of Quick and Easy Weight Loss, avoid desserts and sweet snacks altogether.

COCONUT SPRINKLES
Makes 2 cups • 53 calories per tablespoon

An excellent topping for many desserts, salads, and curries. Coconut Sprinkles are similar to freeze-dried fine-cut coconut (see Resources), which is also crunchy and made naturally sweet by the freeze-drying process.

2 cups unsweetened desiccated coconut   ½ cup maple syrup

Mix coconut with maple syrup in a medium bowl and spread on a stainless-steel baking pan. Bake at low temperature (about 200°F) until coconut is dried out. Break up with hands and store in an airtight container.

AMBROSIA
Serves 8 • 165 calories per serving

---

8 large navel oranges   1 cup **Coconut Sprinkles** (previous recipe) or
¼ cup Grand Marnier   freeze-dried fine-cut coconut

Peel and slice oranges. Place in a serving bowl and sprinkle on Grand Marnier and Coconut Sprinkles. Chill well before serving.

AKWADU
Serves 6 • 225 calories per serving

Coconut, lemon, and orange distinguish this banana dessert that comes from Ghana.

6 medium bananas   3 tablespoons Sucanat, Rapadura, or maple
1 tablespoon butter   sugar
Juice of 2 small oranges   ⅔ cup **Coconut Sprinkles** (see above) or freeze-
Juice of 1 lemon   dried fine-cut coconut

Preheat oven to 375°F. Cut bananas crosswise into halves; cut each half lengthwise into halves and arrange in a greased 9-by-13-inch Pyrex dish. Dot with butter and drizzle with orange and lemon juice. Top with sweetener and sprinkle with Coconut Sprinkles. Bake for 8 to 10 minutes, or until coconut is golden.

THAI BANANA DESSERT IN COCONUT MILK
Serves 4 • 376 calories per serving

This authentic Thai recipe is adapted from *It Rains Fishes: Legends, Traditions and the Joys of Thai Cooking* by Kasma Loha-Unchit.

4 large red bananas, fully ripened
1 can whole coconut milk
¼ cup coconut sugar

¼ teaspoon sea salt
Few drops of mali (Thai jasmine) essence
(optional), available in Asian markets

If red bananas are unavailable, use regular yellow ones. Peel bananas just before you are ready to cook. Cut in half lengthwise, then cut each half into 4 pieces crosswise. Heat coconut milk in a large saucepan, over medium heat. Add sugar, salt, and mali essence, if using. When mixture is hot and smooth, add bananas and simmer about 5 minutes, or until bananas are cooked but still in whole pieces. Serve warm.

BAKED PEARS IN COCONUT MILK
Serves 4 • 547 calories per serving

---

4 ripe Bartlett pears
Juice of 1 lemon
1 can whole coconut milk
4 tablespoons butter
½ cup chopped **Crispy Walnuts** or
Pecans (page 259)

½ cup freeze-dried fine-cut coconut or **Coconut
Sprinkles** (page 214)
2 tablespoons Rapadura, Sucanat, or maple
sugar

Preheat oven to 350°F. Cut pears in half lengthwise, peel, core, and brush with lemon juice. Arrange in a buttered baking dish just large enough to hold pears. Pour coconut milk over pears and bake about 15 minutes. Remove from oven, cool to room temperature, then place in refrigerator to chill. Meanwhile, warm butter in a small skillet over medium heat. Add chopped nuts, coconut, and sweetener and sauté until lightly browned, about 5 minutes. To serve, place 2 pear halves in a bowl, spoon coconut milk over pears, and sprinkle with nut-coconut mixture.

COCONUT CUSTARD
Serves 4 • 302 calories per serving

Another recipe adapted from *It Rains Fishes: Legends, Traditions and the Joys of Thai Cooking* by Kasma Loha-Unchit.

1 cup coconut cream
½ cup coconut sugar

5 eggs
½ teaspoon pure vanilla extract

Heat coconut cream and sugar in a medium saucepan just long enough to dissolve sugar and blend with cream into a smooth mixture. Allow to cool to room temperature. While cream is cooling, preheat oven to 350°F. Beat eggs well and mix in with cooled sweetened coconut cream. Stir in vanilla. Divide mixture among 4 buttered custard cups. Set cups in a pan of hot water and bake for about 30 minutes, or until custard sets and a toothpick comes out clean. Chill well before serving. This dish is delicious served with tropical fruits.

COCONUT MILK ICE CREAM
Serves 6 • 320 calories per serving

½ cup coconut sugar
4 egg yolks
1 tablespoon coconut rum

1 can whole coconut milk
1 cup heavy cream, preferably raw

In a large bowl, beat together sugar and egg yolks until pale in color, about 5 minutes. Whisk in rum, coconut milk, and cream. Freeze in an ice cream maker according to manufacturer's instructions. Serve immediately or store in the freezer.

EASY COCONUT PUDDING
Serves 6 • 570 calories per serving

2 cans whole coconut milk

2 cups freeze-dried coconut

Stir together coconut milk and dried coconut in a bowl and refrigerate overnight. The pudding will be ready in the morning. Added sugar is not necessary in this recipe because of the natural sweetness of the freeze-dried coconut.

COCOA-COCONUT CREAM
Serves 6 • 295 calories per serving

2 cups ricotta cheese, softened
⅓ cup unsweetened cocoa powder
½ cup Sucanat, Rapadura, or maple sugar
½ teaspoon pure vanilla extract
2 tablespoons coconut oil, softened

2 egg yolks
Pinch of sea salt
1 tablespoon coconut rum
¼ cup **Coconut Sprinkles** (page 214) or freeze-dried coconut, for garnish

Place ricotta in a food processor and process until very smooth. Gradually add other ingredients (except Coconut Sprinkles or freeze-dried coconut), processing until smooth. Divide among 6 bowls or parfait glasses and top with Coconut Sprinkles or freeze-dried coconut.

COCONUT MACAROONS
Makes about 15 • 163 calories per macaroon

No sugar is needed in this recipe because of the natural sweetness of the freeze-dried coconut. This is a good way to use up egg whites left over from recipes calling for egg yolks.

4 egg whites
Pinch of sea salt

About 2½ cups freeze-dried fine-cut coconut

Preheat oven to 300°F. Line a baking sheet with buttered parchment paper. Beat egg whites with salt in a bowl until they form stiff peaks. Fold in enough coconut so mixture forms balls, but not so much that mixture is crumbly. Place balls on baking sheet and bake for 30 minutes. Reduce oven temperature to 200°F and bake another hour or so until macaroons are chewy. (If you like your macaroons crisper, bake several hours more.) Remove from oven and let cool completely before removing from parchment paper. Store in an airtight container.

WHIPPED COCONUT CREAM
Makes 2 cups • 33 calories per tablespoon

Coconut cream will whip just like dairy cream, but it takes longer.

1½ cups coconut cream
2 tablespoons Rapadura,
    Sucanat, or maple sugar

1 teaspoon pure vanilla extract

Place cream in a large bowl and whip with an electric mixer at highest speed for several minutes until cream thickens. Add sweetener and vanilla and whip a minute more.

COCONUT BARS
Makes 16 • 208 calories per serving

¾ cup **Crispy Almonds** (page 259)
¼ cup butter or coconut oil, softened
½ cup plus 2 tablespoons arrowroot
¼ cup Rapadura, Sucanat, or maple sugar
1 teaspoon pure vanilla extract
2 pinches of sea salt
1 egg

¼ cup crème fraîche or sour cream
½ cup maple syrup
1 tablespoon pure vanilla extract
Grated rind of 1 lemon
1½ cups **Coconut Sprinkles** (page 214) or
    freeze-dried fine-cut coconut

Preheat oven to 300°F. Place almonds in a food processor and process to a fine powder. Add butter, ½ cup of arrowroot, 1 teaspoon vanilla, sweetener, and a pinch of salt and process until smooth. Press into a well-oiled 9-by-9- or 7-by-11-inch Pyrex pan. Bake 20 minutes. Remove from oven and let cool. Increase oven temperature to 325°F.

In a large bowl, beat egg with cream, maple syrup, 1 tablespoon vanilla, lemon rind, remaining 2 tablespoons arrowroot, and pinch of salt. Stir in Coconut Sprinkles and spread over almond pastry. Bake for about 25 minutes, or until filling is set. Let cool slightly before cutting into bars. Let cool completely before removing bars from the pan.

COCONUT PIE CRUST
Serves 8 • *293 calories per serving for the pie crust itself*

2 cups desiccated coconut
¼ cup Rapadura, Sucanat, or maple sugar

½ cup melted butter or coconut oil

Preheat oven to 300°F. Mix coconut, sweetener, and butter together in a small bowl. Transfer to a buttered and floured 9-inch pie pan and press firmly and evenly against the bottom and sides. Bake for 30 minutes, or until crust is a dark golden color. Allow to cool to room temperature.

COCONUT MOUSSE PIE
Serves 8 • *546 calories per serving*

4 egg yolks, at room temperature
½ cup Rapadura, Sucanat, or
   maple sugar
1 teaspoon pure vanilla extract
1 tablespoon coconut rum
1 cup heavy cream, preferably raw,
   well chilled

1 tablespoon gelatin dissolved in 2 tablespoons warm
   water
4 egg whites, at room temperature
Pinch of sea salt
1 cup grated fresh coconut, 1 cup **Coconut Sprinkles**
   (page 214), or 1 cup freeze-dried coconut
1 recipe **Coconut Pie Crust** (previous recipe), baked

Place egg yolks and sweetener in a large bowl and beat with an electric mixer for several minutes until a pale ribbon forms. Blend in vanilla, rum, cream, and melted gelatin. In a separate bowl, beat egg whites with salt until stiff. Fold egg yolk mixture and coconut into egg white mixture. Pour into pie shell and chill well.

COCONUT CUSTARD PIE
Serves 8 • *542 calories per serving*

3 eggs
½ cup Rapadura, Sucanat, or maple sugar
1 can whole coconut milk
1 teaspoon pure vanilla extract
1 tablespoon coconut rum

Pinch of nutmeg
1 recipe **Coconut Pie Crust** (see above) or **Flaky
   Pie Crust** (page 259), unbaked
1 cup **Whipped Coconut Cream** (page 217) or
   whipped cream

Preheat oven to 350°F. Place eggs and sweetener in a large bowl and beat until well blended. Beat in coconut milk, vanilla, coconut rum, and nutmeg. Pour into pie shell and bake for about 45 minutes, or until a toothpick inserted in center comes out clean. Remove from oven and let cool. Spread whipped cream over pie and chill well.

COCONUTTY TART
Serves 8 • 514 calories per serving

1 recipe **Flaky Pie Crust** (page 259), unbaked
1⅓ cup **Crispy Walnuts** or **Pecans** (page 259)
4 tablespoons butter, melted
⅓ cup Rapadura, Sucanat, or maple sugar
2 eggs

2 tablespoons brandy
1 tablespoon coconut rum
½ teaspoon sea salt
1 cup **Coconut Sprinkles** (page 214) or freeze-dried fine-cut coconut

Preheat oven to 350°F. Line a 10-inch French-style tart pan with removable bottom with Flaky Pie Crust dough. Process nuts in a food processor to a fine powder. Add remaining ingredients except Coconut Sprinkles to processor and process until smooth. Add Coconut Sprinkles and pulse a few times until mixed in. Pour into tart shell and bake for about 40 minutes, or until a toothpick comes out clean.

FLOURLESS COCOA-COCONUT CAKE
Serves 10 • 321 calories per serving

Thanks to Katherine Czapp of the Weston A. Price Foundation's Ann Arbor chapter for this delicious recipe.

7 tablespoons sifted arrowroot powder, plus more for dusting
⅓ cup sifted unsweetened cocoa powder
⅛ teaspoon ground cinnamon
4 egg whites, at room temperature
Pinch of sea salt
⅜ cup Rapadura, Sucanat, or maple sugar

4 egg yolks, at room temperature
1 teaspoon pure vanilla extract
¼ cup Rapadura, Sucanat, or maple sugar
1 cup freeze-dried coarse-cut coconut, plus more to top cake
2 cups **Whipped Coconut Cream** (page 217) or whipped cream

Preheat oven to 350°F. Butter a 9-inch springform cake pan and dust with arrowroot. Sift together arrowroot, cocoa, and cinnamon. In a very clean glass or stainless-steel bowl, beat egg whites with a pinch of salt until frothy. Gradually add ⅜ cup sweetener. Whip whites until glossy and smooth. Set aside.

In another large bowl, beat egg yolks with vanilla until pale in color, about 3 minutes. Gradually add ¼ cup sweetener and beat until yolks are pale and a thick ribbon falls from the beaters, 6 to 7 minutes.

With a rubber spatula, fold about ⅓ of whites into yolks. Sprinkle about ¼ cup of dry ingredients on the yolk batter and fold in gently. Continue to alternately fold in egg whites and dry ingredients. Finally, quickly fold in the coconut.

Turn batter into prepared pan, gently smooth top, and place in oven. Bake 30 minutes, or until cake pulls away from sides of pan and middle springs back if gently pressed. Let cool on a rack about 10 minutes. Release sides and wait another 10 minutes before removing cake. Place on a serving plate and chill well. Ice with whipped cream and gently press freeze-dried coconut into top and sides of cake.

COCONUT CARROT CAKE
Serves 20 • *444 calories per serving*

2½ cups freshly ground spelt, kamut, or whole-wheat flour
1 cup crème fraîche or sour cream
1 cup whole yogurt
1 cup butter or coconut oil, softened
¾ cup Rapadura, Sucanat, or maple sugar
4 eggs
2 teaspoons baking soda
1 teaspoon ground cinnamon
2 teaspoons pure vanilla extract

1 teaspoon sea salt
8-ounce can water-packed crushed pineapple
2 cups finely grated carrots
1 cup freeze-dried coarse-cut coconut
½ cup chopped **Crispy Pecans** (page 259)

For the Icing
2 cups cream cheese, softened
½ cup butter, softened
1 tablespoon pure vanilla extract
½ cup raw honey

Mix together flour, yogurt, and cultured cream in a large bowl. Cover and leave in a warm place for 12 to 24 hours. Preheat oven to 300°F. Butter a 9 by 13-inch Pyrex pan, coat it with unbleached flour, then line it with buttered parchment paper and coat the paper with unbleached flour. Cream butter with sweetener. Beat in eggs, baking soda, cinnamon, vanilla, and salt. Gradually add flour mixture. Fold in pineapple (with juice), carrots, coconut, and nuts. Pour into pan and bake for about 2 hours or until a toothpick comes out clean. Let cool slightly and turn onto a platter or tray.

To make icing, place cream cheese, butter, vanilla, and honey in a food processor and blend until smooth. Generously ice top and sides of cake. Decorate with flowers.

Beverages and Tonics

COCONUT MILK TONIC
Makes 4 cups • *213 calories per cup*

Our Coconut Milk Tonic contains the same amount of calories and calcium as milk. It's an excellent substitute if you can't obtain raw milk or are allergic to milk.

1 can whole coconut milk
1¾ cups water
2 tablespoons maple syrup

1 teaspoon pure vanilla extract
1 teaspoon dolomite powder (see Resources)

Mix all ingredients together in a medium saucepan over medium-low heat, and heat until warm and dolomite is dissolved.

Quick and Easy Weight Loss version: Use a pinch of stevia powder instead of maple syrup (189 calories per cup).

COCONUT LIME COOLER
Makes about 4 cups • *245 calories per cup*

1 can whole coconut milk
4 tablespoons maple syrup

½ cup fresh lime juice
1 cup ice

Place all ingredients in a blender and process until ice is broken up.

COCONUT ORANGE JULIUS
Makes 4 cups • *272 calories per cup*

1 can whole coconut milk
2 egg yolks

2 cups fresh orange juice

Place all ingredients in a blender and process until frothy.

COCONUT COCOA
Makes 3 cups • *303 calories per cup*

1 can whole coconut milk
1 cup water
2 tablespoons maple syrup

2 tablespoons unsweetened cocoa powder
1 teaspoon pure vanilla extract
¾ teaspoon dolomite powder (optional)

Place all ingredients in a medium saucepan over medium-low heat and warm, stirring with a whisk, until ingredients are blended.

COCONUT EGGNOG
Makes 2 cups • *276 calories per ½ cup*

1 can whole coconut milk
4 egg yolks
1 teaspoon pure vanilla extract
¼ teaspoon ground nutmeg

¼ teaspoon ground cinnamon
1 tablespoon maple syrup
2 tablespoons brandy

Place all ingredients in a blender or food processor and blend until frothy.

COCONUT FRUIT SHRUB
Makes 2 quarts   •   35 calories per ½ cup

This easy beverage from colonial times is surprisingly good. The vinegar taste disappears after two days at room temperature, leaving complex sweet-and-sour fruit flavors. Our thanks to Liz Pitfield for her adaptation using coconut vinegar.

2 cups crushed fruit, such as raspberries,   1 cup coconut vinegar
    blackberries, or very ripe peaches   5 cups water

Mix all ingredients together in a glass container. Cover tightly and leave at room temperature for 2 days. Strain and store in the refrigerator. To serve, mix ½ cup shrub with 1 to 2 cups sparkling water and add a pinch of sea salt.

COCONUT KEFIR
Makes 2 quarts   •   70 calories per cup

Coconut juice is widely valued for its medicinal properties and is considered especially beneficial for the kidneys and for digestion. When fermented with kefir powder or grains (see Resources), it makes a tart, bubbly drink loaded with minerals, enzymes, and beneficial bacteria.

2 quarts packaged coconut water   1 package kefir powder or ¾ cup water kefir
    (see Resources) or juice of about   grains
    6 green coconuts

If using green coconuts, pierce coconuts with an ice pick, screwdriver, or electric drill and allow juice to drain through a non-metallic strainer into a glass bowl. Place coconut juice in a glass container and stir in kefir powder or grains. Seal the top of the container. Leave at room temperature for 48 hours.

Store the coconut kefir in the original glass container in the refrigerator, or, for extra bubbly results, transfer to glass beer or soda bottles capped with wire-held cap (see Resources).

Note: Do not store kefir in decorative vinegar bottles that have wire-held stoppers; these have a tendency to explode and can be quite dangerous!

You can reuse the grains immediately to make more coconut kefir, or store them in the refrigerator in a small glass jar with ½ to 1 cup coconut kefir or water plus 1 tablespoon Sucanat or Rapadura. The grains double in size every time you use them, so you can give them to your friends.

If you have used the powder, reserve about ½ cup of the finished kefir and use it instead of powder to inoculate the next batch of coconut kefir. The reserved coconut kefir will work for 5 to 6 batches before you need to use powder again.

Chapter Ten

Traditional Recipes

In this chapter, you'll learn how to make a variety of traditional foods, as well as basics like stocks and lacto-fermented condiments, that you can incorporate into a wide range of nourishing and satisfying recipes.

*Note: Many of our recipes call for **Mary's Oil Blend** (page 188). It's a good idea to make a large batch, so you'll have it on hand whenever you need it.*

Stocks

Given our hectic modern lifestyle, it may seem that preparing stocks from scratch is just too much trouble. Remember, though, that stocks are key, not only to good health, but to delicious food. Bone broths or stocks are the basis of wonderful sauces, soups, and gravies. They also provide minerals—especially calcium—in an easily absorbable form, as well as digestion-enhancing gelatin.

The easiest stock to make is chicken stock. You can make it from raw whole chicken or raw chicken parts, or you can use the bones left over from a chicken meal. Either way, you're making use of the whole animal. If you've never made stock before, one try should convince you that it's really not very difficult, and the health and culinary benefits will be very gratifying!

If making stock just doesn't fit into your busy schedule—especially beef stock, which is more complicated—you can buy good-quality frozen stock in certain specialty stores and through the Internet (see Resources). Be aware, though, that this is an expensive alternative. If you're on Health Recovery, which calls for stock with almost every meal to provide minerals and help heal the digestive system, you will find it much more economical to make your own. **Quick Chicken Stock** (page 224) is a less than ideal alternative to regular homemade or frozen stock, but **Quick Fish Stock** (page 226) is an excellent easy, traditional stock that is nutritionally equivalent to the more classic **Fish Stock** recipe (page 226).

Conveniently, stock can be made in bulk and stored until needed. Clear stock will keep about five days in the refrigerator, longer if reboiled, and several months in the freezer. You may find it useful to store stock in pint- or quart-sized plastic containers in order to have appropriate amounts on hand for sauces and stews. (Be sure to let it cool completely before transferring it to plastic containers.)

If space is at a premium in your freezer, you can reduce the stock by boiling it down for several hours until it becomes very concentrated and syrupy. This reduced, concentrated stock—called *fumet* or *demi-glace*—can be stored in small containers or ziplock bags. Frozen *fumet* in bags is easily thawed by putting the bags under warm running water. Add water to thawed *fumet* to turn it back into stock. Be sure to mark which kind of stock you are storing with stick-on labels—they all look alike when frozen.

Calorie count: Stock provides about 15 calories per cup (30 calories per cup if reduced by half).

RICH CHICKEN STOCK

Making stock is the best way to use the bony parts of a chicken, or the bones left over from a chicken meal. If you want a lot of leftover meat, to make chicken salad, for example, start with a whole chicken. Whenever possible, use pasture-fed and/or organic chicken. If you buy chicken directly from a farmer, be sure to ask for the head and feet and use these in the stock—they contain a lot of gelatin. (In France, when you buy a chicken from a butcher, the head and feet are always included, precisely for stock making.)

Neck, back, and wings from 1 chicken plus head and feet (optional), or carcass or bones from 1 baked or roasted chicken, or 1 whole raw chicken	¼ cup vinegar (any type) 3 stalks celery, chopped 2 onions, chopped 2 carrots, peeled and chopped
4 quarts cold filtered water	1 teaspoon dried green peppercorns, crushed

Preheat oven to 400°F. Place chicken parts in a large stainless-steel pan and brown for about ½ hour. (Omit this step if you are making stock with a whole chicken.) Place chicken in a stockpot and add remaining ingredients. Leave 1 hour. Place on the stove and heat over medium heat. When stock starts to simmer, reduce heat to lowest setting. Stock should gently simmer, not boil. Simmer for at least 2 hours, or as long as 24 hours. Remove chicken pieces and strain stock. Remove any additional meat from backs, neck, and wings and use in soups and salads. (If you are using a whole chicken, separate the meat from the bones and the skin after it cooks. The bones may be used to make stock a second time.)

Chill strained stock and remove any fat that congeals at the top. (There is nothing wrong with this fat, but the best clear sauces are made with chicken stock from which the fat has been removed.)

QUICK CHICKEN STOCK
Makes 1 quart

Two 14-ounce cans Health Valley chicken stock   1 teaspoon dolomite powder (see Resources)

Place stock and dolomite in a medium saucepan over medium heat, and heat until dolomite is dissolved.

BEEF STOCK

Beef stock is more difficult to make than chicken stock—but not that difficult. And it's the first step in producing delicious pot roasts and meat sauces. Whenever possible, use grass-fed and/or organic meat and bones.

About 4 pounds beef marrow and
    knuckle bones
1 calf's foot, cut into pieces (optional)
½ cup vinegar (any type)
4 or more quarts cold filtered water
3 pounds meaty rib or neck bones

3 onions, coarsely chopped
3 carrots, coarsely chopped
3 celery sticks, coarsely chopped
Several sprigs of fresh thyme, tied together
    (optional)
1 teaspoon dried green peppercorns, crushed

Preheat oven to 400°F. Place marrow and knuckle bones and calf's foot, if using, in a very large pot. Add vinegar and cover with water. Let stand for 1 hour. Meanwhile, place meaty bones in a roasting pan, place in oven, and bake until well browned, about 1 hour. Add meaty bones to pot, then add vegetables. Pour fat out of roasting pan, add cold water to pan, set over high heat, and bring to a boil, stirring with a wooden spoon to loosen coagulated juices. Add this liquid to pot. Add additional water, if necessary, to cover the bones, but liquid should come no higher than within 1 inch of rim of pot, since volume expands slightly during cooking. Bring to a boil. A large amount of scum will come to the top, and it is important to remove this with a spoon. After you have skimmed, reduce heat and add thyme and crushed peppercorns. Simmer stock for at least 12 hours and as long as 72 hours.

Remove bones with tongs or a slotted spoon. Remove any meat and use in soups and salads. Strain stock into a large bowl. Let cool in the refrigerator and remove congealed fat that rises to the top. Transfer to smaller containers and to the freezer for long-term storage.

FISH STOCK

"Fish broth will cure anything" is a South American proverb. Fish broth is the basic ingredient for nourishing fish soups, sauces, and stews. Use only heads and carcasses of non-oily fish, since oily fish may become rancid, with off-flavors.

2 tablespoons butter	¼ cup vinegar (any type) or white wine
2 onions, coarsely chopped	Several sprigs of fresh thyme (optional)
1 carrot, coarsely chopped	Several sprigs of fresh parsley
½ cup dry white wine or vermouth	1 bay leaf
1 to 4 whole carcasses, including heads, of	About 3 quarts cold filtered water
non-oily fish such as sole, turbot, rockfish,	
or snapper, depending on size of fish	

Melt butter in a large stainless-steel pot over low heat. Add onions and carrot and cook, about ½ hour, until soft. Add wine, raise heat to high, and bring to a boil. Add fish carcasses and cover with cold filtered water. Add vinegar. Bring to a boil and skim off scum and impurities as they rise to the top. Tie herbs together and add to pot. Reduce heat, cover, and simmer for at least 2 hours or as long as 24 hours. Remove carcasses with tongs or a slotted spoon and strain liquid into pint-sized storage containers for refrigerator or freezer. Chill well in refrigerator and remove any congealed fat before transferring to the freezer for long-term storage.

QUICK FISH STOCK
Makes 2 quarts

This is an easy version of fish stock from Japan.

1 cup bonito flakes (shaved dried fish;	2 quarts cold filtered water
see Resources)	¼ cup vinegar (any type)

Place all ingredients in a large stainless-steel pot, bring to a boil, and skim. Lower heat, cover, and simmer for 2 to 3 hours. Let stock cool and strain into storage containers.

Lacto-Fermented Condiments

We've described the magic of lacto-fermented foods in Chapter 5. These foods involve a partnership between the cook and the microscopic world. They're not just easy but fun to make. And if you've never made lacto-fermented condiments before, you'll be amazed at how well the foods are preserved and how wonderful they taste. Lacto-fermented vegetables, such as sauerkraut, will keep up to a year in the refrigerator, and lacto-fermented fruit, such as chutneys, will keep at least two months.

Lacto-fermentation requires two basic pieces of equipment and two basic ingredients. For equipment, you will need quart-sized, widemouthed mason jars, available at any hardware store, along with some kind of pusher or pounder, such as a small meat mallot that you would use to tenderize meat.

The two ingredients are good-quality unrefined sea salt and homemade whey. The whey acts as an inoculant, a source of lactic acid–producing bacteria, and the salt preserves the foods until enough lactic acid is produced to take over that role. *Do not use powdered whey*—bacteria are killed by the powdering and drying process. Fresh whey is easy to make (see following recipe) and lasts a long time in the refrigerator. (For recipes that don't contain fruit, you can omit whey and double the amount of salt.)

Whenever possible, we suggest you eat fruits and vegetables that have been grown organically; but for lacto-fermentation, organic fruits and vegetables are a must. Pesticides can inhibit the fermentation process, and if the food is of poor quality, the lactic acid–producing bacteria cannot proliferate. The better the quality of the food you are fermenting, the better your results will be.

If you feel you don't have time to lacto-ferment foods, we're happy to report that commercial lacto-fermented condiments are now becoming available, especially the more common ones like sauerkraut and pickles. Authentic, nonpasteurized kimchi (Korean sauerkraut) can be purchased at Asian markets (but look for a brand that does not contain MSG). See Resources for sources of these products.

HOMEMADE WHEY
Makes 2½ cups whey and 1½ cups cream cheese

1 quart good-quality plain whole yogurt or kefir or

1 quart raw milk that has been allowed to sour and separate

Note: To separate and sour raw milk, place in a glass container, cover, and leave at room temperature for several days—it may take up to 5 days—until the milk has clearly separated into curds and whey.

Line a colander or large strainer with a kitchen towel and set it over a bowl. Place yogurt, kefir, or separated raw milk in the towel-lined colander or strainer, cover with a towel or plate, and leave overnight. The whey will drip into the bowl. The next day, tie up the ends of the towel with string and suspend it by tying it to a spoon set across a deep container. Transfer the whey that has already accumulated in the bowl to a jar and refrigerate. Additional whey will drip out of the towel over the next day or two—add this to the jar. Remove the cream cheese from the towel and store in the refrigerator. The whey will keep for many months, and the cream cheese will keep for about 2 weeks.

SAUERKRAUT
Makes 1 quart   •   8 calories per ¼ cup

1 medium head organic cabbage,   1 tablespoon sea salt
  cored and finely shredded   ¼ cup **Homemade Whey** (previous recipe)
1 tablespoon caraway seeds

Note: If you don't use whey, use 2 tablespoons sea salt.

In a large bowl, mix cabbage with caraway seeds, salt, and whey. Pound with a wooden pounder or meat hammer for about 10 minutes to release juices. Let sit for 30 minutes or so to allow cabbage to wilt. Pound again for a few minutes and stuff into a quart-sized, widemouthed mason jar, pressing down firmly with a pounder or meat hammer until juices cover top of the cabbage. The top of the cabbage should be at least 1 inch below the top of the jar, since it will expand somewhat during fermentation. Cover tightly and keep at room temperature for about 3 days before transferring to the refrigerator. The sauerkraut should bubble when you first open the jar. It may be eaten immediately, but it improves with age.

KIMCHI
Makes 2 quarts   •   10 calories per ¼ cup

1 head Napa cabbage, cored and shredded   3 cloves garlic, peeled and minced
1 bunch green onions, chopped   ½ teaspoon dried chile flakes
1 cup carrots, grated   1 tablespoon sea salt
½ cup daikon radish, grated (optional)   ¼ cup **Homemade Whey** (page 227)
1 tablespoon grated fresh ginger

Note : If you are not using whey, use 2 tablespoons sea salt.

Place vegetables, ginger, chile flakes, salt, and whey in a large bowl and pound with a wooden pounder or meat hammer to release juices. Let sit for half an hour to allow the cabbage to wilt. Pound again for a few minutes and stuff into a quart-sized, widemouthed mason jar. Press down firmly with a pounder or meat hammer until juices come to the top of the cabbage. The top of the vegetables should be at least 1 inch below the top of the jar. Cover tightly and keep at room temperature for about 3 days before transferring to the refrigerator.

PICKLED CUCUMBERS
Makes 1 quart   •   About 10 calories per pickle

4 to 5 pickling cucumbers or   1 tablespoon sea salt
  15 to 20 gherkins   ¼ cup **Homemade Whey** (page 227)
1 tablespoon brown mustard seeds   1 cup filtered water
2 tablespoons fresh dill, snipped

Note: If you are not using whey, use 2 tablespoons sea salt.

Wash cucumbers well and place in a quart-sized, widemouthed mason jar. Combine remaining ingredients and pour over cucumbers, adding more water if necessary to cover cucumbers. The top of the liquid should be at least 1 inch below the top of the jar. Cover tightly and keep at room temperature for about 3 days before transferring to the refrigerator.

PINEAPPLE CHUTNEY
Makes 1 quart   •   About 20 calories per ¼ cup

This chutney goes well with meat and with various coconut curries.

1 small pineapple	2 tablespoons fresh lime juice
1 bunch fresh cilantro, coarsely chopped	2 teaspoons sea salt
1 tablespoon grated fresh ginger	¼ cup **Homemade Whey** (page 227)
1 jalapeño chile, seeded and finely chopped (optional)	½ cup filtered water

In a large bowl, mix together pineapple, cilantro, ginger, and jalapeño, if using. Place in a quart-sized, widemouthed mason jar. Press down lightly with a wooden pounder or meat hammer. Mix together lime juice, salt, whey, and water and pour over pineapple, adding more water if necessary to cover the pineapple. The chutney should be at least 1 inch below the top of the jar. Cover tightly and keep at room temperature for 2 days before transferring to refrigerator. This should be eaten within 2 months.

PEACH CHUTNEY
Makes 1 quart   •   About 40 calories per ¼ cup

This spicy chutney is delicious with Indian-style curries.

½ cup filtered water	½ cup chopped **Crispy Pecans** (page 259)
Juice of 2 lemons	½ cup dark raisins
Grated rind of 2 lemons	1 teaspoon ground cumin
2 tablespoons Rapadura, Sucanat, or maple sugar	½ teaspoon red pepper flakes
2 teaspoons sea salt	½ teaspoon dried green peppercorns, crushed
¼ cup **Homemade Whey** (page 227)	½ teaspoon dried thyme
3 to 5 fresh peaches, enough to make about 3 cups chopped	1 teaspoon whole fennel seeds
	1 teaspoon whole coriander seeds

In a large bowl, mix together water, lemon juice, lemon rind, sweetener, salt, and whey. Peel peaches and cut up into the lemon juice mixture. Mix in nuts, raisins, herbs, and spices and place in a quart-sized, widemouthed mason jar.

Press down lightly with a wooden pounder or a meat hammer, adding more water if necessary to cover the fruit. The mixture should be at least 1 inch below the top of the jar. Cover tightly and keep at room temperature for 2 days before transferring to refrigerator. This should be eaten within 2 months.

PAPAYA OR MANGO CHUTNEY
Makes 1 quart • About 20 calories per ¼ cup

Another great accompaniment for curries and other coconut dishes.

3 cups peeled and cubed ripe papaya
  or mango
1 tablespoon grated fresh ginger
1 red pepper, seeded and cut into julienne
1 small onion, chopped
1 jalapeño chile, seeded and chopped
  (optional)

½ cup chopped fresh mint leaves
1 bunch fresh cilantro, chopped
2 tablespoons Rapadura, Sucanat, or maple sugar
½ cup fresh lime juice
2 teaspoons sea salt
¼ cup **Homemade Whey** (page 227)
½ cup filtered water

In a large bowl, mix together papaya or mango, ginger, pepper, onion, jalapeño, if using, mint, and cilantro and place in a quart-sized, widemouthed mason jar. Press down lightly with a wooden pounder or meat hammer. Mix together remaining ingredients and pour into jar, adding more water if necessary to cover fruit. The chutney should be at least 1 inch below the top of the jar. Cover tightly and leave at room temperature for 2 days before transferring to refrigerator. Eat within 2 months.

CORN RELISH
Makes 1 quart • About 20 calories per ¼ cup

---

3 cups fresh corn kernels
1 small tomato, peeled, seeded, and diced
1 small onion, finely diced
½ green pepper, seeded and diced

2 tablespoons chopped fresh cilantro leaves
¼ to ½ teaspoon red pepper flakes
1 tablespoon sea salt
4 tablespoons **Homemade Whey** (page 227)

In a large bowl, mix together all ingredients. Pound lightly with a wooden pounder or a meat hammer to release juices. Place in a quart-sized, widemouthed mason jar and press down with a pounder or meat hammer until juices cover the relish. The top of the vegetables should be at least 1 inch below the top of the jar. Cover tightly and keep at room temperature for about 3 days before transferring to the refrigerator.

BREAD AND BUTTER PICKLES
Makes 2 quarts • *About 20 calories per ¼ cup*

This wonderful recipe comes from Weston A. Price Foundation chapter leader Kim Lockard.

7 cups thinly sliced pickling cucumbers
  or gherkins
1 cup thinly sliced mild onion
1 cup fresh lemon juice
⅓ cup **Homemade Whey** (page 227)

1 cup honey or maple syrup
3 tablespoons sea salt
1 to 2 tablespoons whole celery seeds
2 teaspoons turmeric
1 tablespoon yellow mustard seeds

In a large bowl, mix cucumbers with onion and place in 2 quart-sized, wide-mouthed mason jars, pressing down lightly with a pounder or meat hammer. Combine remaining ingredients and pour over cucumbers, adding more water if necessary to cover. Keep the top of the liquid 1 inch below the top of the jar. Cover tightly and keep at room temperature for about 2 days before transferring to the refrigerator.

CILANTRO SALSA
Makes 1 quart • *About 20 calories per ¼ cup*

Thanks to Bonnie Kinningham for this easy and delicious recipe for lacto-fermented salsa.

28-ounce can organic whole peeled
  tomatoes, liquid drained off
¼ large onion, coarsely chopped
2 cloves garlic, coarsely chopped
1 serrano chile, seeded and coarsely chopped
1 teaspoon sea salt

½ teaspoon dried oregano
Juice of 1 lemon or 2 limes
¼ cup **Homemade Whey** (page 227)
1 large bunch fresh cilantro, coarsely
  chopped

Place all ingredients except cilantro in a food processor and process until smooth. Stir in cilantro. Place in a quart-sized, widemouthed mason jar. The top of the vegetables should be at least 1 inch below the top of the jar. Cover tightly and keep at room temperature for about 3 days before transferring to the refrigerator.

Soups

CREAM OF VEGETABLE SOUP
Serves 8   •   130 calories per 1 cup serving

This is the basic recipe for creamed vegetable soup. It's easy to prepare when you use a handheld blender so you can blend the soup right in the pot. Add the raw or cultured cream to the bowls when serving, so the enzymes are not destroyed.

4 tablespoons butter	1½ quarts chicken stock
3 medium onions, peeled and chopped, or 2 leeks, washed and sliced	Several sprigs of fresh thyme, tied together
2 carrots, peeled and chopped	½ teaspoon dried green peppercorns, crushed
3 medium baking potatoes or 6 red potatoes, cut into pieces	4 small zucchinis, trimmed and sliced
	Sea salt and freshly ground black pepper
	1 cup sour cream or crème fraîche

Melt butter in a large stainless-steel pot over low heat. Add onions and carrots, cover, and cook over lowest possible heat for at least 30 minutes, or until vegetables soften but don't burn. Add potatoes and stock, raise heat, bring to a rapid boil and skim. Reduce heat and add thyme sprigs and crushed peppercorns. Cover and simmer until potatoes are soft. Add zucchini and cook until just tender, 5 to 10 minutes. Remove thyme sprigs. Puree soup with a handheld blender. If soup is too thick, thin with filtered water. Season with salt and pepper. Ladle into heated bowls and garnish with 1 tablespoon sour cream or crème fraîche per bowl.

BEEF VEGETABLE SOUP
Serves 8   •   315 calories per 1 cup serving

This soup makes its own stock—no need to have any on hand.

2 pounds beef ribs	Several sprigs of fresh thyme, tied together
2 quarts cold filtered water	½ cup red wine
½ cup vinegar (any type)	½ cup Eden whole-grain or rice noodles broken into 1-inch pieces
1 can tomato paste	
1 clove garlic, crushed	2 cups diced mixed fresh or frozen vegetables
1 teaspoon dried green peppercorns, crushed	Sea salt to taste
	Naturally fermented soy sauce or miso

If possible, have the butcher cut ribs into 1-inch pieces. Preheat oven to 400°F. Strew ribs in a stainless-steel baking pan and bake for about 45 minutes, or until meat is well browned. Remove with tongs to a large pot and add cold water and vinegar. Add a little water to the pan, bring to a boil, and deglaze, then add this liquid to the pot. Let soak for 1 hour, then bring to a simmer and skim any scum that rises to the surface.

Add tomato paste, garlic, peppercorns, thyme, and red wine and simmer for 2 to 3 hours, until meat is very tender. Remove bones, along with meat and thyme. Let bones cool and remove meat from bones. (You should have about 2 cups of meat.) Chop up meat and add to soup, along with noodles and vegetables. Simmer until noodles and vegetables are tender, about 15 minutes. Season with salt and soy sauce.

MISO SOUP WITH CABBAGE
Serves 4 • *56 calories per 1 cup serving*

1 quart **Quick Fish Stock** (page 226)
1 tablespoon naturally fermented
  soy sauce
2 tablespoons naturally fermented miso

1 onion, sliced
2 cups green or Chinese cabbage, coarsely
  shredded
1 tablespoon Thai fish sauce

Bring stock to a boil in a medium pot, skim and whisk in miso. Add remaining ingredients, lower heat, and simmer until vegetables are soft, about 10 minutes.

MEDITERRANEAN FISH SOUP
Serves 6 • *213 calories per serving*

3 tablespoons extra-virgin olive oil
  or **Mary's Oil Blend** (page 188)
2 onions, peeled and chopped
4 tablespoons tomato paste
1½ quarts **Fish Stock**
  or **Quick Fish Stock** (page 126)
½ cup red wine or brandy
3 cloves garlic, mashed

¼ teaspoon cayenne pepper
Several sprigs of fresh thyme and
  rosemary, tied together
1 pound fish (any type), skinned and
  cut into chunks
¾ pound shelled shrimp or crabmeat
Sea salt or Thai fish sauce and freshly
  ground black pepper to taste

Warm oil in a large pot over medium heat. Add onions and sauté until soft and golden. Stir in tomato paste. Add fish stock and wine, raise heat, bring to a boil, and skim. Reduce heat, add garlic, cayenne, and herbs, and simmer about 30 minutes. Add fish and shrimp and simmer 10 minutes more. Season with salt or Thai fish sauce and pepper. Remove thyme and rosemary before serving.

CREAMY ONION SOUP
Serves 4 • *286 calories per serving*

4 tablespoons butter or **Mary's Oil Blend**
  (page 188)
2 large onions, thinly sliced
4 cups beef stock
¼ cup brandy

1 cup sour cream or crème fraîche
1 teaspoon dried thyme
Sea salt and freshly ground black pepper
  to taste

Melt butter in a medium pot over low heat. Add onions and sauté until golden. Add brandy, raise heat, bring to a boil, and skim. Add remaining ingredients and simmer about 10 minutes, or until flavors amalgamate.

Appetizers and Lunch Dishes

STEAK TARTARE
Makes 2 cups • 209 calories per ¼ cup

Use only the best-quality organic and/or grass-fed beef and be sure to freeze it for 14 days before you use it to kill any pathogens or parasites.

1 pound ground sirloin or fillet,
  frozen 14 days and thawed
2 egg yolks
1 medium yellow onion, finely minced
¼ cup finely chopped fresh parsley
Sea salt and freshly ground black pepper to taste

Cayenne pepper to taste
3 tablespoons Dijon-style mustard
1 red onion, finely chopped, for serving
Capers, for serving
Butter, for serving

In a large bowl, mix beef with egg yolks, yellow onion, mustard, and parsley and season with salt, pepper, and cayenne. Form into a mound on a platter. Surround meat with whole-grain crackers and serve with chopped red onion, capers, and butter.

OYSTER SHOOTERS
Serves 4 • 40 calories per serving

---

8 raw oysters
4 tablespoons good-quality ketchup
  (see Resources)

1 tablespoon horseradish sauce

Place 1 oyster in each of 8 shot glasses. In a small bowl, mix together ketchup and horseradish sauce. Place a dollop of sauce on each oyster.

CHICKEN LIVER PATÉ
Makes 2 cups • 150 calories per ¼ cup serving

---

2 tablespoons butter
2 tablespoons olive oil or
  Mary's Oil Blend (page 188)
1 pound chicken livers, preferably organic
¼ cup brandy or cognac
1 cup chicken or beef stock
½ teaspoon dry mustard

½ teaspoon dried rosemary
1 teaspoon dried green
  peppercorns, crushed
2 cloves garlic, crushed
4 tablespoons (½ stick) butter, softened
Sea salt to taste

Warm butter and oil in a large saucepan over medium heat. Add chicken livers and sauté until browned, about 10 minutes. Add brandy, stock, mustard, rosemary, green peppercorns, and garlic. Bring to a boil, then boil vigorously until most of liquid has evaporated. Transfer to a food processor along with softened butter and process until smooth. Season with salt. Transfer to a crock or small soufflé dish, cover, and refrigerate.

COD'S LIVER SPREAD
Makes 1 cup • 245 calories per ¼ cup

Cod's liver actually tastes like tuna! And save the oil—it's cod-liver oil!

4¼-ounce can smoked cod's liver
3 tablespoons **Mayonnaise** (page 238)

Sea salt and freshly ground black pepper to taste

Remove cod's liver from oil and place in a food processor. Add mayonnaise and process until smooth. Season with salt. Serve with whole-grain crackers or **Coconut Crackers** (page 209).

SALMON ROE ON TOAST
Serves 3 • 186 calories per serving

---

3 slices sourdough whole-grain bread
3 tablespoons **Mary's Oil Blend**
(page 188) or melted butter

2 ounces (¼ cup) fresh or canned salmon roe caviar
Finely snipped fresh dill, for garnish

Preheat oven to 300°F. Remove crusts from bread and slice on diagonal to make 2 triangles out of each piece. Place on baking sheet, brush with oil blend, and bake for 30 minutes, or until bread is lightly browned and crisp. Spread salmon roe on bread and top with fresh dill.

FISH ROE SPREAD
Makes 1 cup • 370 calories per ⅓-cup serving

Spreads made from fish roe, or *tarama*, are popular throughout the Mediterranean area. This is a particularly delicious way to prepare this wonderful superfood. Use fresh salmon roe or canned preserved salmon or carp roe (caviar). (See Resources for recommended brands.) This recipe is adapted from *Bulgarian Rhapsody: The Best of Balkan Cuisine* by Linda Joyce Forristal.

2 ounces fresh salmon roe or
canned salmon or carp caviar
1 small onion, minced
½ cup **Mary's Oil Blend** (page 188)

Juice of 1 large lemon
2 teaspoons cold water
Sea salt to taste

Place roe and onion in a food processor and process until well blended. With motor running, add oil blend, drop by drop, forming a thick emulsion. Add lemon juice in the same manner, then the 2 teaspoons water. Season with salt. (If you are using canned roe, you may not need any added salt.)

QUESADILLAS
Serves 4 • 505 calories per serving

Quesadillas are delicious served with **Cilantro Salsa** (page 231) and sliced avocados or **Coconut Avocado Dip** (page 190).

4 sprouted whole-wheat tortillas
   (Alvarado bakery brand)
2 cups grated raw jack or cheddar cheese
1 small jar green chiles, chopped

About 1 cup shredded leftover chicken, turkey, or
   duck meat (optional)
2 tablespoons finely chopped fresh cilantro
About ¼ cup lard

Warm lard in a medium cast-iron skillet over medium heat. Place 1 tortilla in skillet and put ½ cup cheese, 1 tablespoon green chiles, ¼ cup leftover meat, if using, and 1½ teaspoons cilantro on one side of tortilla. Fold other side over. Repeat so that you have 2 quesadillas in the pan at the same time. Fry until brown on one side, turn, and brown on the other side.

SALMON CREAM CHEESE ROLLS
Serves 2 • 247 calories per serving

6 tablespoons cream cheese
2 tablespoons chopped fresh dill,
   or 1 teaspoon dried

Sea salt and freshly ground black pepper to taste
4 ounces sliced smoked salmon, preferably wild

In a small bowl, mix cream cheese with dill and season with salt and pepper. Spread mixture over salmon slices and roll up. Chill well. Slice into ½-inch rounds. Serve with toothpicks.

SEVICHE
Serves 4 • 329 calories per serving

1 pound sea bass, whitefish,
   or mackerel fillets
½ cup fresh lime juice
2 tablespoons **Homemade Whey**
   (page 227), optional
2 medium tomatoes, peeled, seeded,
   and diced
1 small red onion, finely chopped

2 jalapeño chiles, seeded and finely chopped
¼ cup extra-virgin olive oil or **Mary's Oil Blend**
   (page 188)
2 tablespoons finely chopped fresh cilantro
Sea salt to taste
1 avocado, cut into wedges
1 lemon, cut into wedges

Cut fish into ½-inch cubes and place in a large bowl. Stir in lime juice and whey, if using, and marinate in the refrigerator for 4 to 6 hours, stirring occasionally, until fish becomes opaque or "cooked." Remove fish from marinade with a slotted spoon and place in another bowl. Add tomatoes, onion, jalapeños, oil, and cilantro and marinate in the refrigerator another hour. Season with salt. Serve with avocado and lemon wedges.

Quick and Easy Weight Loss version: Omit avocado (248 calories per serving).

Dressings and Sauces

BASIC SALAD DRESSING
Makes about ¾ cup   •   87 calories per tablespoon

If you are on Quick and Easy Weight Loss or Health Recovery, use **Mary's Oil Blend**, rather than olive oil, to increase your intake of lauric acid from coconut oil and to avoid overconsumption of monounsaturates (which can promote weight gain). The flax oil adds omega-3 fatty acids to help redress the omega-6/omega-3 imbalance so prevalent in modern diets. Two teaspoons of flax oil is enough since it's possible to create an imbalance in the other direction, of too much omega-3. Be sure to store your flax oil in the refrigerator. (For recommended brands of raw wine vinegar, see Resources.)

About 1 teaspoon smooth or grainy
  Dijon-style mustard
2 tablespoons plus 1 teaspoon raw wine
  vinegar

½ cup extra-virgin olive oil or **Mary's Oil Blend**
  (page 188)
2 teaspoons expeller-expressed flax oil

Dip a fork into jar of mustard and transfer about 1 teaspoon to a small bowl. Add vinegar and mix. Add oil in a thin stream, stirring all the while with the fork, until oil is well mixed or emulsified. Add flax oil and use immediately or store in refrigerator.

Variation: Balsamic Salad Dressing
  Use balsamic vinegar in place of raw wine vinegar.

Variation: Creamy Salad Dressing
  Add 2 tablespoons cream to the dressing.

CAESAR SALAD DRESSING
Makes about ¾ cup • 92 calories per tablespoon

About 1 teaspoon smooth or grainy
 Dijon-style mustard
2 tablespoons plus 1 teaspoon raw wine vinegar
1 egg yolk

1 glove garlic, crushed
½ cup extra-virgin olive oil or **Mary's Oil**
 Blend (page 188)
2 teaspoons expeller-expressed flax oil

Dip a fork into jar of mustard and transfer about 1 teaspoon to a small bowl. Add vinegar and mix. Add egg yolk and garlic. Add olive oil in a thin stream, stirring all the while with the fork, until oil is well mixed or emulsified. Add flax oil and use immediately or store in refrigerator.

ASIAN SALAD DRESSING
Makes about 1¼ cups • 74 calories per tablespoon

4 tablespoons rice vinegar
2 tablespoons naturally fermented soy sauce
2 teaspoons grated fresh ginger
2 teaspoons toasted sesame oil
2 teaspoons finely chopped green onions or chives

1 clove garlic, mashed (optional)
1 teaspoon raw honey
⅔ cup **Mary's Oil Blend** (page 188)
2 teaspoons expeller-expressed flax oil

Place all ingredients in a jar and shake vigorously. Store in refrigerator.

MAYONNAISE
Makes about 1 cup • 99 calories per tablespoon

Mary's Oil Blend is perfect for mayonnaise—it provides the benefits of coconut oil, including firmness when refrigerated, and does not have the strong taste of olive oil. If you do not want to make your own mayonnaise, an excellent commercial brand is Delouis Fils, available in the refrigerated section of many specialty stores and gourmet markets. Note that commercial mayonnaise is about 110 calories per tablespoon; by using Mary's Oil Blend with coconut oil, we reduce the caloric value slightly, since coconut oil contains fewer calories than regular vegetable oil or olive oil.

1 whole egg, at room temperature
1 egg yolk, at room temperature
1 teaspoon Dijon-style mustard
1½ tablespoons fresh lemon juice

1 tablespoon **Homemade Whey** (page 227),
 optional
Sea salt and freshly ground black pepper to taste
¾ cup **Mary's Oil Blend** (page 188)

Place egg, egg yolk, mustard, salt, pepper, lemon juice, and whey in a food processor. Process until well blended, about 30 seconds. With the motor running, add oil blend, drop by drop (some food processors have a hole at the bottom of the cylindrical part that does this automatically). Taste and check seasoning. You may want to add more salt and lemon juice. If you have added whey, let mayonnaise sit at room temperature, well covered, for 7 hours before refrigerating. With whey added, mayonnaise will keep several months and will become firmer over time. Without whey, mayonnaise will keep, refrigerated, for about 2 weeks.

CURRIED MAYONNAISE
Makes about 2 cups • 74 calories per tablespoon

This curried mayonnaise has a slightly sweet taste. It is delicious as a dip or used in chicken salad.

1 cup **Mayonnaise** (page 238) or good-quality purchased mayonnaise such as Delouis Fils brand (see Resources)
½ cup sour cream or crème fraîche
3 tablespoons **Mary's Oil Blend** (page 188) or extra-virgin olive oil

3 tablespoons raw coconut, rice, wine, or apple cider vinegar
3 tablespoons curry powder
1 tablespoon tomato paste
1 teaspoon Sucanat, Rapadura, or maple sugar

In a medium bowl, whisk together all ingredients.

TERIYAKI SAUCE
Makes ¾ cup • 23 calories per tablespoon

1 tablespoon grated fresh ginger
3 garlic cloves, crushed
1 tablespoon toasted sesame oil

1 tablespoon rice vinegar
1 tablespoon raw honey
½ cup naturally fermented soy sauce

In a medium bowl, whisk together all ingredients.

BARBEQUE SAUCE
Makes 1½ cups • 19 calories per tablespoon

¾ cup **Teriyaki Sauce** (previous recipe)   ¾ cup naturally sweetened ketchup (see Resources)

In a medium bowl, whisk together all ingredients.

SWEET-AND-SOUR SOY SAUCE
Makes 1 cup • 11 calories per tablespoon

From *The Vietnamese Cookbook* by Diana My Tran.

2 cloves garlic, finely minced
2 tablespoons coconut or maple sugar
2 tablespoons fresh lime or lemon juice

½ cup warm water
7 tablespoons naturally fermented soy sauce
Cayenne pepper to taste (optional)

Mix together garlic, sugar, lime juice, water, and soy sauce in a small bowl until sugar is completely dissolved. Add cayenne, if using.

PARSLEY BUTTER SAUCE
Makes about ½ cup • *80 calories per tablespoon*

This is a delicious, easy, and healthy sauce that goes with any type of meat. Use fish stock if you are serving the sauce with fish, chicken stock for chicken, and beef stock for red meat.

3 tablespoons minced shallots or
  green onions
2 tablespoons sherry vinegar
¼ cup dry white wine
1 cup fish, chicken, or beef stock

½ cup sour cream or crème fraîche
3 tablespoons butter, softened
1 tablespoon coarse-grain mustard
Sea salt to taste
2 tablespoons finely chopped fresh parsley

Combine shallots, vinegar, wine, stock, and cream in a medium saucepan over high heat, bring to a boil, and reduce to about half, or until sauce thickens slightly. Reduce heat and whisk in butter and mustard. Season with salt. Just before serving, stir in parsley.

PESTO
Makes 1 cup • *90 calories per tablespoon*

Pesto is normally used on pasta, but it is delicious as an accompaniment to fish and meat, or even spread on corn on the cob!

2 cups packed fresh basil leaves
3 cloves garlic
½ teaspoon sea salt
¼ cup toasted pine nuts or
  Crispy Walnuts (page 259)

2 ounces good-quality grated Parmesan
  cheese
¼ to ½ cup **Mary's Oil Blend** (page 188) or
  extra-virgin olive oil

Place basil in a food processor. Pulse until well chopped. Add garlic, salt, pine nuts, and Parmesan and blend well. Using attachment for adding liquids drop by drop, and with motor running, add oil blend to form a thick paste. Pesto will keep several days, well sealed, in refrigerator, or it may be frozen.

HE-MAN SAUCE
Makes 1 cup • *32 calories per tablespoon*

This is a great substitute for commercial steak sauce, to serve with steaks, chops, or roasts.

½ cup naturally sweetened ketchup
(see Resources)
1 tablespoon coarse-grain mustard
1 tablespoon fresh lemon juice
3 tablespoons butter

2 tablespoons dry sherry
1 teaspoon Thai fish sauce
Dash of Tabasco sauce
¼ teaspoon sea salt
¼ teaspoon freshly ground black pepper

Place all ingredients in a glass or ceramic container set in simmering water. Stir occasionally until butter is melted and sauce is warmed through.

Salads

ASIAN CHEF'S SALAD WITH NOODLES
Serves 4 • 623 calories per serving

---

8 cups salad greens
3 medium tomatoes, diced
1 red onion, finely chopped
2 cups diced cooked turkey, chicken,
or duck meat

1 cup Eden rice or other whole-grain noodles
broken into 2-inch pieces, cooked and drained
4 tablespoons lard, goose fat, or
Mary's Oil Blend (page 188)
½ cup **Asian Salad Dressing** (page 238)

Place salad greens in a large bowl and strew tomato and onions over greens. Warm 2 tablespoons lard in a large skillet over medium heat. Add meat and sauté 8 minutes or until well browned. Transfer to salad bowl using a slotted spoon. Add remaining 2 tablespoons lard to skillet and sauté cooked noodles until golden brown, about 5 minutes. Transfer to a paper towel to soak up excess oil. Toss over salad. Pour on dressing, toss salad, and serve immediately.

Quick and Easy Weight Loss version: Do not sauté meat in oil and omit the noodles (406 calories per serving).

SALADE NIÇOISE
Serves 2 • 435 calories per serving

See Resource section for brands of tuna that do not contain hydrolyzed protein, a source of MSG.

2 small red potatoes
1 cup French beans, ends removed and
cut into 1-inch lengths
2 cups baby salad greens
2 small ripe tomatoes, cup into wedges

6 small black olives
1 small can water-packed tuna
4 tablespoons **Basic Salad Dressing** (page 237)
1 tablespoon finely chopped fresh parsley

Plunge potatoes into a large pot of boiling water. When potatoes are half tender, add beans to water and cook until tender (about 8 minutes for the beans). Pour into a colander and rinse immediately with cold water.

Divide salad greens between 2 large plates. Garnish with tomatoes, potatoes, beans, and olives. Flake tuna and arrange over salad greens. Dribble dressing over salad, sprinkle with parsley, and serve.

WILD SALMON SALAD
Serves 4 • 420 calories per serving

2 cups leftover cooked wild salmon or
   2 small cans wild salmon
4 stalks celery, finely chopped
4 tablespoons finely chopped onion

2 tablespoons finely chopped fresh dill or cilantro
½ cup **Mayonnaise** (page 238)
4 tablespoons toasted pine nuts
Sea salt to taste

Place salmon in a large bowl and break up with a fork. Mix in remaining ingredients and season with salt.

Quick and Easy Weight Loss version: Omit pine nuts (376 calories per serving).

SHRIMP SALAD WITH PAPAYA
Serves 4 • 231 calories per serving

2 cups cooked baby shrimp
6 to 8 green onions, chopped
2 tablespoons finely chopped fresh cilantro

½ cup **Basic** or **Asian Salad Dressing** (pages 237, 238)
2 small papayas, cut lengthwise and seeds removed

In a medium bowl, mix together shrimp, onions, cilantro, and dressing. Place half of a papaya on each of 4 plates and fill with shrimp salad.

CAESAR SALAD
Serves 4 • 275 calories per serving

2 hearts of romaine lettuce
¼ cup best-quality Parmesan cheese,
   freshly grated

½ cup **Caesar Salad Dressing** (pages 237)
8 anchovies

Cut lettuce into 1-inch slices. Place in a large bowl and mix with Parmesan and Caesar Salad Dressing. Divide among 4 plates and place 2 anchovies over each salad.

Variation: Chicken, Duck, or Shrimp Caesar Salad

Add 2 cups chicken, duck meat, or shrimp sautéed in 2 tablespoons lard, goose fat, or **Mary's Oil Blend** (page 188) and drained on paper towels (558 calories per serving).

PAPAYA GRAPEFRUIT SALAD
Serves 4   •   242 calories per serving

1 small papaya, skin and seeds removed and cut into strips	4 tablespoons **Basic Salad Dressing** (page 237)
1 grapefruit, skin removed and sectioned	½ teaspoon poppy seeds
1 medium tomato, cut into thin wedges	4 tablespoons finely chopped onion
1 avocado, cut into thin strips	1 tablespoon chopped fresh cilantro

Arrange papaya, grapefruit, tomato, and avocado on 4 plates. Mix dressing with poppy seeds and dribble over fruit. Sprinkle onion and cilantro over salad.

WATERCRESS SALAD
Serves 4   •   262 calories per serving

2 bunches watercress, stems removed	1 small red onion, thinly sliced
4 heads Belgium endive	2 tablespoons toasted pine nuts
1 head radicchio or ¼ head red cabbage, finely shredded	½ cup **Balsamic Salad Dressing** (page 237)
	2 ounces blue cheese, crumbled

Wash and dry watercress. Remove outer leaves of endive and slice at ¼-inch intervals. In a large bowl, mix all ingredients except cheese with dressing and divide among 4 plates. Sprinkle cheese over salad and serve.

CUCUMBER RAITA
Serves 4   •   69 calories per serving

This is a delicious, refreshing salad with hot Indian curries and spicy food.

2 cucumbers, peeled, seeded, and finely chopped	1 small red onion, peeled and finely chopped
Sea salt	2 cups plain whole yogurt
1 red or green pepper, seeded and finely chopped	½ teaspoon toasted cumin seeds

Place chopped cucumbers in a colander and mix with sea salt. Let stand for an hour or so. Pat cucumbers dry, place in a large bowl, and mix with remaining ingredients.

GREEK SALAD WITH SALAMI
Serves 2 • 464 calories per serving

4 cups salad greens
2 tablespoons extra-virgin olive oil or
   Mary's Oil Blend (page 188)
1 tablespoon raw wine vinegar
1 teaspoon dried oregano

1 small red onion, finely sliced
4 pieces pickled red pepper
4 ounces feta cheese, crumbled
2 ounces salami, thinly sliced (see Resources for
   recommended brands)

In a large bowl, toss salad greens with oil, vinegar, and oregano. Divide between 2 plates and garnish with onion, red pepper, feta, and salami.

Variation: Greek Salad with Shrimp
Use ½ pound grilled shrimp in place of salami (464 calories per serving).

MESCLUN SALAD
Serves 4 • 329 calories per serving

6 cups mesclun (baby salad greens)
1 tablespoon toasted pine nuts
½ cup **Balsamic Salad Dressing** (page 237)

2 ounces blue cheese
4 **Croutons** (page 258)

In a large bowl, mix greens with pine nuts and dressing and divide among 4 large plates. Garnish each plate with slice of blue cheese and a crouton.

Quick and Easy Weight Loss version: Omit croutons (250 calories per serving).

ASIAN COLESLAW
Serves 6 • 426 calories per serving

½ cup rice or red wine vinegar
½ cup natural peanut butter
1 tablespoon Rapadura, Sucanat, or
   maple sugar
1 tablespoon naturally fermented soy sauce
1 tablespoon **Mary's Oil Blend** (page 188)
1 tablespoon grated fresh ginger
1 tablespoon fresh lime juice

2 cloves garlic, chopped
1 large Napa or savoy cabbage, very thinly sliced
1 large bell pepper, seeded and cut into thin
   julienne
1 red onion, thinly sliced
4 jalapeño chiles, seeded and chopped fine
1 cup chopped **Crispy Peanuts** (page 259)

Make dressing by mixing vinegar, peanut butter, sweetener, soy sauce, oil, ginger, lime juice, and garlic together with a whisk in a bowl. Place cabbage, pepper, onion, jalapeño, and peanuts in a separate bowl and toss with dressing.

Seafood Entrées

SAUTÉED FILLET OF SOLE
Serves 4   •   386 calories per serving

---

1 pound fresh fillet of sole
About ½ cup unbleached flour
½ teaspoon freshly ground black pepper
½ teaspoon sea salt

About ¼ cup clarified butter or ghee
About ¼ cup extra-virgin olive oil or **Mary's Oil Blend** (page 188)

Wipe fillets thoroughly and trim off any ends that are very thin in comparison to the rest of the fillet. You may wish to cut the fillets in half, crosswise. Mix together flour, pepper, and salt on a large plate. Dredge fish well.

In a cast-iron skillet, heat about 2 tablespoons each clarified butter and oil until they foam. Sauté fish fillets until golden brown, a few at a time, over moderately high heat, starting with the flatter side, cooking 3 to 5 minutes per side, depending on the thickness of the fish. Transfer to a heated platter and keep warm in the oven while you prepare the other fillets. You will need to replenish butter and oil between batches.

Serve with **Parsley Butter Sauce** (page 240) or **Curried Mayonnaise** (page 239).

EASY BAKED SALMON
Serves 4   •   332 calories per serving

1⅓ pounds wild salmon fillet
½ lemon
2 tablespoons melted butter

1 tablespoon unbleached flour
¼ teaspoon paprika
½ teaspoon sea salt

Preheat oven to 350°F. Set salmon, skin side down, in a buttered Pyrex baking dish. Squeeze on lemon juice, then brush generously with butter. Sprinkle on flour and spread with a spatula to make a thin, even coat. Sprinkle on paprika and salt. Bake for 10 to 15 minutes, or until salmon is almost, but not quite, cooked through. Place under broiler for about 1 minute, until flour coating becomes browned. Serve plain or with **Hot Coconut Sauce** (page 190), **Parsley Butter Sauce** (page 240), or **Pesto** (page 240).

CRAB CAKES
Serves 4 • 357 calories per serving

2 eggs, lightly beaten
2 small onions, finely minced
1 cup sourdough whole-grain breadcrumbs
2 tablespoons Dijon-style mustard
¼ to ½ teaspoon cayenne pepper
1 bunch fresh cilantro, chopped

1 teaspoon grated lemon rind
Sea salt and freshly ground black pepper to taste
2 cups fresh crabmeat
2 tablespoons or more butter
2 tablespoons or more **Mary's Oil Blend**
(page 188)

In a large bowl, combine eggs with onions, breadcrumbs, mustard, cayenne, cilantro, lemon rind, salt, and pepper. Mix in crab and form into 8 cakes. Warm butter and oil in a large skillet over medium-high heat. Sauté crab cakes, a few at a time, until golden on both sides. Serve with **Coconut Red Pepper Sauce** (page 189), **Curried Mayonnaise** (page 239), or **Parsley Butter Sauce** (page 240).

CAJUN SWORDFISH WITH CORN
Serves 4 • 344 calories per serving

Cajun seasoning contains thyme, cayenne pepper, paprika, and ground celery seed. Use a brand of Cajun seasoning that lists all the ingredients to be sure it doesn't contain MSG (if the label says "spices," MSG is a likely ingredient); otherwise, make your own mixture.

1 teaspoon sea salt
1 tablespoon Cajun seasoning
1 pound swordfish steak, about ½ inch thick
4 tablespoons ghee or clarified butter, melted
1 cup onion, finely chopped

1 cup green pepper, seeded and chopped
1 cup red pepper, seeded and chopped
2 cups corn kernels, freshly removed from the cob

In a small bowl, mix salt with Cajun seasoning. Brush swordfish with melted ghee on both sides and sprinkle on seasoning, reserving any excess. Place remaining ghee in a cast-iron skillet. Cook swordfish over medium-high heat about 5 minutes per side, until a fork pierces it easily. Remove to a platter and keep warm in the oven. Add remaining seasoning and vegetables to the pan. Sauté, stirring constantly, over medium-high heat for about 2 minutes. Strew vegetables around swordfish and serve.

Poultry Entrées

EASY BAKED CHICKEN
Serves 4 • 312 calories per serving

Whenever possible, use farm-raised, pasture-fed chicken or, failing that, organic chicken.

1 whole chicken, including head and feet if possible	Several sprigs of fresh tarragon or thyme, or 1 teaspoon dried
1 tablespoon melted butter	½ cup dry white wine
Salt and freshly ground pepper to taste	4 cups chicken stock

Cut up chicken, reserving backs, wings, neck, head, and feet for chicken stock. (The leftover bones can also be used for making stock.) Place breasts, thighs, and drumsticks skin side up in a stainless-steel baking pan. Brush with butter and sprinkle with salt and pepper. Lay sprigs of herbs over chicken.

Note: Chicken may be prepared the day ahead to this point and reserved, covered, in refrigerator while stock is being made.

To bake chicken, preheat oven to 350°F and bake about 2 hours, until chicken is golden brown. Remove chicken to a heated platter and reserve in a warm oven while making sauce. Deglaze pan with wine and add chicken broth. Boil vigorously until sauce is reduced to about 2 cups.

CHICKEN LIVER SUPREME
Serves 4 • 370 calories per serving

¼ cup unbleached white flour	¼ teaspoon dill
Sea salt and freshly ground black pepper	1 clove garlic, crushed
1 pound chicken livers, cut into ½-inch pieces	½ teaspoon dried crushed rosemary
2 tablespoons clarified butter, lard, or **Mary's Oil Blend** (page 188)	4 small slices sourdough whole-grain bread, crusts removed
¼ cup brandy	2 tablespoons clarified butter, lard, or
¼ cup red wine	**Mary's Oil Blend**
2 cups chicken stock	

Make a mixture of flour, salt, and pepper on a large plate. Pat chicken liver pieces dry and dredge in the flour mixture. Warm 2 tablespoons clarified butter in a large sauté pan over medium heat. Sauté liver in small batches until well browned, removing to a plate with a slotted spoon. Deglaze the pan with brandy and red wine. Add stock, dill, garlic, and rosemary and bring to a rolling boil until sauce reduces by half and thickens. Reduce to a simmer and return chicken livers to the pan. Simmer for 5 to 10 minutes. Meanwhile, fry the bread in remaining clarified butter, lard, or Mary's Oil Blend. To serve, place bread on individual plates and spoon chicken livers with sauce onto the bread.

Quick and Easy Weight Loss version: Omit fried bread (280 calories per serving).

TERIYAKI DUCK BREASTS
Serves 4 • 711 calories per serving

2 large duck breasts ¾ cup **Teriyaki Sauce** (page 239)

Trim excess fat off the duck breasts, score remaining fat, and pound meat part of breast with a meat hammer. Place in a large bowl and marinate in the refrigerator for several hours in Teriyaki Sauce. Pat dry with paper towels and sauté in a heavy skillet over medium-high heat, about 5 minutes per side, starting with the skin side down. To serve, slice thinly across the grain, arrange on individual plates, and dribble marinade over the slices.

Red Meat Entrées

Red meat forms an integral part of a healthy diet. It is an excellent source of protein, minerals (especially zinc), and B vitamins, especially B_{12}. Make an effort to purchase meat that has been pasture-raised; its fat will be rich in vitamin E and CLA, a substance that protects against cancer. Most of these nutrients are in the fat, so be sure to eat the fat with your meat!

If your only choice is meat from a supermarket, red meat is still the best choice. Of all the meats commercially available, beef and lamb are the cleanest.

RIB-EYE STEAK OR LAMB CHOPS
WITH MUSTARD CREAM SAUCE
Serves 4 • 362 calories per serving

Two 6-ounce rib-eye steaks or four 4-ounce 2 tablespoons Thai fish sauce
   lamb chops 1 cup sour cream or crème fraîche
Sea salt and freshly ground black pepper to taste 1 tablespoon mustard
1 tablespoon lard or **Mary's Oil Blend** (page 188)

Rub steaks or lamb chops with salt and pepper. Heat lard in a large cast-iron skillet. Cook steaks or lamb chops for about 5 minutes per side over medium-high heat, until medium rare. Remove to a heated platter and keep in warm oven while making sauce. Deglaze pan with fish sauce and stir in cream and mustard. Bring to a boil and reduce, stirring, until sauce becomes very thick.

BAKED LAMB CHOPS WITH RED PEPPERS AND ONIONS
Serves 4   •   353 calories per serving

You can use the inexpensive cuts of lamb for this delicious dish.

Four 6-ounce lamb shoulder chops	2 to 3 large onions, sliced in half across the equator
Juice of 1 lemon	2 large red peppers, seeded and quartered
¼ cup unbleached white flour	1 tablespoon melted butter, lard, or **Mary's Oil**
Sea salt and freshly ground black pepper	**Blend** (page 188)

In the morning, rub lemon juice into the chops. Cover and leave at room temperature for about 8 hours. Wipe dry and dredge in a mixture of flour, salt, and pepper placed on a large plate. Preheat oven to 350°F. Rub a glass baking pan with a little butter and place chops in pan. Strew onions and peppers in the pan and brush with melted butter. Bake for about 2 hours, turning chops and peppers after 1 hour.

LIVER STIR-FRY
Serves 4   •   565 calories per serving

---

1 pound beef or calf's liver, cut into strips	Sea salt and freshly ground black pepper
Juice of 2 lemons	1 pound sliced bacon, cut into pieces
½ cup unbleached white flour	2 large onions, chopped

Place liver in a large bowl with lemon juice and marinate for several hours in refrigerator. Pat pieces dry and dredge in a mixture of flour, salt, and pepper placed on a large plate. In a cast-iron skillet over medium heat, cook the bacon until crisp. Remove with a slotted spoon to a heated platter. Cook chopped onion in bacon fat until browned. Remove with a slotted spoon to heated platter. Stir-fry liver in remaining fat until browned on all sides. Return onions and bacon to the pan and mix well. Sauté a few minutes more until the liver is medium-rare. Serve immediately.

Quick and Easy Weight Loss version: Use only ½ pound bacon (388 calories per serving).

HEARTY HAMBURGER WITH SAUTÉED ONIONS AND HE-MAN SAUCE
Serves 4   •   432 calories per serving

Heart is an excellent source of co-enzyme Q_{10}, so important for a healthy muscles—including the heart! It adds a slightly sweet taste to the burger. If you don't use heart, use 1 pound ground chuck.

¾ pound ground chuck
¼ pound ground heart (optional)
1 tablespoon very finely chopped onion
1 tablespoon finely chopped fresh parsley

⅛ teaspoon cayenne pepper
Sea salt and freshly ground black pepper
1 large onion, thinly sliced
1 cup **He-Man Sauce** (page 240)

In a large bowl, mix ground meat with chopped onion, parsley, cayenne, salt, and pepper and form into patties. Heat a well-seasoned cast-iron skillet and cook burgers over medium-high heat for about 5 minutes on each side, or until medium-rare. Transfer to a heated platter and keep warm in the oven while cooking onions. Sauté sliced onions in beef fat remaining in pan until soft. Strew over hamburger. Serve with He-Man Sauce.

Quick and Easy Weight Loss version: Omit He-Man Sauce (304 calories per serving).

LEG OF LAMB WITH ROOT VEGETABLES
Makes six 3-ounce servings, with leftovers • *565 calories per serving, including vegetables*

You will need a meat thermometer to cook this roast.

3 cloves garlic
1 onion, sliced
1 small leg of lamb
6 tablespoons melted butter
3 tablespoons smooth or coarse-grain
  Dijon-style mustard
Several sprigs of fresh thyme, rosemary,
  or tarragon, or 1 teaspoon dried

6 new potatoes, cut in half
1 pound carrots, peeled and cut into
  sticks
3 turnips, peeled and cut into quarters
½ cup dry white wine or vermouth
3 to 4 cups beef stock
Sea salt to taste

Preheat the oven to 450°F. Peel garlic cloves but leave them whole. Place garlic and sliced onion in a large stainless-steel roasting pan. Set leg of lamb, fat side up, on a rack in the pan. Thoroughly mix 3 tablespoons of butter with mustard and brush on lamb. Place sprigs of herbs on top and insert meat thermometer. Set in oven and immediately reduce heat to 350°F. Roast until thermometer registers rare or medium-rare, about 15 minutes to the pound. About 1 hour before the roast finishes, strew potatoes, carrots, and turnips around the roast on the rack and brush them with remaining 3 tablespoons butter.

Remove the roast, set on a heated platter, and keep warm in oven while finishing potatoes and making sauce. Remove rack, placing vegetables in bottom of pan. Brush vegetables with drippings and bake another 15 minutes or so, until they are soft. Transfer to heated platter. Pour wine and stock into the pan and bring to a rapid boil, stirring with a wooden spoon to scrape up any accumulated juices. Boil until sauce reduces to about 1 cup, skimming occasionally. Season with salt.

Use leftovers to make **Leftover Red Meat Curry** (page 200).

BARBEQUED BEEF RIBS
Serves 8　•　419 calories per serving

2 large racks beef ribs　　　　　1½ cups **Barbeque Sauce** (page 239)

Brush racks of beef ribs with barbeque sauce and marinate at room temperature for several hours or all day in the refrigerator. Cook on the barbeque with the top down over very low flame for about 30 minutes on each side, brushing occasionally with marinade. Check frequently to ensure ribs do not burn.

PORK AND BROCCOLI STIR-FRY
Serves 4　•　349 calories per serving

1 pound lean pork, cut into thin strips
½ cup vinegar (any type)
1 cup chicken stock
¼ cup naturally fermented soy sauce
¼ teaspoon red chile flakes
1 tablespoon grated fresh ginger
2 cloves garlic, finely chopped
¼ cup rice or red wine vinegar

2 teaspoons Sucanat, Rapadura, or coconut sugar
2 tablespoons lard, goose fat, or **Mary's Oil Blend** (page 188)
1 bunch green onions, cut into 1-inch pieces
2 red peppers, seeded and cut into thin strips
2 cups broccoli florets
1 tablespoon arrowroot dissolved in 1 tablespoon water

Place pork in a large bowl with vinegar and marinate for several hours. Drain and dry well with paper towels. Mix stock, soy sauce, chile flakes, ginger, garlic, rice vinegar, and Sucanat and set aside. Heat lard in a cast-iron skillet or wok over medium-high heat. Stir-fry pork until moisture evaporates and pork browns. Add green onions, peppers, and broccoli and stir-fry for several minutes, until vegetables soften slightly. Add sauce mixture and bring to a boil. Add arrowroot mixture and boil vigorously until sauce thickens. Serve immediately.

BEEF STIR-FRY WITH PINEAPPLE
Serves 4　•　569 calories per serving

1 cup beef stock
¼ cup rice or red wine vinegar
¼ cup naturally fermented soy sauce
¼ teaspoon red pepper flakes
1 tablespoon Rapadura, Sucanat, or coconut sugar
1 teaspoon grated fresh ginger
2 cloves garlic, finely chopped
1 pound skirt or flank steak, cut across the grain into thin strips

2 tablespoons lard, goose fat, or **Mary's Oil Blend** (page 188)
1 cup coarsely chopped **Crispy Peanuts** or **Cashews** (page 259)
1 bunch green onions, sliced on an angle
2 large carrots, peeled and cut into julienne
1 red bell pepper, seeded and cut into julienne
2 cups cubed pineapple
1 tablespoon arrowroot mixed with 1 tablespoon water

In a medium bowl, mix stock with vinegar, soy sauce, pepper flakes, sweetener, ginger, and garlic and set aside. Pat beef with paper towels to dry. In a cast-iron skillet or wok, heat lard and stir-fry beef until moisture evaporates and the beef browns. Add green onions, carrots, bell peppers, cashews or peanuts, and pineapple and stir-fry a few minutes more. Add sauce mixture and bring to a boil. Add arrowroot mixture and boil vigorously until sauce thickens, about 10 minutes. Serve immediately.

EASY POT ROAST
Serves 8   •   464 calories per serving

2 pounds skirt steak or chuck roast
1 cup red wine vinegar
2 cups beef stock
1 small can tomato paste
2 tablespoons balsamic vinegar
1 tablespoon tamarind paste
   (available in Asian markets) or
   several pieces fresh orange peel

2 cloves garlic, mashed
1 teaspoon dried green peppercorns, crushed
Several sprigs of fresh rosemary or thyme
½ pound carrots, peeled and cut into sticks
1½ pounds small red potatoes
Sea salt and freshly ground black pepper

Pound meat lightly with a meat hammer or pierce with a meat tenderizer and marinate several hours at room temperature in a large bowl with red wine vinegar, or overnight in the refrigerator. Dry well, discarding vinegar. Place in an oiled casserole or Dutch oven. Preheat oven to 250°F. Place stock, tomato paste, balsamic vinegar, tamarind paste, garlic, and dried peppercorns in a medium pot over medium heat, and heat until well blended. Pour over meat. Strew herbs over the meat. Cover pan and bake for at least 4 hours, or until meat is very tender. Add carrots and potatoes to pan about 1 hour before serving. When vegetables are tender, transfer meat and vegetables to a platter, remove herbs, and bring sauce to a boil over the stove. Allow to reduce slightly and season with salt and pepper.

Eggs

Eggs from pastured hens are one of Nature's perfect foods, supplying Westerners the same types of nutrients that South Sea Islanders obtained from fish; they are an integral part of our diet plans. It's important to purchase the best-quality eggs you can find, preferably from hens that are on pasture in the outdoors. Second best is organic eggs, but be aware that organic eggs almost always come from hens in confinement.

The yolks of hens on pasture are rich in vitamins A and D, as well as DHA, the long-chain fatty acids so important to neurological function and reproductive health.

If the eggs come from hens on pasture that have not been fed antibiotics and have been carefully handled (see page 81 for a discussion of this), it is perfectly safe to eat the yolks raw or lightly cooked. The whites contain enzyme inhibitors that can interfere with digestion, so are better eaten cooked.

SUPER SCRAMBLE
Serves 2 • 209 calories per serving

2 eggs
2 egg yolks
1 tablespoon cream
1 tablespoon finely chopped fresh parsley (optional)

1 tablespoon butter
Pinch of sea salt

In a medium bowl, beat eggs, egg yolks, cream, and salt with a fork or wire whisk until blended. Stir in parsley, if using. Warm butter in a medium skillet over medium heat, add eggs and cook, stirring, until scrambled.

CHEESE OMELET
Serves 2 • 305 calories per serving

2 eggs
2 egg yolks
2 tablespoon water
Dash of Tabasco sauce

2 ounces grated cheddar or Parmesan cheese
1 tablespoon chopped fresh parsley or chives
1 tablespoon butter

In a medium bowl, beat eggs, egg yolks, water, and Tabasco together with a fork or wire whisk until blended. Melt butter in a cast-iron skillet over medium heat until it foams. Pour in egg mixture and sprinkle on cheddar cheese and chopped parsley or chives. Cook several minutes, then fold over half the omelet. Transfer to a heated platter and serve.

ENGLISH BREAKFAST
Serves 2 • 445 calories per serving

2 ounces additive-free sausage
   or no-nitrate bacon
2 slices sourdough whole-grain bread

1 tablespoon lard or **Mary's Oil Blend** (page 188)
4 eggs
1 tomato, thickly sliced

Cook the sausage or bacon in a cast-iron skillet over medium-high heat. Transfer to a heated platter and keep warm in the oven. Place bread in skillet and then turn so that both sides soak up the fat. Transfer to platter. Add lard to pan, fry eggs to desired doneness, and transfer to platter. Raise heat and cook tomato slices on both sides until browned. Transfer to platter. Return bread to pan and cook on both sides until nicely browned. To serve, place a slice of bread on each of 2 heated plates. Place eggs on bread and surround with tomato and sausage or bacon.

SPANISH OMELET
Serves 2   •   359 calories per serving

4 eggs
Sea salt and freshly ground black pepper
2 ounces grated jack or cheddar
 cheese

1 tablespoon finely chopped fresh parsley
1 tablespoon lard or **Mary's Oil Blend** (page
 188)
2 medium potatoes, thinly sliced

In a medium bowl beat eggs with salt and pepper. Stir in cheese and parsley. Heat lard in a cast-iron skillet over medium heat. Fry potatoes in lard until golden, about 10 minutes, until lightly browned. Spread out potatoes in the pan. Pour in egg mixture, cover, and cook over medium heat until egg sets, about 5 minutes. Turn out onto a large plate. Slice in wedges and serve.

Vegetables

SLOW-BAKE TOMATOES
Serves 4   •   141 calories per serving

2 tablespoons extra-virgin olive oil or
 Mary's Oil Blend (page 188)
12 Roma tomatoes

1 tablespoon Sucanat, Rapadura, or maple
 sugar

Preheat oven to 250°F. Place oil in a Pyrex baking dish and brush to cover sides and corners. Add tomatoes and brush oil on tomatoes. Bake for several hours. Thirty minutes before serving, sprinkle with sweetener and raise oven temperature to 300°F.

STUFFED TOMATOES
Serves 6   •   66 calories per serving

3 large tomatoes
Sea salt and freshly ground black pepper to taste
2 slices whole-grain bread

2 tablespoons butter, softened
2 tablespoons grated Parmesan cheese
½ teaspoon fines herbs

Preheat oven to 350°F. Slice tomatoes in half around the equator, remove seeds, and place cut side up in a buttered baking dish. Sprinkle with a little salt and pepper. Process bread in a food processor to make fine crumbs. Add butter, Parmesan, and herbs and pulse a few times until well blended. Spread a spoonful of stuffing over each tomato half. Bake for about 30 minutes, or until lightly browned.

STEAMED SPINACH
Serves 4   •   69 calories per serving

9 ounces (4 cups, lightly packed)   About ½ cup water
    fresh spinach   2 tablespoons butter

Place spinach and water in a large pot over medium heat and steam until completely wilted. Use a slotted spoon to transfer to a serving bowl. Press out additional liquid with spoon. (Liquid may be saved and added to gravies or discarded.) Top with butter and place in a warm oven until ready to serve.

STEAMED BROCCOLI
Serves 4   •   74 calories per serving

2 cups broccoli florets   2 tablespoons butter

Place broccoli in top portion of a two-part vegetable steamer. Steam for about 5 minutes, until broccoli turns bright green and is just tender. Transfer to a serving bowl and dot with butter. Place in a warm oven until ready to serve.

STEAMED ASPARAGUS
Serves 4   •   75 calories per serving

1 bunch asparagus   2 tablespoons melted butter
Juice of half a lemon

Trim asparagus and place in top portion of a two-part vegetable steamer. Steam for about 5 minutes, until asparagus turns bright green and is just tender. Transfer to a serving bowl. Meanwhile, melt butter with lemon juice in a small skillet over medium heat and pour over asparagus. Place in a warm oven until ready to serve.

STEAMED BRUSSELS SPROUTS
Serves 4   •   81 calories per serving

2 cups Brussels sprouts   2 tablespoons melted butter

Cut the ends off the Brussels sprouts, then cut an X into the remaining stem end. (This will help them cook evenly.) Place in top portion of a two-part vegetable steamer. Steam for about 10 minutes, until Brussels sprouts are tender. Transfer to a serving bowl and pour melted butter over them. Place in a warm oven until ready to serve.

STEAMED CABBAGE
Serves 4 • 69 calories per serving

---

1 medium cabbage, core removed and   1 tablespoon butter
   sliced very thinly   Sea salt and freshly ground black pepper
½ cup water

Place cabbage and water in a large pan and dot top with butter. Sprinkle on salt
and a generous amount of pepper. Steam for about 5 minutes, until cabbage is
limp. Use a slotted spoon to transfer to a serving bowl.

GREEN BEANS WITH BUTTER
Serves 2 • 104 calories per serving

---

2 cups green beans or French beans   1 tablespoon melted butter

Remove ends and strings from the beans. Green beans should be cut lengthwise (this can be done by hand or in a food processor). Cut beans into 1-inch
lengths. Plunge into a pot of boiling water and cook until tender, 6 to 8 minutes.
Pour into a colander and immediately rinse with cold water. Toss with melted
butter and keep in a warm oven until ready to serve.

HASH BROWN POTATOES
Serves 4 • 113 calories per serving

---

2 large potatoes, washed but not peeled   1 tablespoon butter
Filtered water   1 tablespoon extra-virgin olive oil or **Mary's**
¼ cup **Homemade Whey** (page 227) or   **Oil Blend** (page 188)
   vinegar (any type)   Freshly ground black pepper to taste
1 tablespoon sea salt, plus more to taste

Use food processor to cut potatoes into a small julienne. Immediately place in a
bowl with water, whey, and salt. Press potatoes down so that they are entirely covered with water, cover bowl, and soak overnight. Pour out water, skim off top
layer of potatoes (which will have turned brown), place remainder of the potatoes
in a tea towel, and wring out thoroughly.

Melt butter and oil in a large, heavy skillet. Place potatoes in pan and press
down firmly. Sprinkle with salt and pepper, cover pan, and cook over medium
heat for about 5 minutes. Turn potatoes and cook, covered, another 5 minutes or
so, or until potatoes are well browned on both sides.

SAUTÉED SWEET POTATO
Serves 2   •   329 calories per serving

---

1 large sweet potato   Sea salt to taste
3 tablespoons lard or **Mary's Oil Blend** (page 188)

Peel sweet potato, cut into quarters lengthwise, and cut into small slices. Warm lard in a medium skillet over medium heat. Add sweet potatoes and sauté about 15 minutes, or until golden, and season with a generous amount of salt.

Grains

All our recipes for wheat and oats are soaked overnight in warm acidulated water, a process that activates numerous enzymes that neutralize the many anti-nutrients and irritants in whole grains. Even people who are sensitive to grains can usually tolerate grains that have been carefully soaked and then cooked. However, our **Breakfast Cereal** (page 258) is best for those who digest grains more easily.

BASIC OATMEAL
Serves 4   •   100 calories per serving

Oatmeal is a delicious, warming, nourishing breakfast food. Serve with several of the following: butter, cream, a natural sweetener, **Coconut Sprinkles** (page 214), or freeze-dried coconut, raisins, chopped dates, or chopped **Crispy Nuts** (page 259).

Note: You can cook a large amount of oatmeal, store it in the refrigerator, and reheat a portion as needed, adding a little water to prevent burning.

1 cup rolled oats   1 teaspoon sea salt
1 cup warm water   1 cup water
2 tablespoons fresh lemon juice, vinegar
  yogurt, **Kefir** (page 261), or **Homemade
  Whey** (page 227)

In a medium bowl, mix oats in 1 cup warm water and 2 tablespoons lemon juice, vinegar, yogurt, or whey. Cover and leave at room temperature overnight. In the morning, bring 1 cup water to boil in a medium pot. Add salt and soaked oats and bring to a boil. Reduce heat and simmer 1 to 2 minutes, until oatmeal thickens.

Variation: Ginger Oatmeal   *Serves 4   •   144 calories per serving*
Add 1 tablespoon grated ginger and ¼ cup pine nuts to oatmeal while cooking.

CROUTONS
Serves 6   •   119 calories per serving

A few croutons in a soup or salad can turn an ordinary dish into an extraordinary one.

4 slices whole-grain sourdough bread,   4 tablespoons lard or **Mary's Oil Blend** (page 188)
    crusts removed   Sea salt to taste

Cut bread into small cubes and sauté in lard with a generous dash of sea salt until golden. You may also cut the bread on the diagonal to make 2 triangles, sprinkle with salt, and sauté on both sides in lard or oil until golden.

BREAKFAST CEREAL
Makes about 10 cups   •   383 calories per cup

This ingenious soaked-grain recipe was developed by Laurie Smith of the Weston A. Price Foundation. As it bakes it fills the house with a heavenly aroma. The final product is dry and crunchy and so sweet it requires no added sweetener.

6 cups freshly ground whole-wheat or   ¼ cup melted coconut oil or butter
    spelt flour   ½ cup maple syrup
3 cups whole milk, preferably raw   1 teaspoon sea salt
1 cup water   1 teaspoon pure vanilla extract
¼ cup **Homemade Whey** (page 227)   1 teaspoon ground cinnamon
2 teaspoons baking soda   1 teaspoon pure maple flavoring

In a large bowl, mix flour with milk, water, and whey, cover, and leave at room temperature overnight. In the morning add the remaining ingredients and more water, if needed, to make a pourable batter. Preheat oven to 350°F. Prepare two 9-by-13-inch baking pans with coconut oil and pour half the batter into each. Bake for 35 to 45 minutes, or until a toothpick inserted in the center comes out clean. Remove from oven and lower oven temperature to 200°F. Allow cereal to cool and then crumble up onto baking sheets. Bake until completely dry and hard, about 1 hour. To get a uniform size, process briefly in batches in a food processor. Store in airtight containers at room temperature.

To serve, add raw milk or cream diluted with water and raisins or fresh fruit. Allow cereal to soften in the milk or cream slightly before eating.

Nuts

CRISPY NUTS
Makes 4 cups   •   200 to 250 calories per ¼ cup

Many recipes in this book call for Crispy Nuts, and they are also great to eat plain as a nutritious snack. Crispy pecans, almonds, macadamias, peanuts, and cashews can be stored in an airtight container at room temperature; the omega-3 content of walnuts makes them susceptible to rancidity, so store walnuts in an airtight container in the refrigerator. We recommend skinless almonds, as the skins can be irritating to the digestive tract, even when soaked.

4 cups raw pecans, walnut halves, almonds   1 tablespoon sea salt
   (whole skinless, slivered, or sliced),   Filtered water
   macadamias, peanuts, or cashews

Place nuts in a bowl with salt and cover with water. Cover loosely and leave at room temparature about 8 hours. *(Note: Soak cashews for 6 hours, no longer.)* Drain in a colander and strew onto a stainless-steel baking pan or cookie sheet. Place in an oven set at 150°F and let them dehydrate for 12 to 24 hours or until completely dry and crisp. (You may also use a dehydrator.)

Desserts

FLAKY PIE CRUST
Serves 10, when used in a pie   •   About 152 calories per serving of crust alone

---

For this pie crust, we cheat a little and allow unbleached white flour, to ensure that the crust is very light and the taste does not interfere with the taste of the filling. When you use a food processor, the results are foolproof.

1⅓ cups unbleached white flour   ½ cup (1 stick) frozen butter
Pinch of sea salt   2 egg yolks
Pinch of stevia powder   3 tablespoons cold water

Sift flour, salt, and stevia powder into food processor. Place butter on a board and cut into about 16 pieces using a sharp knife. Distribute butter over flour. Pulse processor several times until butter is broken into pea-sized pieces and is well distributed. Beat egg yolks briefly with a fork, dribble over flour mixture, and pulse once or twice. Have cold water ready. Turn on processor and immediately pour water in. Stop processor at once. (Butter should still be visible as pea- and seed-sized pieces.)

Turn crust onto waxed paper, wrap up, and squeeze together, forming a ball. Refrigerate several hours. Roll out on a pastry cloth, using unbleached white flour to keep dough from sticking.

For a French-style tart pan (with removeable bottom), press dough firmly into sides of pan and drape over the top. Roll a rolling pin over the top to trim crust evenly. For an American-style pie pan, line pan with dough and pinch edges to make a fluted edge.

Prick dough several times with a fork. Place in a cool oven and turn on heat. (Gradual warming will prevent excessive shrinking of dough.) Bake at 300°F for 15 minutes for a partially baked pastry and 25 minutes for a fully baked pastry.

WHIPPED CREAM
Makes 2 cups • About 35 calories per tablespoon

2 cups good-quality heavy cream, preferably raw, not ultrapasteurized
1 teaspoon pure vanilla extract

1 tablespoon maple sugar or pinch of stevia powder

Beat cream in a glass bowl with a whisk or an electric beater. When cream makes soft folds, beat in vanilla and maple sugar or stevia powder.

STEWED FRUIT
Makes about 1 quart • 75 calories per ½ cup

Stewed fruit is an old-fashioned dessert, but satisfying and healthy. Use the juice from stewed fruit for making **Kefir Fruit Soda** (page 262) or add a small amount to sparkling water to make a spritzer. Serve stewed fruit with **Coconut Sprinkles** (page 214), **Whipped Cream** (previous recipe), **Whipped Coconut Cream** (page 217), or **Vanilla Ice Cream** (following recipe).

About 4 pounds organic fresh fruit, such as apricots, peaches, plums, or nectarines, or a mixture

Several slices of fresh ginger
½ cup Rapadura, Sucanat, or maple sugar
Filtered water

Cut fruit in half and remove the pits. You may peel fruit, but it is not necessary if fruit is organic. Place in a large pot with ginger and sweetener and cover with filtered water. Bring to a boil, reduce heat, and simmer, covered, for about 1 hour. Allow to cool and remove fruit with a slotted spoon to a serving bowl.

VANILLA ICE CREAM
Makes 1 quart • 294 calories per ½ cup

With the new small ice cream makers that include a double-walled canister you can keep in the freezer, ice cream making is very easy. Now you can have ice cream made with natural sweeteners, egg yolks, and pure cream, and without all the additives (many of which are not listed on the label). These ice creams are very dense in calories, but so satisfying that it is difficult to eat more than half a cup.

Homemade ice cream will be quite hard when you take it out of the freezer. (Commerical ice cream remains soft enough to scoop, even when frozen, because a compound akin to anti-freeze is added.) If you store ice cream in a shallow container and remove it from the freezer about 5 minutes before serving, it will be soft enough to cut or spoon. Adding 2 tablespoons of vodka or other liqueur will also help keep the ice cream soft.

6 egg yolks	3 cups heavy cream, preferably raw, not
½ cup Rapadura, Sucanat, or maple sugar	ultrapasteurized
1 tablespoon pure vanilla extract	2 tablespoons vodka (optional)

In a large bowl, beat egg yolks with sweetener for several minutes until pale and thick. Beat in vanilla, cream, and vodka, if using. Prepare in the ice cream maker according to manufacturer's directions.

Beverages and Tonics

In addition to our versatile **Raw Milk Tonic** (an important part of Health Recovery) and homemade milk **Kefir**, you'll find below several easy-to-make and delicious soft drinks made with water kefir grains or kefir powder (see Resources). You will be amazed at how simple it is to make these delicious, healthy fizzy drinks.

Other lacto-fermented drinks in this section include **Beet Kvass** (page 263; important in Health Recovery), which uses **Homemade Whey** (page 227) as an inoculant, and **Kombucha** (page 264).

RAW MILK TONIC
Makes 2 cups • 311 calories per cup

2 egg yolks	1¾ cups raw milk
2 tablespoons molasses	

In a large glass, beat egg yolks with molasses and stir in milk. Sip slowly.

KEFIR
Makes 1 quart • 200 calories per cup

1 quart whole milk, preferably raw but not ultrapasteurized	½ cup kefir grains or 1 package kefir powder (see Resources)

Place milk in a glass or ceramic container and add kefir grains or powder. Cover tightly and leave at room temperature overnight or until desired tartness is obtained. If you are using kefir grains, strain out the grains using a non-metallic strainer, rinse them with water, and either use again or store in a jar in the refrigerator with about ½ cup milk.

KEFIR SODAS
Makes 2 quarts   •   About 40 calories per cup

Easy-to-make, delicious kefir sodas are a wonderful alternative to commercial sodas. Instead of creating health problems, like modern soft drinks, our kefir sodas contribute to easy digestion and overall good health. Thanks to Sarah Pope, Weston A. Price Foundation chapter leader for Tampa, Florida, for her pioneering work in developing these delicious drinks.

You can use either water kefir grains or kefir powder (see Resources). Use about ¾ cup grains or 1 packet powder for 2 quarts of soda. Place all ingredients in a 2-quart glass container, add water kefir grains or powder, fill with water to make 2 quarts, cover tightly, and leave at room temperature for 48 hours. Strain the liquid through a non-metallic strainer.

If using grains, rinse them with water and either use again or store in a jar in the refrigerator with about ½ cup water mixed with 1 tablespoon Rapadura, Sucanat, or maple sugar. If using the powder, reserve about ½ cup liquid as a starter for the next batch—this will work for about 5 to 6 batches, then you will need to use powder again.

Store the soda in the original glass container in the refrigerator, or, for extra bubbly results, transfer to glass beer or soda bottles capped with wire-held caps. (See Resources.)

Note: Do not store soda in decorative vinegar bottles that have wire-held stoppers; these have a tendency to explode and can be quite dangerous!

Kefir Cream Soda
½ cup Rapadura, Sucanat, or maple sugar   Slices of organic lemon, lime, or orange
1 tablespoon pure vanilla extract   (optional)

Kefir Ginger Ale
4 tablespoons coarsely chopped fresh ginger   ½ cup Rapadura, Sucanat, or maple sugar
Juice of 4 limes

Kefir Lemonade
1 cup fresh lemon juice   ½ cup Rapadura, Sucanat, or maple sugar

Kefir Limeade with Mint
1 cup fresh lime juice   Several sprigs of fresh mint
½ cup Rapadura, Sucanat, or maple sugar

Kefir Fruit Soda
2 cups juice left over from making   ¼ cup Rapadura, Sucanat, or maple sugar
Stewed Fruit (page 260)

Kefir Berry Soda

This soda is slightly more complicated, but well worth the effort. (Use kefir powder, not grains, to make this soda, as the grains tend to favor an alcoholic fermentation when the fructose content is high.) Make 2 cups puree of organic fresh berries (strawberries, raspberries, blackberries, etc.) in a food processor. Pass through a strainer (to remove seeds) into a bowl. Add ½ cup Rapadura, Sucanat, or maple sugar, enough water to make 2 quarts, and 1 package powder. Cover with a towel and leave at room temperature 48 hours. Carefully skim off any foam that has risen to the top. Strain into bottles with wire-held caps. Leave at room temperature for 48 hours and then store in the refrigerator. To avoid large amounts of fizz, open bottles carefully while very cold.

BEET KVASS
Makes 2 quarts • About 50 calories per cup

This drink is essentially medicinal. You wouldn't serve it to guests—but it has extraordinary healing powers. We've had more positive testimonials about beet kvass than about any other beverage in our book *Nourishing Traditions*.

Beets are loaded with nutrients. One 4-ounce glass of beet kvass, morning and night, is an excellent blood tonic, promotes regularity, aids digestion, alkalizes the blood, cleanses the liver, and is a good treatment for kidney stones.

The quality of the beets has a profound effect on the results. The final product should be somewhat thick and slightly bubbly. However, even if the drink is thin and not particularly bubbly, it will still provide many healing benefits.

Note: Do not use grated beets to make beet tonic. When grated, beets exude too much juice, resulting in too-rapid fermentation that favors production of alcohol rather than lactic acid. The beets should be coarsely chopped by hand.

3 medium or 2 large organic beets, peeled   1 tablespoon sea salt
   and coarsely chopped   Filtered water
¼ cup **Homemade Whey** (page 227)

Place beets, whey, and salt in a 2-quart glass container. Add filtered water to fill the container. Stir well and cover securely. Keep at room temperature for 2 days before transferring to refrigerator. To serve, pour through a strainer.

When most of the liquid has been drunk, you can fill up the container with water and keep it at room temperature another 2 days. The resulting brew will be slightly less strong than the first. After the second brew, discard the beets and start again. You may, however, reserve some of the liquid and use this as your inoculant instead of the whey.

KOMBUCHA
Makes 3 quarts   •   About 40 calories per cup

3 quarts filtered water
1 cup sugar
1 tablespoon sea salt (optional)
4 organic black tea bags

½ cup kombucha from a previous culture
(this can be the liquid that the mushroom
comes in)
1 kombucha mushroom (see Resources)

Bring 3 quarts filtered water to boil in a large pot. Add sugar and salt, if using, and simmer until dissolved. Remove from heat, add tea bags, and allow tea to steep until water has completely cooled. Remove tea bags. Pour cooled liquid into a 4-quart Pyrex bowl and add ½ cup kombucha from previous batch. Place the mushroom on top of the liquid.

Make a crisscross over the bowl with masking tape, cover loosely with a cloth or towel, and transfer to a warm, dark place, away from contaminants and insects. In about 7 to 10 days the kombucha will be ready, depending on the temperature. It should be rather sour and possibly fizzy, with no taste of tea remaining. Transfer to covered glass containers and store in the refrigerator.

Note: Do not wash kombucha bowls in the dishwasher; however, you can wash the glass containers you store it in.

When the kombucha is ready, your mushroom will have grown a second spongy pancake. This can be used to make other batches or given away to friends. Store fresh mushrooms in the refrigerator in a glass or stainless-steel container—never plastic. A kombucha mushroom can be used dozens of times. If it begins to turn black, or if the resulting kombucha doesn't sour properly, it's a sign that the culture has become contaminated. When this happens, it's best to throw away all your mushrooms and order a new clean one.

Note: White sugar, rather than honey or Rapadura, and black tea, rather than flavored teas, give the highest amounts of beneficial organic acids. Non-organic tea is high in fluoride, a known thyroid depressant, so always use organic tea.

A word of caution: Some people may have an allergic reaction to kombucha. If you have allergies, start with a small taste to observe any adverse effects. If you react badly, use **Beet Kvass** (page 263) for several weeks to detoxify, then try again.

Chapter Eleven

Resources

Depending on where you live, you'll find most of the items listed below widely available in health food stores, specialty stores, upscale markets, or Asian markets. Below we've listed the brands you're likely to find in stores, and even some national chains that carried them at the time of this writing. And if you can't find particular products in your area, or your local retailers don't carry our preferred brands, we've also listed mail-order sources for everything. Phone numbers, Internet addresses, and availability of products may change after this writing.

Coconut Products

Coconut Oil

We recommend virgin coconut oil, which is produced locally using low-tech, traditional processes, for all the recipes in this book.

Most commercial coconut oil is refined, bleached, and deodorized (RBD). The coconuts are transported great distances to a refining factory, where they are opened up and laid in the sun to dry. The dried coconut meat—called copra—becomes brown and rancid and may develop mold. Next, the meat is put into a huge press that extracts the oil at temperatures over 200°F (and this is called "cold-pressing"!) or treated with solvents and subjected to even higher temperatures. The oil then goes through a "refining" process that involves adding lye or caustic soda. After this it's bleached, usually by passing it through acid and alkaline clays. Refining and bleaching deplete vitamin E and other nutrients. The final step involves deodorizing the oil, to remove any burnt or metallic taste, by heating the oil and bubbling gas through it while a vacuum pulls off the vapors. The result is a tasteless, odorless coconut oil that may contain solvent and lye residues. This highly industrialized process brings profits to large companies, not small producers. Even though deodorized, much industrially processed coconut oil has a burnt or metallic taste.

A particularly natural method for extracting the oil involves letting coconut milk stand in a covered bucket for about 24 hours. After 24 to 36 hours, the oil naturally separates from the water fraction, producing a pure oil with all the coconut scent. Brian Shilhavy of Tropical Traditions has been instrumental in reviving this traditional method and supporting artisanal coconut oil producers in the Philippines by importing the oil and providing it to consumers in the United States.

Virgin coconut oil is extracted from pressed fresh coconut meat by a variety of methods, including gentle heating, fermentation, refrigeration, enzymes, and mechanical centrifuge. Throughout, the temperature does not exceed about 170°F. Virgin coconut oil is white or cream colored and has a mild coconut flavor. Most virgin coconut oil is organic, but in any case, coconut palms are rarely sprayed. (For further information on coconut oil processing, visit tropicaltraditions.com.)

In stores: Garden of Life (sold in the vitamin section)
   Omega Nutrition (sold in the vitamin section)
   Spectrum unrefined coconut oil (sold in the vitamin section)

Mail order: Tropical Traditions (highly recommended), tropicaltraditions.com, (866) 311-2626
   Wilderness Family Naturals, wildernessfamilynaturals.com, (866) 936-6457
   Radiant Life, radiantlifecatalog.com, (888) 593-8333
   Coconut Oil Online, coconutoil-online.com, (800) 922-1744
   Beyond a Century, beyond-a-century.com, (800) 777-1324

Coconut Milk

Canned coconut milk is widely available in stores and on the Internet. Unfortunately, most brands available in stores contain either an emulsifier, to keep the milk from separating, or a preservative. If you are making authentic Thai dishes or want to use the separated cream, you will need coconut milk without emulsifiers. Be sure to purchase *whole* coconut milk, not lite—lite coconut milk has most of the valuable fatty acids removed!

In stores: Native Forest (contains guar gum, an emulsifier, yet it usually separates)
   Thai Kitchen (contains guar gum, an emulsifier)
   Mae Ploy, in Asian markets (contains a preservative but no emulsifier)
   Chaokoh, in Asian markets (contains a preservative but no emulsifier)

Mail order: Wilderness Family Naturals, wildernessfamilynaturals.com, (866) 936-6457; carries the Coco Gem brand (contains no emulsifiers or preservatives)
   Chef Shop, chefshop.com (877) 337-2491; carries its own brand (contains no emulsifiers or preservatives)

Pacific Rim Gourmet, pacificrim-gourmet.com, (800) 910-WOKS; carries Mae Ploy and Chaokoh brands

Asian Food Grocer, asianfoodgrocer.com, (877) 360-1855; carries Orchids brand

Coconut Cream

This is the thick creamy part that rises to the top of coconut milk. It actually can be whipped, like whipped cream.

In stores: Usually available under various brand names at Asian markets.

Mail order: Wilderness Family Naturals, wildernessfamilynaturals.com, (866) 936-6457

Coconut Oil Online, coconutoil-online.com, (800) 922-1744

Creamed Coconut

This is made by grinding coconut meat very finely, pressing it into blocks, and refrigerating. It resembles hard white butter. It can be reconstituted by gently melting with a small amount of water. You can use reconstituted creamed coconut like coconut milk, although it has a slightly gritty texture. Unfortunately, most brands contain sodium metabisulfate, a preservative.

In stores: Usually available under various brand names at Asian markets.

Mail order: Tropical Traditions, tropicaltraditions.com, (866) 311-2626

Available by the case from P. A. Tropical Products, (718) 763-5888.

Desiccated Coconut

Look for a product that does not contain preservatives.

In stores: Widely available in health food stores and specialty markets

Mail order: Coconut Oil Online, coconutoil-online.com, (800) 922-1744

Freeze-Dried Coconut

This delicious product is made by freeze-drying fresh coconut meat. It is naturally sweet and absolutely delicious. Comes in both coarse and fine cut.

In stores: Balducci's markets (New York and Washington, D.C.); sold as "fancy" coconut

Mail order: Wilderness Family Naturals, wildernessfamilynaturals.com (866) 936-6457

Coconut Sugar

A wonderful natural sweetener made from the sap of coconut flowers. Also called "palm sugar," it is less sweet than other natural sweeteners. It comes as a pale paste. Use in coconut desserts and soups, since (unlike other natural sweeteners) it won't turn the white coconut milk brown.

In stores: Available in Asian markets under various brand names.

Mail order: Temple of Thai, templeofthai.com, (877) 811-8773
Taste of Asia, tasteofasia.com

Coconut Juice (Coconut Water)

The watery juice inside the immature coconut. It's not hard to extract the water, as the immature coconuts are relatively soft, although you will need a good tool, such as a hammer and punch or a drill.

In stores: Many upscale and Asian markets carry immature coconuts.

Mail order: Best Oriental Produce, Los Angeles, primafresh.com, (213) 662-9385, sells immature coconuts by the case.
Wilderness Family Naturals, wildernessfamilynaturals.com, (866) 936-6457, sells packaged coconut water very reasonably in cases of 36 (200-ml) containers.
Glaser Organics, glaserorganicfarms.com, (305) 238-7954, ships fresh organic coconut water throughout the United States

Coconut Vinegar

In stores: Available in Asian markets under various brand names.

Mail order: Taste of Asia, tasteofasia.com

Coconut Rum

In stores: Sold in most liquor stores.

Dolomite

A very inexpensive and useful calcium supplement for adding to Coconut Milk Tonic, quick broths, and other beverages. Be sure to purchase the powder, not the pills. One teaspoon contains the calcium provided by one quart of milk.

In stores: KAL dolomite powder at Vitamin Shoppe stores

Mail order: KAL dolomite powder at vitaminshoppe.com, (800) 223-1216

Raw Milk

For local sources and availability in your state, visit realmilk.com or contact a local chapter of the Weston A. Price Foundation, listed at westonaprice.org, (202) 333-HEAL.

In stores: Claravale Dairy raw whole cow's milk (California)
Organic Pastures raw whole cow's milk (California)
Note: Organic Pastures raw milk may be available in health food stores in many states under the label SuperLeche.
Golden Fleece raw goat's and cow's milk (Florida)
Sweetwoods Dairy raw whole goat's milk (New Mexico)

Mail order: Organic Pastures, (559) 846-9732, organicpastures.com and mercola.com

Eggs and Meat Products, Pasture-Raised

See classified ads in *Wise Traditions*, the journal of the Weston A. Price Foundation, (202) 333-HEAL, or contact a local chapter, listed at westonaprice.org. See also eatwild.com.

In stores: Lamb from New Zealand or Iceland
Coleman's beef and lamb
Prather Ranch beef
Niman Ranch pork
Welsh Family meats
Sunflower Field meats
Organic Pastures beef
Shelton's poultry
Rocky chicken
Rosie chicken
Pollo Real chicken
Diestal turkey

Mail order: Tropical Traditions, tropicaltraditions.com, (866) 311-2626
Real Foods Market, realfoodsmarket.com, (866) 284-7325
Fox Fire Farms lamb, (970) 563-4675
White Egret Farm natural meats, whiteegretfarm.com, (512) 276-7408
Peaceful Pastures grass-fed meats, peacefulpastures.com, (615) 683-4291
Meadow Raised grass-fed meats, (607) 278-5602
Grassland grass-fed beef, grasslandbeef.com, (877) 383-0051
Greatbeef, greatbeef.com
Ranch Foods Direct beef (not grass-fed, but naturally raised), ranchfoodsdirect.com, (866) 866-6328

Lacto-Fermented Beverage Supplies

You can make our fermented beverages using either kefir grains or kefir powder. The following products are available by mail order:

Milk Kefir Grains

Mail order: G.E.M. Cultures, gemcultures.com, (707) 964-2922
Marilyn Jardembski, (419) 237-3095

Water Kefir Grains
For water-based beverages

Mail order: Marilyn Jardembski, (419) 237-3095

Kefir Powder
For either milk or water-based beverages

Mail order: Body Ecology, bodyecologydiet.com, (800) 511-2660
Wilderness Family Naturals, wildernessfamilynaturals.com, (866) 936-6457

Kombucha Mushrooms

Mail order: Laurel Farms, (941) 351-2233
G.E.M. Cultures, gemcultures.com, (707) 964-2922
A. F. Kombucha, kombucha2000.com, (877) 566-2824

Kombucha (ready-made)

In stores: Portland Brewing Co. kombucha drinks
Pro Natura kombucha tea

Mail order: A. F. Kombucha, kombucha2000.com, (877) 566-2824

Bottles with Wire Stoppers
Mountain Homebrew & Wine Supply, mountainhomebrew.com, (425) 803-3996

Lacto-Fermented Condiments

In stores: Real Pickles (sauerkraut, Asian sauerkraut, pickles)
Garden of Life lacto-fermented foods
Rejuvenative Foods cultured vegetables
Deep Root lacto-fermented vegetables
Sanga's kimchi

Mail order: Deep Root lacto-fermented vegetables, biolact.com

Wellspring Farm of Vermont sauerkraut, wellspringfarmvt.com, (802) 426-3890

Real Pickles, realpickles.com

Goldmine sauerkraut, goldminenaturalfood.com, (858) 537-9830

Rejuvenative Foods, rejuvenative.com, (800) 805-7957

Grain and Salt Society, celtic-seasalt.com, (800) 867-7258

Hawthorne Valley, hawthornevalleyfarm.com, (518) 672-7500

Stock

Many upscale markets make their own stock (chicken, fish, beef, and veal) and sell it frozen. Likewise, some farmers who sell grass-fed meats also make stock with the bones and sell it directly to consumers. To locate farmers who sell stock, contact a local chapter of the Weston A. Price Foundation, weston aprice.org, (202) 333-HEAL. You may also purchase canned stock (see brand names listed below) and add dolomite (see recipe for **Quick Chicken Stock,** page 225). For sources of bonito flakes (for making **Quick Fish Stock,** recipe page 226, see below). We do not recommend stock sold in boxes.

In stores: Rich Addition (beef, fish, and chicken)

Just Take Stock/Copper Stockpot (fish, beef, chicken, and turkey)

Hay Day Country Market

Health Valley canned chicken and beef broth

Shelton's canned chicken and beef broth

Mail order: Just Take Stock/Copper Stock Pot, copperstockpot.com, (877) 827-8625

Sweeteners

In addition to the products below, check out Coconut Sugar on page 267.

Honey, Raw

Be sure the label specifies "raw" honey; honey labeled "unheated" has actually been heated!

In stores: Really Raw Honey

Honey in the Rough

Natural Rush honey

Famous Questa virgin clover honey

Mail order: Really Raw Honey, (800) REALRAW
   Walt's Swarmbusting honey, (611) 384-2384
   Apitherapy raw honey, (802) 985-5852

Dehydrated Cane Sugar Juice

In stores: Sucanat
   Rapadura

Mail order: Rapadura, rapunzel.com, (800) 207-2814
   Organic Mascava Sugar, matefactor.com, (800) 656-3668

Maple Syrup
   Be sure to purchase organic maple syrup—non-organic maple syrup is extracted using formaldehyde. Use Grade B, if you can find it—it contains more nutrients and is usually less expensive.

In stores: Shady Maple Farms organic maple syrup
   Spring Tree organic maple syrup
   Russell organic maple syrup

Mail order: Grain & Salt Society, (828) 299-9005
   Coombs Vermont Gourmet, maplesource.com, (888) 266-6271

Maple Sugar
   Maple sugar is dehydrated maple syrup. This is an excellent sweetener, loaded with nutrients and without the strong taste of dehydrated cane sugar juice. It comes granulated or as a fine powder.

In stores: Shady Maple Farms maple sugar granules

Mail order: Mother Linda's maple sugar powder, motherlindas.com
   Coombs Vermont Gourmet maple granules and powder, maplesource.com, (888) 266-6271

Stevia Powder
   Be sure to use the green powder, which is simply the ground-up herb, rather than the white powder, which is the extracted compound.

In stores: Often sold as a bulk herb.
   Planetary Formulas

Mail order: Body Ecology, bodyecologydiet.com, (800) 511-2660
   Stevia.com

Superfoods

Acerola powder and Amla tablets (natural vitamin C)

Mail order: Radiant Life, radiantlifecatalog.com, (888) 593-8333

Bitters, Swedish

In stores: Available at most health food stores.

Mail order: Life's Vigor, lifesvigor.com, (661) 589-1818

Butter Oil, High-Vitamin (X-Factor)

Mail order: Radiant Life, radiantlifecatalog.com, (888) 593-8333
    Green Pastures Products, greenpasture.org, (402) 338-5551

Cod-Liver Oil, Regular

In stores: Garden of Life (available in health food stores)

Cod-Liver Oil, High-Vitamin

Mail order: Radiant Life, radiantlifecatalog.com, (888) 593-8333
    Green Pastures Products, greenpasture.org, (402) 338-5551

Desiccated Liver

In stores: Solgar desiccated liver

Mail order: J. R. Carlson Laboratories, carlsonlabs.com, (800) 323-4141

Ox Bile

Mail order: Organic Pharmacy, organic-pharmacy.com, (800) 819-6742
    Natural Health Consultants, naturalhealthconsult.com, (888) 852-4993

Wheat Germ Oil

In stores: NOW brand wheat germ oil

Mail order: DNE and NOW brands at Shopping.com
   Iherb.com, (888) 792-0028

Yeast Flakes, Nutritional
We recommend Frontier brand. Most other brands contain additives or are processed in such a way that MSG is formed.

Mail order: Frontier brand, frontierherb.com, (800) 669-3275
   Radiant Life, radiantlifecatalog.com, (888) 593-8333

Other Food Products

Arrowroot Powder
Arrowroot powder makes an excellent thickener in Asian dishes; it is also an ingredient in **Coconut Almond Cookies** (page 212), **Flourless Cocoa-Coconut Cake** (page 219), **Coconut Bars** (page 217).

In stores: Some health food stores carry arrowroot in packages or spice bottles.

Mail order: Radiant Life, radiantlifecatalog.com, (888) 593-8333
   Natural Lifestyle, (800) 752-2775
   Bob's Red Mill, bobsredmill.com, (503) 654-3215
   Azure Standard, azurestandard.com, (541) 467-2230
   Frontier, frontierherb.com, (800) 669-3275

Bonito Flakes
Used for making **Quick Fish Stock** (page 226).

In stores: Eden bonito flakes

Mail order: Chef Shop, chefshop.com, (877) 337-2491

Bread

In stores: Shiloh Farms breads
   Pacific Bakery breads
   Food for Life bread
   Nature's Path manna bread
   Cloud Cliff Aged Nativo bread
   Cybros sprouted bread products

Traditional pumpernickel breads from Germany
Alvarado Bakery sprouted whole-wheat tortillas

Mail order: Grindstone bread, grindstone@pon.net
Mountain Eagle Bakery, (406) 222-3617
Grain & Salt Society, (800) 867-7258
Miller's Bakery, (530) 532-6384.
Natural Bridge Bakery breads, bakedaze@madison.nc.us
Berkshire Mountain Bakery, (866) 274-3664
O Bread Bakery, (802) 985-8771

Butter, Grass-Fed

For local sources, see classified ads in *Wise Traditions*, journal of the Weston A. Price Foundation, or contact a local chapter of the Weston A. Price Foundation, westonaprice.org, (202) 333-HEAL.

In stores: Organic Pastures raw butter (California)
Kerry Goldbutter
Straus Family Creamery butter
Vermont Butter and Cheese Company butter
Organic Valley cultured butter
Trickling Springs Creamery butter
Natural by Nature organic whipped butter
Traderspoint Creamery butter (Indiana)
Trader Joe's organic sweet cream butter

Mail order: Organic Pasture raw butter from grass-fed cows, organicpastures.com

Cheese

Many wonderful raw cheeses, both domestic and European, are available in upscale markets and on the Internet (see realmilk.com).

In stores: Brunkow Dairey
Rogue Gold
Bravo
Meadow Creek Dairy
Giving Nature
Hawthorne Valley
Maytag blue cheese
Salemville Amish blue cheese
Ruminano Parmesan
Redwood Hill goat cheese

Mail order: Tropical Traditions, tropicaltraditions.com, (866) 311-2626

Zingerman's, zingermans.com, (888) 636-8162
Robert's Food Page, rrich.com/revrawcheese
Hendricks Farm, (267) 718-0219
Green Pastures Dairy, greenpasturesdairy.com, (218) 384-4513
Westminster Dairy, (802) 387-4412
White Egret Farm raw goat cheese, whiteegretfarm.com, (512) 276-7408
Peaceful Pastures raw cheese, peacefulpastures.com, (615) 683-4291
Mercola.com
Organicpastures.com

Condiments Without MSG

In stores: Hain's mustard
  Westbrae mustard
  Grey Poupon mustard
  Anton Kozkil's mustard
  Eden toasted sesame oil
  Busha Browne's Planters steak sauce
  Seeds of Change ketchup
  Tree of Life ketchup
  Muir Glen ketchup
  The Wizard's organic Worchestershire sauce

Crackers

Unfortunately, at this writing, no commercial crackers contain coconut oil. We look forward to the availability of bakery products containing coconut oil in the near future.

In stores: Ak Mak crackers
  Wasa sourdough rye crackers
  Kavli flat breads
  Aunt Gussie's cracker flats
  Finn Crisp
  Late July organic crackers (made with palm oil)
  Hol-Grain rice crackers

Cream

See classified ads in *Wise Traditions*, journal of the Weston A. Price Foundation, or contact a local chapter of the Foundation, westonaprice.org, (202) 333-HEAL.

In stores: Organic Pastures raw cream (California)
  Claravale Dairy raw cream (California)

Butterworks pasteurized cream (New England)
Natural by Nature pasteurized cream (East Coast)
Chrome Dairy pasteurized cream (East Coast)
Lewes Dairy pasteurized cream (East Coast)
Straus Family Creamery pasteurized cream (California)
Traderspoint Creamery pasteurized cream (Indiana)

Mail order: Organic Pastures raw cream, organicpastures.com

Curry Paste

In stores: Thai Kitchen red and green curry pastes
Mae Ploy green curry paste (in Asian markets)

Eggs
Genuinely pastured eggs usually need to be purchased directly from a farmer, either through a co-op or at a farmers' market. For sources, contact a local chapter of the Weston A. Price Foundation, westonaprice.org, (202) 333-HEAL. The brands listed below are organic and/or free-range.

In stores: Shelton's
Gold Circle Farm
Happy Hen
Rock Island
Judy's Family Farm
Organic Valley
Trader Joe's Fertile
Giving Nature

Fish Eggs
Many good fish sellers sell fresh salmon roe in season. High-quality canned roe also is available.

In stores: Romanoff Red (salmon) caviar
Krinos Tarama (carp roe caviar)

Mail order: Krinos Tarama, 3e.com

Fish Sauce, Thai
Look for higher-grade sauce in glass bottles, sold in both upscale markets and Asian markets.

In stores: Thai Kitchen fish sauce

Flax Oil

In stores: Omega Nutrition
    Barlean's

Mail order: Omega Nutrition, omeganutrition.com, (800) 661-3529

Ghee

In stores: Purity Farms organic ghee

Mail order: Grain and Salt Society, celtic-seasalt.com, (800) 867-7258
    Wilderness Family Naturals, wildernessfamilynaturals.com, (800) 945-3801

Grains, Organic

In stores: Widely available in health food stores

Mail order: Natural Lifestyle, (800) 752-2775
    Community Mill and Bean, (800) 755-0554

Goose Fat
Canned goose fat often is available in upscale markets. It can be used interchangeably with lard for sautéing, especially in Asian dishes.

In stores: Rougie

Mail order: Mother Linda's, motherlindas.com
    Edouard Artzner, chefshop.com, (877) 337-2491

Lard
Lard without preservatives is rarely available in stores, although you can often find it at farmers' markets. For locally produced lard from pastured pigs, contact a local chapter of the Weston A. Price Foundation, westonaprice.org, (202) 333-HEAL, or check the classified ads in *Wise Traditions,* the foundation's quarterly magazine.

Mail order: Mother Linda's, motherlindas.com
    Dietrich's lard, (610) 756-6344

Macadamia Nuts, Raw

In stores: Trader Joe's

Macaroons

In stores: Jennie's macaroons (produced by Red Mill Farms of Brooklyn, NY)

Mail order: jenniesmacaroons.com, (718) 384-4814

Meats, Processed

In stores: Primo Naturale salami
Applegate Farms deli meats
Beeler's pork products
Citterio salami
Yorkshire Farms bacon
Niman Ranch pork sausage
Niman Ranch bacon

Mail order: Zingerman's (for bacon), zingermans.com, (888) 636-8162
Dietrich's deli meats (610) 756-6344
Green Pastures Dairy summer sausage, greenpasturesdairy.com, (218) 384-4513

Mayonnaise

In stores: Delouis Fils mayonnaise (sold in refrigerated section of upscale markets)
Hain's safflower mayonnaise (second choice)

Miso

In stores: Eden miso
South River miso

Mail order: South River miso, southrivermiso.com, (413) 369-4057

Olive Oil

In stores: Soler Romero extra-virgin organic olive oil

Mail order: Pietro del Marco, (914) 723-5850
Bariani Olive Oil, Radiant Life, radiantlifecatalog.com, (888) 593-8333
Tiburtini Olive Oil, zingermans.com, (888) 636-8162

Paté, Liverwurst, Fresh

In stores: Trois Petits Cochons
D'Artagnan

Mail order: Dietrich's liverwurst, (610) 756-6344
 Chef Shop, chefshop.com, (877) 337-2491

Peanut Butter, Natural

In stores: Crazy Richard's peanut butter
 Walnut Acres peanut butter
 Whole Foods organic peanut butter
 Arrowhead Mills peanut butter

Salt
 Use only unrefined sea salt or mined salt.

In stores: Real Salt

Mail order: Grain & Salt Society, celtic-seasalt.com, (800) 867-7258
 Radiant Life, radiantlifecatalog.com, (888) 593-8333
 Tribal Trading Company, (800) 656-3668, www.matefactor.com

Seafood, Canned
 Read labels carefully. Many brands of tuna contain hydrolyzed protein, a source of MSG.

In stores: Skansen canned cod liver
 Roland canned smoked cod liver
 Officer canned smoked cod liver
 Natural Value tuna and sardines in olive oil
 King Oscar sardines
 Season sardines
 Bela-Olhao sardines
 Crown Prince tuna in water
 Deep Sea tuna in water
 Trader Joe's Tongol tuna in water
 Natural Sea tuna
 Bumble Bee Alaskan sockeye red salmon
 Natural Sea sockeye salmon
 Seabear smoked salmon paté
 Polar anchovies in olive oil
 Cento anchovies and sardines in olive oil
 Crown Prince oysters in water
 Dave's albacore fillets and fancy salmon
 Brunswick Canadian sardines in spring water

Seafood, Wild, Fresh, or Smoked

FDA regulations stipulate that fish sellers must label their fresh seafood as wild or farmed. Whenever possible, purchase wild fresh seafood.

In stores: Arctic Pride frozen shrimp
  Sea Bear Alaskan salmon products
  Wildcatch salmon products
  Spence & Co. wild smoked king salmon
  Raincoast wild salmon

Mail order: Arctic Pride frozen shrimp, (207) 772-2299
  Vital Choice, wild salmon, vitalchoice.com (800) 608-4825

Sesame Oil, expeller-expressed

In stores: Spectrum sesame oil

Mail order: Omega Nutrition, omeganutrition.com, (800) 661-3529

Soups

The following two brands of soup are naturally made with real stock and carried in some upscale markets and restaurants. Check their websites for availability.

In stores: Kettle Cuisine, kettlecuisine.com, (877) 302-SOUP
  Copper Stockpot, copperstockpot.com, (877) 827-8625

Soy Sauce

In stores: Ohsawa Nama Shoyu unpasteurized soy sauce
  Eden naturally fermented soy sauce
  San-J naturally fermented soy sauce
  Westbrae naturally fermented soy sauce

Mail order: South River soy sauce, southrivermiso.com, (413) 369-4057

Spices and Herbs (non-irradiated)

In stores: Spice Hunter herbs and spices
  Frontier herbs and spices
  Morton & Bassett spices

Mail order: Frontier, frontierherb.com, (800) 669-3275

Tomato Products, Canned

In stores: Muir Glen tomato products
   Bionaturae tomato products

Vegetables, Frozen

In stores: Sno-Pac frozen vegetables
   Cascadian Farms frozen vegetables and berries

Vinegar

In stores: Eden raw wine, apple cider, and rice vinegars
   Bragg's raw, organic apple cider vinegar
   Omega organic apple cider and balsamic vinegars
   Bionaturae organic balsamic vinegar
   Dessinaux wine vinegar

Yogurt

In stores: Seven Stars Farm
   Brown Cow
   Erivan
   Stonyfield Farms
   Butterworks
   Hawthorne Valley
   Pequea Valley Farm
   Coach Farm goat yogurt
   Redwood Hill goat yogurt
   Old Chatham sheep yogurt

Specialty Items

These products usually are only available at Asian markets.
Coconut sugar (also by mail order, see page 268)
Galangal (Thai ginger), fresh or frozen
Jasmine essence
Kaffir lime leaves, fresh or frozen
Lemongrass, fresh
Tamarind paste (also at chefshop.com)

Coconut Oil for Beautiful Skin

Coconut is more than a fabulous food—it's also one of the great beauty secrets of the tropics. The lovely, velvety skin so characteristic of tropical peoples, despite their spending so much time in the sun, comes from the combination of a healthy diet, rich in coconut oil and vitamin A from seafood, plus liberal use of coconut oil on the skin.

Westerners who try coconut oil on their skin report a new softness, magically reduced pores and wrinkles, and even the disappearance of rashes, fungal infections, scars, and warts. Acne blemishes dry up quickly, and the skin heals well.

When you first try coconut oil, you may notice an initial outbreak of small pimples, but this is actually a cleansing effect, and it soon clears up. For skin care, be sure to use virgin coconut oil that has not been processed with harsh chemicals.

Several coconut oil–based cosmetic products are available from Tropical Traditions, tropicaltraditions.com, (866) 311-2626, if you don't feel like making your own.

Bath Oil

For dry skin, add coconut oil to your bath. If you like, toss in a few drops of essential oils as well. After the bath, apply more coconut oil directly to your skin to make it soft and beautiful, especially during the driest times of the year.

Acne

People who suffer from serious acne have told us that the following recipe greatly decreases their blemishes and scarring:

1 cup virgin coconut oil   ¼ cup aloe vera gel

Apply to skin several times per day. This also works wonders on stretch marks! Remember that getting off processed foods and taking cod-liver oil is a must for treating acne. Pharmaceutical acne preparations are based on synthetic vitamin A, which can have some serious side effects. Much better to get natural vitamin A from cod-liver oil.

Wrinkles

Virgin coconut oil is the perfect wrinkle preventer. Free of harmful additives and chemicals, it is well absorbed and never makes the face look greasy. Coconut oil not only protects against new wrinkles, but also helps existing small wrinkles disappear. The combination of coconut oil applied nightly to the skin plus coconut oil and cod-liver oil in the diet is the recipe for beautiful skin right into advanced old age.

Hair

In the Philippines, women soak their hair in coconut oil for 30 minutes before shampooing. Sometimes they apply a very small amount of coconut oil after washing their hair, starting with the ends and working it back toward the scalp. If you swim in chlorinated pools, be sure to apply coconut oil to your hair before going in the water to keep it soft and shiny.

Psoriasis and Eczema

Here's an excellent remedy for these stubborn skin conditions. Very often, severe cases of psoriasis and eczema clear up with just a few applications.

1 cup unrefined coconut oil   10 drops lavender essential oil

Fungal Infections

This excellent remedy works wonders with fungal infections and rashes.

1 cup unrefined coconut oil   1 teaspoon tea tree oil

Apply to the feet for athlete's foot, as well as to any rash that may be fungal in origin.

Arthritis and Joint Pains

Traditional native massage therapists of the Philippines use coconut oil for swollen joints, muscle pains, and even broken bones. Often the oil is infused with local herbs, including cayenne, a native wild hot pepper. So we offer you this recipe, to use on your own aches and pains.

1 cup unrefined coconut oil   1 tablespoon organic cayenne pepper

Set the coconut oil in a glass container in simmering water. When the oil is thoroughly melted, add the cayenne. Let it sit in simmering water for about half an hour, until the cayenne has thoroughly released its various healing compounds. Let it cool and then massage it into painful joints or sprained muscles.

Warts

Apply coconut oil to warts several times per day—they often will disappear!

Deodorant

Coconut oil is an excellent deodorant. You can add an essential oil to it if you want some fragrance, but it works wonders used straight, even when you are doing manual labor. And it doesn't stain your clothes!

Insect Repellent

Many people are concerned about using insect repellent containing insecticides such as DEET. A mixture of coconut oil and essential oils makes an excellent insect repellent without the dangers of harsh pesticides. In a 2001 study reported on CNN and posted at ScienceDaily.com, catnip oil proved highly effective against mosquitoes. Several excellent commercial formulations are available from Tropical Traditions, tropicaltraditions.com, (866) 311-2626, or you can make your own:

1 cup virgin coconut oil

1 teaspoon catnip oil

1 teaspoon other essential oil, such as citronella, lemongrass, peppermint, or tans

Index